Advances in Physiologic Pacing

Editors

KENNETH A. ELLENBOGEN
PUGAZHENDHI VIJAYARAMAN
SANTOSH PADALA

CARDIAC ELECTROPHYSIOLOGY CLINICS

www.cardiacEP.theclinics.com

Consulting Editors
RANJAN K. THAKUR
ANDREA NATALE

June 2022 • Volume 14 • Number 2

ELSEVIER

1600 John F. Kennedy Boulevard • Suite 1800 • Philadelphia, Pennsylvania, 19103-2899

http://www.theclinics.com

CARDIAC ELECTROPHYSIOLOGY CLINICS Volume 14, Number 2
June 2022 ISSN 1877-9182, ISBN-13: 978-0-323-98711-0

Editor: Joanna Collett
Developmental Editor: Hannah Almira Lopez

Cardiac Electrophysiology Clinics (ISSN 1877-9182) is published quarterly by Elsevier Inc., 360 Park Avenue South, New York, NY 10010-1710. Months of issue are March, June, September, and December. Subscription prices are $247.00 per year for US individuals, $525.00 per year for US institutions, $259.00 per year for Canadian individuals, $549.00 per year for Canadian institutions, $315.00 per year for international individuals, $549.00 per year for international institutions and $100.00 per year for US, Canadian and international students/residents. To receive student/resident rate, orders must be accompanied by name of affilliated institution, date of term, and the signature of program/residency coordinator on institution letterhead. Orders will be billed at individual rate until proof of status is received. Foreign air speed delivery is included in all Clinics subscription prices. All prices are subject to change without notice. **POST-MASTER:** Send address changes to Cardiac Electrophysiology Clinics, Elsevier Health Sciences Division, Subscription Customer Service, 3251 Riverport Lane, Maryland Heights, MO 63043. **Customer Service: 1-800-654-2452 (US and Canada). From outside of the US and Canada, call 314-477-8871. Fax: 314-447-8029. E-mail: JournalsCustomer-Service-usa@elsevier.com (for print support); JournalsOnlineSupport-usa@elsevier.com (for online support).**

Reprints. For copies of 100 or more of articles in this publication, please contact the Commercial Reprints Department, Elsevier Inc., 360 Park Avenue South, New York, NY 10010-1710. Tel.: 212-633-3874; Fax: 212-633-3820; E-mail: reprints@elsevier.com.

Cardiac Electrophysiology Clinics is covered in *MEDLINE/PubMed (Index Medicus)*.

Contributors

CONSULTING EDITORS

RANJAN K. THAKUR, MD, MPH, MBA, FHRS
Professor of Medicine and Director, Arrhythmia Service, Thoracic and Cardiovascular Institute, Sparrow Health System, Michigan State University, Lansing, Michigan, USA

ANDREA NATALE, MD, FACC, FHRS
Executive Medical Director, Texas Cardiac Arrhythmia Institute, St. David's Medical Center, Austin, Texas, USA; Consulting Professor, Division of Cardiology, Stanford University, Palo Alto, California, USA; Adjunct Professor of Medicine, Heart and Vascular Center, Case Western Reserve University, Cleveland, Ohio, USA; Director, Interventional Electrophysiology, Scripps Clinic, San Diego, California, USA; Senior Clinical Director, EP Services, California Pacific Medical Center, San Francisco, California, USA

EDITORS

KENNETH A. ELLENBOGEN, MD
Kimmerling Professor of Medicine, Director, Cardiac Electrophysiology Laboratory, VCU School of Medicine, Virginia Commonwealth University/Pauley Heart Center, Richmond, Virginia, USA

PUGAZHENDHI VIJAYARAMAN, MD
Associate Professor of Medicine, Geisinger Commonwealth School of Medicine, Program

Director, CCEP Fellowship, Scranton, Pennsylvania, USA; Director, Cardiac Electrophysiology, Geisinger Heart Institute, Wilkes-Barre, Pennsylvania, USA

SANTOSH PADALA, MD
Associate Professor of Medicine, VCU School of Medicine, Richmond, Virginia, USA

AUTHORS

ANGELO AURICCHIO, MD, PhD
Director of Electrophysiology Unit, Cardiocentro Ticino Institute, Ente Ospedaliero Cantonale, Lugano, Switzerland

ENRICO BARACCA, MD
Arrhythmia and Electrophysiology Unit, Division of Cardiology, Department of Specialistic Medicine, Santa Maria della Misericordia General Hospital, Rovigo, Italy

TIMOTHY R. BETTS, MD
Consultant Cardiologist and Professor of Cardiovascular Medicine, Oxford Biomedical

Research Centre; Oxford Heart Centre, John Radcliffe Hospital, Oxford University Hospitals NHS Foundation Trust, Oxford, United Kingdom

PIERRE BORDACHAR, MD, PhD
Bordeaux University Hospital (CHU), Cardio-Thoracic Unit, Pessac, France; IHU Liryc, Electrophysiology and Heart Modeling Institute, fondation Bordeaux Université, Pessac-Bordeaux, France

HARAN BURRI, MD
Department of Cardiology, University Hospital of Geneva, Geneva, Switzerland

MARCO CENTIONI, MD
Arrhythmia and Electrophysiology Unit, Division of Cardiology, Department of Specialistic Medicine, Santa Maria della Misericordia General Hospital, Rovigo, Italy

KENNETH A. ELLENBOGEN, MD
Kimmerling Professor of Medicine, Director, Cardiac Electrophysiology Laboratory, VCU School of Medicine, Virginia Commonwealth University/Pauley Heart Center, Richmond, Virginia, USA

MARK K. ELLIOTT, MBBS
School of Biomedical Engineering and Imaging Sciences, King's College London, Department of Cardiology, Guy's and St Thomas' NHS Foundation Trust, London, United Kingdom

MICHAEL E. FIELD, MD
Department of Medicine, Medical University of South Carolina, Charleston, South Carolina, USA

DARREL P. FRANCIS, MD
Professor, National Heart and Lung Institute, Imperial College London, Hammersmith Hospital, London, United Kingdom

MICHAEL R. GOLD, MD, PhD
Department of Medicine, Medical University of South Carolina, Charleston, South Carolina, USA

ZAIN S. GOWANI, MD
Department of Medicine, Medical University of South Carolina, Charleston, South Carolina, USA

PEREGRINE G. GREEN, BMBCh
Department of Physiology, Anatomy and Genetics, University of Oxford; Oxford Centre for Clinical Magnetic Resonance Research (OCMR), University of Oxford; Oxford Heart Centre, John Radcliffe Hospital, Oxford University Hospitals NHS Foundation Trust, Oxford, United Kingdom

LUUK HECKMAN, MD
Department of Physiology, Cardiovascular Research Institute Maastricht (CARIM), Maastricht University, the Netherlands

NEIL HERRING, DPhil
Associate Professor, Department of Physiology, Anatomy and Genetics, University of Oxford; Oxford Heart Centre, John Radcliffe Hospital, Oxford University Hospitals NHS Foundation Trust, Oxford, United Kingdom

BENGT HERWEG, MD, FACC, FHRS
Department of Cardiovascular Sciences, University of South Florida Morsani College of Medicine, Tampa General Hospital, Tampa, Florida, USA

WEIJIAN HUANG, MD
Department of Cardiology, The First Affiliated Hospital of Wenzhou Medical University, The Key Lab of Cardiovascular Disease of Wenzhou, Wenzhou, China

SANDEEP K. JAIN, MD
Professor of Medicine, Director, Cardiac Electrophysiology, Heart and Vascular Institute, University of Pittsburgh Medical Center, Pittsburgh, Pennsylvania, USA

MAREK JASTRZĘBSKI, MD, PhD
Professor, First Department of Cardiology, Interventional Electrocardiology and Hypertension, Jagiellonian University Medical College, Jagiellonian University in Krakow, Kraków, Poland

NANDITA KAZA, MBChB
National Heart and Lung Institute, Research Fellow, Imperial College London, Hammersmith Hospital, London, United Kingdom

DANIEL KEENE, PhD
National Heart and Lung Institute, Clinical Senior Lecturer in Cardiology (Clinical Electrophysiology), Imperial College London, Hammersmith Hospital, London, United Kingdom

JUSTIN LUERMANS, MD, PhD
Department of Cardiology, Cardiovascular Research Institute Maastricht (CARIM), Maastricht University Medical Centre (MUMC+), the Netherlands; Department of Cardiology, Radboud University Medical Centre (RadboudUMC), Nijmegen, the Netherlands

JOOST LUMENS, PhD
Department of Biomedical Engineering,
Cardiovascular Research Institute Maastricht
(CARIM), Maastricht University, the
Netherlands

LINA MARCANTONI, MD
Arrhythmia and Electrophysiology Unit,
Division of Cardiology, Department of
Specialistic Medicine, Santa Maria della
Misericordia General Hospital, Rovigo, Italy

VISHAL S. MEHTA, MBBS
School of Biomedical Engineering and Imaging
Sciences, King's College London, Department
of Cardiology, Guy's and St Thomas'
NHS Foundation Trust, London, United
Kingdom

ALEJANDRA A. MIYAZAWA, MBChB
National Heart and Lung Institute, Imperial
College London, Hammersmith Hospital,
London, United Kingdom

TARDU ÖZKARTAL, MD
Consultant Cardiologist, Electrophysiology
Unit, Cardiocentro Ticino Institute,
Ente Ospedaliero Cantonale, Lugano,
Switzerland

GIANNI PASTORE, MD
Arrhythmia and Electrophysiology Unit,
Division of Cardiology, Department of
Specialistic Medicine, Santa Maria della
Misericordia General Hospital, Rovigo,
Italy

SYLVAIN PLOUX, MD, PhD
Bordeaux University Hospital (CHU), Cardio-
Thoracic Unit, Pessac, France; IHU Liryc,
Electrophysiology and Heart Modeling
Institute, fondation Bordeaux Université,
Pessac-Bordeaux, France

**SHUNMUGA SUNDARAM PONNUSAMY,
MD**
Associate Professor, Department of
Cardiology, Velammal Medical College
Hospital and Research Institute, Madurai, India

FRITS PRINZEN, PhD
Department of Physiology, Cardiovascular
Research Institute Maastricht (CARIM),
Maastricht University, the Netherlands

JOHN RICKARD, MD, MPH
Staff Physician, Section of Cardiac
Electrophysiology, Department of
Cardiovascular Medicine, Heart, and Vascular
Institute, Cleveland Clinic, Cleveland, Ohio,
USA

JESSE RIJKS, MD
Department of Cardiology, Cardiovascular
Research Institute Maastricht (CARIM),
Maastricht University Medical Centre
(MUMC+), the Netherlands

CHRISTOPHER A. RINALDI, MD, FHRS
School of Biomedical Engineering and Imaging
Sciences, King's College London, Department
of Cardiology, Guy's and St Thomas'
NHS Foundation Trust, London,
United Kingdom

SAMIR SABA, MD
Professor of Medicine, Division Chief,
Cardiology, Co-Director, Heart and Vascular
Institute, University of Pittsburgh Medical
Center, Pittsburgh, Pennsylvania, USA

MARC STRIK, MD, PhD
Bordeaux University Hospital (CHU), Cardio-
Thoracic Unit, Pessac, France; IHU Liryc,
Electrophysiology and Heart Modeling
Institute, fondation Bordeaux Université,
Pessac-Bordeaux, France

LAN SU, MD
Department of Cardiology, The First Affiliated
Hospital of Wenzhou Medical University, The
Key Lab of Cardiovascular Disease of
Wenzhou, Wenzhou, China

BRETT TOMASHITIS, MD
Department of Medicine, Medical University of
South Carolina, Charleston, South Carolina,
USA

JEREMY S. TREGER, MD, PhD
The University of Chicago Medicine, Center for
Arrhythmia Care, Heart and Vascular Center,
Chicago, Illinois, USA

GAURAV A. UPADHYAY, MD, FACC, FHRS
Heart and Vascular Center, Associate
Professor of Medicine, Director, Heart Station,
Section of Cardiology, Center for Arrhythmia
Care, The University of Chicago Medicine,
Chicago, Illinois, USA

ANTONIUS M.W. VAN STIPDONK, MD, PhD
Department of Cardiology, Cardiovascular
Research Institute Maastricht (CARIM),
Maastricht University Medical Centre
(MUMC+), the Netherlands

NIRAJ VARMA, MA, MD, PhD, FRCP
Professor of Medicine, Cardiac Pacing and
Electrophysiology, Heart and Vascular
Institute, Cleveland Clinic, Cleveland, Ohio,
USA

KEVIN VERNOOY, MD, PhD
Department of Cardiology, Cardiovascular
Research Institute Maastricht (CARIM),
Maastricht University Medical Centre
(MUMC+), the Netherlands; Department of
Cardiology, Radboud University Medical
Centre (RadboudUMC), Nijmegen, the
Netherlands

PUGAZHENDHI VIJAYARAMAN, MD
Associate Professor of Medicine, Geisinger
Commonwealth School of Medicine, Program
Director, CCEP Fellowship, Scranton,
Pennsylvania, USA; Director, Cardiac
Electrophysiology, Geisinger Heart Institute,
Wilkes-Barre, Pennsylvania, USA

CHAU N. VO, MD
Cardiac Electrophysiology Fellow, Department
of Medicine, Medical University of South
Carolina, Charleston, South Carolina, USA

ALLAN WELTER-FROST, MD, MPH
Department of Cardiovascular Sciences,
University of South Florida Morsani College of
Medicine, Tampa General Hospital, Tampa,
Florida, USA

**ZACHARY I. WHINNETT, BM, BS, FRCP,
PhD**
Reader in Cardiac Electrophysiology, National
Heart and Lung Institute, Imperial College
London, Hammersmith Hospital, London,
United Kingdom

DAVID R. WILSON II, MD
Department of Cardiovascular Sciences,
University of South Florida Morsani College of
Medicine, Tampa General Hospital, Tampa,
Florida, USA

**FRANCESCO ZANON, MD, FESC, FHERA,
FHRS**
Arrhythmia and Electrophysiology Unit,
Division of Cardiology, Department of
Specialistic Medicine, Santa Maria della
Misericordia General Hospital, Rovigo, Italy

ALWIN ZWEERINK, MD, PhD
Department of Cardiology, University Hospital
of Geneva, Geneva, Switzerland; Department
of Cardiology and Amsterdam Cardiovascular
Sciences (ACS), Amsterdam University
Medical Centers (AUMC), Location VU Medical
Center, Amsterdam, the Netherlands

Contents

> Pacing therapy aims to improve overall cardiac function by normalizing cardiac electrical activation. Although hemodynamic measurements allow the impact of cardiac pacing on cardiac function to be quantified, the protocol is crucial to minimize the effect of noise and achieve greater precision. Multiple steps can be undertaken to optimize accuracy of hemodynamic measurements. These include comparing with a reference state, using an average of a set number of beats, making repeated measurements, ensuring all beats are included, and pacing at faster heart rates. These measurements can aid comparison between different pacing modalities and guide optimal programming.

> His Bundle Pacing (HBP) is a form of physiologic pacing achieved through implantation of a pacing electrode into the His bundle. HBP began 20 years ago without any dedicated tools. As specific tools became available HBP quickly spread and proved to be a viable alternative to traditional right ventricle pacing. HBP is reliable and effective in preserving the physiologic ventricular synchrony with clinical benefits particularly evident when a high percentage of pacing is required. Unipolar signals from the lead tip guide the implant. 3D electroanatomical mapping could further assist the procedure.

> His bundle (HB) pacing is an increasingly popular method of physiologic ventricular pacing. The electrocardiographic hallmark of physiologic pacing is the preservation or restoration of physiologic activation times in the left ventricle—a principle of paramount diagnostic importance. The current review focuses on the differentiation between 3 possible capture types when the pacing lead is placed in the HB region: selective HB capture when only HB is activated, nonselective HB capture when there is simultaneous activation of the adjacent right ventricular septal (RVS)

myocardium, and selective RVS capture when HB is not activated at all but only septal myocardium.

Left Bundle Branch Pacing: How I Do It?   165

Lan Su, Kenneth A. Ellenbogen, and Weijian Huang

Since the first case of left bundle branch pacing (LBBP) achieved via the transventricular septal approach in 2017, LBBP has rapidly evolved into clinical practice with a high success rate and satisfactory pacing/sensing parameters compared with His bundle pacing (HBP). In this article, we review the criteria of LBB capture, standardized testing methods of LBBP. We focus on the determination of the initial lead entry site in the right side of the interventricular septum for LBBP, deep fixation of the lead tip into the left ventricular septal sub-endocardium, avoidance of lead septal perforation and solutions to challenging cases.

Physiology of Left Ventricular Septal Pacing and Left Bundle Branch Pacing   181

Jesse Rijks, Justin Luermans, Luuk Heckman, Antonius M.W. van Stipdonk, Frits Prinzen, Joost Lumens, and Kevin Vernooy

Following the recognition of the adverse effects of right ventricular pacing, alternative permanent pacing strategies aiming to maintain a synchronous ventricular contraction have been sought. The quest for the optimal pacing site has recently led to several promising and rapidly emerging new pacing strategies, such as left ventricular septal pacing and left bundle branch pacing. In both animal and human studies, these pacing strategies seem to maintain electrical and mechanical activation of the left ventricle to a (near)physiologic level. However, more studies on the long-term effects of both strategies are needed.

Evaluation of Criteria for Left Bundle Branch Capture   191

Shunmuga Sundaram Ponnusamy and Pugazhendhi Vijayaraman

Left bundle branch pacing (LBBP) provides electrical and mechanical synchrony at low and stable pacing output and effectively corrects distal conduction system disease. The criteria for differentiating LBBP from LV septal pacing has not been validated in large trials. There are several electrocardiography-based and intracardiac electrogram-based criteria to confirm LBB capture. In this section, the authors review these criteria and their overall accuracy.

What Intracardiac Tracings Have Taught Us About Left Bundle Branch Block   203

Jeremy S. Treger and Gaurav A. Upadhyay

Current electrocardiogram (ECG) criteria for left bundle branch block (LBBB) are largely based on early work in animal models or on mathematical models of cardiac activation. The resulting criteria have modest specificity, and up to one-third of patients who meet current ECG criteria for LBBB may have intact conduction through their His-Purkinje systems. Intracardiac tracings offer the ability to accurately discriminate between LBBB and other causes of delayed activation, which may facilitate the development of more accurate ECG criteria. Assessing these distinctions are particularly salient to applications for conduction system pacing.

What Body Surface Mapping Has Taught Us About Ventricular Conduction Disease Implications for Cardiac Resynchronization Therapy and His Bundle Pacing   213

Marc Strik, Sylvain Ploux, and Pierre Bordachar

The degree and pattern of conduction disease seem determinant when assessing potential cardiac resynchronization therapy (CRT) candidates. In the present review, the authors discuss the available noninvasive techniques that can be used to acquire ventricular activation time maps. They describe what body surface mapping has taught us about left bundle branch block, right bundle branch block, intraventricular conduction delay, and right ventricular pacing and discuss the ability of derived parameters of electrical dyssynchrony to predict long-term clinical response to CRT or His bundle pacing.

Pacing Optimized by Left Ventricular dP/dt$_{max}$ 223

Mark K. Elliott, Vishal S. Mehta, and Christopher A. Rinaldi

Left ventricular (LV) dP/dt$_{max}$ provides a sensitive measure of the acute hemodynamic response to cardiac resynchronization therapy (CRT) and can predict reverse remodeling on echocardiography. Its use to guide LV lead placement has been shown to improve outcomes in a multicenter randomized trial. Given the invasive protocol required for measurement, it is unlikely to be universally beneficial for patients undergoing CRT but may be useful for patients who do not respond to conventional CRT, or in those who have borderline indications or risk factors for nonresponse. In such cases, LV dP/dt$_{max}$ may help guide LV lead placement, optimize device programming, and select the best alternative method of delivering CRT, such endocardial LV pacing or conduction system pacing.

Role of Electrical Delay in Cardiac Resynchronization Therapy Response   233

Zain S. Gowani, Brett Tomashitis, Chau N. Vo, Michael E. Field, and Michael R. Gold

Traditionally, left ventricular (LV) lead position was guided by anatomic criteria of pacing from the lateral wall of the LV. However, large trials showed little effect of LV lead position on outcomes, other than noting worse outcomes with apical positions. Given the poor correlation of cardiac resynchronization therapy (CRT) outcomes with anatomically guided LV lead placement, focus shifted toward more physiologic predictors such as targeting the areas of delayed mechanical and electrical activation. Measures of left ventricular delay and interventricular delay are strong predictors of CRT response.

Programming Algorithms for Cardiac Resynchronization Therapy   243

Niraj Varma

Current cardiac resynchronization therapy (CRT) implant guidelines emphasize the presence of electrical dyssynchrony (left bundle branch block (LBBB) and QRS > 150 ms) yet have modest predictive value for response and have not reduced the 30% nonresponse rate. Optimized programming to optimize CRT delivery has promised much but to date has largely been ineffective. What is missing is the understanding of LV paced effects (which are unpredictable) and optimal paced AV interval (that can be conserved during physiologic variations) that then can be incorporated into an individualized programming prescription. Automatic device-based algorithms that deliver electrical optimization and maintain this during ambulatory fluctuations in AV interval are discussed.

success, resulting in widely variable clinical response. Limitations of conventional bi-ventricular pacing evolve around myocardial scar, fibrosis, and inability to effectively stimulate diseased tissue. Several observational and acute hemodynamic studies have demonstrated improved electrical resynchronization and echocardiographic response with conduction system pacing. This article provides a systematic review of conduction system pacing as a physiologic alternative to conventional CRT, which is currently undergoing rigorous investigation.

His-Optimized and Left Bundle Branch-Optimized Cardiac Resynchronization Therapy: In Control of Fusion Pacing   311

Alwin Zweerink and Haran Burri

Fusion pacing, which exploits conduction via the intrinsic His-Purkinje system, forms the basis of recent cardiac resynchronization therapy (CRT) optimization algorithms. However, settings need to be constantly adjusted to accommodate for changes in AV conduction, and the algorithms are not always available (eg, depending on the device, in case of AV block or with atrial fibrillation). His-optimized cardiac resynchronization therapy (HOT-CRT), and left-bundle branch optimized cardiac resynchronization therapy (LOT-CRT) which combines conduction system pacing with ventricular fusion pacing, provide constant fusion with ventricular activation (irrespective of intrinsic AV conduction). These modalities provide promising treatment strategies for patients with heart failure, especially in those with chronic atrial fibrillation who require CRT (in whom the atrial port is usually plugged and can be used to connect the conduction system pacing lead).

Status and Update on Cardiac Resynchronization Therapy Trials   323

Angelo Auricchio and Tardu Özkartal

After decades of clinical use, cardiac resynchronization therapy (CRT) can be considered an established therapy. However, there are multiple open questions to be addressed that shall further improve the proportion of patients responding to CRT. Progress in better understanding the relationship between electrical and mechanical disorder in patients with heart failure with ventricular conduction abnormalities is important. This article presents and discusses ongoing studies in different areas of CRT research, including patient selection by novel diagnostic tools, extension of clinical criteria, left ventricular lead positioning and pacing site selection, optimization of CRT delivery and programming, and selection of device type.

Generating Evidence to Support the Physiologic Promise of Conduction System Pacing: Status and Update on Conduction System Pacing Trials   345

Nandita Kaza, Daniel Keene, and Zachary I. Whinnett

Conduction system pacing avoids the potential deleterious effects of right ventricular pacing in patients with bradycardia and provides an alternative approach to cardiac resynchronization therapy. We focus on the available observational and randomized evidence and review studies supporting the safety, feasibility, and physiologic promise of conduction system approaches. We evaluate the randomized data generated from the available clinical trials of conduction system pacing, which have led to the recent inclusion of CSP in international guidelines. Future randomized trials will build on the physiologic promise of conduction system pacing approaches and importantly, offer information on clinical endpoints.

CARDIAC ELECTROPHYSIOLOGY CLINICS

THE CLINICS ARE AVAILABLE ONLINE!
Access your subscription at:
www.theclinics.com

Foreword
Advances in Physiologic Pacing

As our island of knowledge grows, so does the shore of our ignorance.
—John Archibald Wheeler, twentieth century physicist

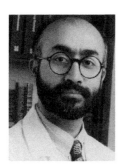 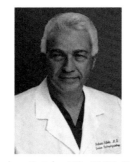

Ranjan K. Thakur, MD, MPH, MBA, FHRS   Andrea Natale, MD, FACC, FHRS

Consulting Editors

We are pleased to introduce this issue of the *Cardiac Electrophysiology Clinics* focused on advances in physiologic pacing, but we are also saddened by the unexpected and sudden demise of one of the coeditors, Dr Santosh Padala. Quite appropriately, the other two coeditors, Dr Kenneth Ellenbogen and Dr Pugazhendhi Vijayaraman, have memorialized this issue by dedicating it to their promising, young colleague. We offer our heartfelt condolences to Dr Padala's colleagues and young family.

Since the advent of ventricular pacing in the 1950s, it soon became clear that while this was a life-saving therapy, it was nonphysiologic and left much room for advancements. Physiologic cardiac pacing has been the paragon we've been seeking since the advent of pacing more than 60 years ago. These advances required improvement in our understanding of physiology of cardiac pacing and technical advances developed by industry. There have been many advancements, such as dual chamber pacing, cardiac resynchronization, and most recently in ascendancy, conduction system pacing.

Although His-bundle pacing was initially described by Dr Pramod Deshmukh 25 years ago, it took the electrophysiology community many years to realize its potential. Initially there were very few practitioners of His-bundle pacing due to its technical challenges. However, in the last decade, there has been a worldwide resurgence. This has led to excellent research and development of new concepts. One such example is the realization that the target pacing site may not be limited to the bundle of His, but also includes the proximal left bundle; hence, it may be more accurate to talk about conduction system pacing and not just His-bundle pacing.

We congratulate the editors of this issue, which offers a contemporary perspective on a six-decades-old challenge. Like all issues in science, what's new and unexplored today will become

Card Electrophysiol Clin 14 (2022) xiii–xiv
https://doi.org/10.1016/j.ccep.2022.04.001
1877-9182/22/© 2022 Published by Elsevier Inc.

settled within a few years, for as our island of knowledge grows, so will the shore of our ignorance, and we will be revisiting future advances once again. In the meantime, we hope the readership will find the current issue helpful in furthering their understanding of the contemporary issues.

Ranjan K. Thakur, MD, MPH, MBA, FHRS
Sparrow Thoracic and Cardiovascular Institute
Michigan State University
1440 East Michigan Avenue; Suite 400
Lansing, MI 48912, USA

Andrea Natale, MD, FACC, FHRS
Texas Cardiac Arrhythmia Institute
Center for Atrial Fibrillation at
St. David's Medical Center
1015 East 32nd Street, Suite 516
Austin, TX 78705, USA

E-mail addresses:
thakur@msu.edu (R.K. Thakur)
andrea.natale@stdavids.com (A. Natale)

Preface
The Next Revolution in Cardiac Pacing

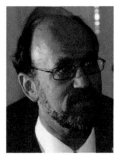

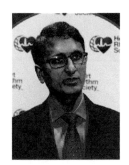

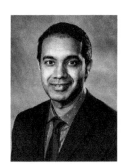

Kenneth A. Ellenbogen, MD   Pugazhendhi Vijayaraman, MD   Santosh Padala, MD

Editors

If the first revolution of cardiac pacing was physiologic pacing, defined as dual-chamber pacing, then the second revolution was cardiac resynchronization pacing with use of the coronary sinus lead to achieve more physiologic resynchronization of the heart, while the third revolution in cardiac pacing is conduction system pacing. Over the last 4 years since *Cardiac Electrophysiology Clinics* published an issue on His bundle pacing, much has been accomplished and published by many groups. Conduction system pacing has expanded from His bundle pacing to include left bundle branch area pacing comprising direct left bundle branch pacing and left ventricular septal pacing.

In the current issue, we bring together experts from all over the world in conduction system pacing. The pace of developments in this field is truly amazing, so we look forward to updating this subject again in 4 years. The field and our understanding of conduction system pacing, both anatomy and physiology, have now advanced to the point of designing both small and large clinical trials. This issue provides the expert and the novice of conduction system pacing an in-depth understanding of the field, where it has been and where it is going.

We are grateful to have an incredibly talented group of authors and experts contribute to this issue. We appreciate all the time and effort they put into their work. We look forward to being able to provide a foundation for a much better understanding of this field and to participating in its development.

Kenneth A. Ellenbogen, MD
411 Wishart Court
Henrico, VA 23229-7082, USA

Pugazhendhi Vijayaraman, MD
16 Mallard Way
Mountain Top, PA 18707, USA

Santosh Padala, MD
4314 Bon Secours Parkway, Unit B
Henrico, VA 23233, USA

E-mail addresses:
ken.ellenbogen@gmail.com
kenneth.ellenbogen@vcuhealth.org
(K.A. Ellenbogen)
pvijayaraman@gmail.com
pvijayaraman1@geisinger.edu (P. Vijayaraman)
santoshpadala@gmail.com
santosh.padala@vcuhealth.org (S. Padala)

Preface

The Next Revolution in Cardiac Pacing

  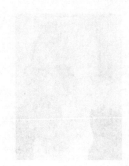

Santosh Padala, MD   Pugazhendhi Vijayaraman, MD   Kenneth A. Ellenbogen, MD

Editors

In the first cardiac pacemakers, pacing of the physiologic cavity served as dual-chamber pacing, then the second revolution was cardiac resynchronization pacing with use of the coronary sinus lead to achieve more physiologic resynchronization of the heart, while the third revolution in cardiac pacing is conduction system pacing. Over the last 4 years since Cardiac Electrophysiology Clinics published its review on His bundle pacing, much has been accomplished and published by many groups. Conduction system pacing has expanded from His bundle pacing to include left bundle branch area pacing comprising other left bundle branch pacing and left ventricular septal pacing.

In the current issue, we bring together experts from all over the world in conduction system pacing. The pace of developments in this field is truly amazing, so we look forward to updating this subject again in 4 years. The field and our understanding of conduction system pacing, both anatomy and physiology, have now advanced to the point of designing both small and large clinical trials. This issue provides the expert and the novice of conduction system pacing an in-depth understanding of the field, where it has been and where it is going.

We are excited to have an incredible international group of authors and experts contribute to this issue. We appreciate all the time and effort they put into their work. We look forward to seeing them provide a foundation for a much better understanding of this field and to participating in its development.

Kenneth A. Ellenbogen, MD
VCU Health
Virginia

Pugazhendhi Vijayaraman, MD
Geisinger Heart Institute
Wilkes Barre, PA 18711, USA

Santosh Padala, MD
VCU Health
Richmond, VA 23298, USA

E-mail addresses:
kenellenbogen@gmail.com;
kenneth.ellenbogen@vcuhealth.org
(K.A. Ellenbogen);
pvijayaraman1@gmail.com;
pvijayaraman1@geisinger.edu (P. Vijayaraman);
santoshpadala@gmail.com;
santosh.padala@vcuhealth.org (S. Padala)

Card Electrophysiol Clin 14 (2022)xv
https://doi.org/10.1016/j.ccep.2021.12.017
1877-9182/22/© 2021 Published by Elsevier Inc.

Dedication

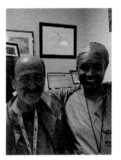

Santosh Padala, MD (1982-2021)

This issue is dedicated to our friend and colleague, Santosh Padala, MD, who died much too young. We both had the privilege of working with him over a number of years as he trained in electrophysiology and then joined the VCU faculty. Over the last seven years, his contributions to the field of electrophysiology and pacing were substantial and will far outlast his all too brief life. Each day and every patient he touched were made better by that interaction. He was a truly outstanding clinician, clinical researcher, teacher, and human being. Not only his patients but also all health care providers who came into contact with him were changed through his sheer joy and enthusiasm for learning, teaching, and healing his patients. His constant amazement and joy in everything he did continue to inspire each of us every day. He was beloved by so many, including his large extended family and friends. We hope his memory will be a source of inspiration for all.

Kenneth A. Ellenbogen, MD
VCU School of Medicine
Richmond, VA, USA

Pugazhendhi Vijayaraman, MD
Geisinger Heart Institute
Wilkes-Barre, PA, USA

E-mail addresses:
ken.ellenbogen@gmail.com
kenneth.ellenbogen@vcuhealth.org
(K.A. Ellenbogen)
pvijayaraman@gmail.com
pvijayaraman1@geisinger.edu (P. Vijayaraman)

Basic Principles of Hemodynamics in Pacing

Alejandra A. Miyazawa, MBChB, Darrel P. Francis, MD, Zachary I. Whinnett, BM, BS, FRCP, PhD*

KEYWORDS

- Hemodynamics • Optimization • Cardiac resynchronization therapy • Pacing

KEY POINTS

- The aim of pacing therapy is to improve cardiac function by correcting electrical conduction abnormalities.
- Hemodynamic measurements can be used to assess and quantify the impact of cardiac pacing on cardiac function.
- When using hemodynamic measures to assess the impact of pacing, it is important to use a protocol that minimizes the impact of noise, so that the required level of precision can be achieved.
- Hemodynamic measurements can be used to compare different pacing modalities within the same patient.
- Hemodynamic measurements have the potential to guide optimal programming.

BACKGROUND

Introduction

Pacemakers were first developed to treat the severe hemodynamic compromise occurring as a result of bradycardia in patients with advanced conduction system disease. As the delivery of pacing therapy has become more sophisticated and the indications have expanded, the fundamental aim has remained the same: to improve cardiac function by normalizing cardiac electrical activation in patients with conduction system disease.

Throughout the history of developing pacing therapy, hemodynamic assessment has provided a useful tool in guiding the development of new pacing approaches. Investigators have used hemodynamic measurements because they allow acute changes in cardiac function to be determined and quantified.

The first pacemakers had a single lead in the right ventricle. This allowed treatment of asystole and complete heart block. Even with this simple design, there were immediate hemodynamic improvements with the onset of pacing therapy.[1,2]

Going beyond simply delivering sufficient ventricular activation, the first "physiologic pacing" was sequential atrioventricular (AV) pacing.[3] Again, hemodynamic assessment demonstrated improvements in cardiac function.[4,5]

When cardiac resynchronization therapy, delivered using biventricular pacing, was being developed, it was the improvements observed in acute hemodynamic measurements with temporary pacing that encouraged the investigators to proceed to implant a permanent pacemaker with a coronary sinus lead.[6,7]

Hemodynamic measurements can also guide optimal programming of pacemakers because hemodynamics are a final common pathway through which cardiac function expresses itself.

However, hemodynamic measurements are not static. They fluctuate in response to numerous biological phenomena, including respiration and other autonomic phenomena. These processes are numerous, continuous, and variable and make the identification of the hemodynamic consequences of a change in pacing configuration more challenging. Because we are not able to

National Heart and Lung Institute, Imperial College London, Hammersmith Hospital, Du Cane Road, London W12 0HS, UK
* Corresponding author.
E-mail address: z.whinnett@imperial.ac.uk

Card Electrophysiol Clin 14 (2022) 133–140
https://doi.org/10.1016/j.ccep.2021.12.001

measure and subtract the contributions of these background biological phenomena on hemodynamics, they are best treated as "noise."

Measurement of pacing efficacy is therefore an exercise in reliably separating the signal from the noise. The signal is the element that is consistent on every instance a pacing configuration is tested, and the noise is the remainder, which varies between repeated measurements. When an average of multiple measurements of a pacing effect is taken, the impact of noise consistently shrinks with the square root of the number of repeat measurements.

In this review, the authors assess the potential role of hemodynamic measurements as (i) a method for assessing new pacing approaches or indications, (ii) a method for personalizing programming, and (iii) potential hemodynamic measures and protocols for minimizing the effect of noise.

Does the Hemodynamic Acquisition Protocol Matter?

Because the early studies[1,2] examined bradycardia pacing, the effect size was so large (**Fig. 1**) that it dwarfed the biological noise, and there was no need for repeated measurements to separate signal from noise.

Nevertheless, on close inspection, the blood pressure values before and after onset of pacing show considerable natural variability.

When biventricular pacing is delivered to patients with left bundle branch block (LBBB), the hemodynamic benefit is again large enough[8] to confidently distinguish from the background noise, for example, an increase in systolic blood pressure of 7.8 mm Hg[9] when compared with AAI pacing and an 11% increase in left ventricular (LV) dP/dt$_{max}$.[10]

The benefits of performing studies assessing the hemodynamic effect of novel pacing approaches are that they allow these new approaches to be tested efficiently in relatively small cost-effective studies. This means the potential new treatments can be efficiently investigated, and only the most promising require further evaluation in much more costly trials, which examine the impact on longer-term outcomes. However, it is important that the protocols used in the hemodynamic studies are sufficiently robust, so that they are not adversely affected by the impact of noise.

NOISE + SELECTION = UPWARD BIAS

Noise alone does not generate false positive results. In fact, where there is a comparison between

2 prespecified settings, noise favors false negative results, because the statistical tests are assessing whether the observed results are easily explainable from the amount of noise seen.

However, upward bias occurs if the study design means the optimal pacing configuration is selected using a noisy measurement, and then the *same* measurement is used to identify how much better that pacing configuration is compared with the other tested configurations. This is not necessarily obvious to clinicians, and the authors therefore describe an example of a study that was limited by this problem.

Multipoint pacing was developed as a potential alternative to standard bipolar LV pacing, in patients with heart failure and LBBB. Investigators set about performing an acute hemodynamic study to assess whether multipoint pacing provided greater hemodynamic improvements.[11] The study used invasive LV dP/dt$_{max}$ measurements and compared the tested pacing intervention with AAI pacing. Each participant underwent measurements with standard biventricular pacing, and 4 different multipoint pacing configurations. The multipoint pacing configuration that gave the highest value was considered the personalized optimum. This doomed the trial to be positive. There were inevitably fluctuations in all the measurements because of biological variability (and not because of differences in pacing configuration). Furthermore, multipoint pacing had *four* chances to produce a reading higher than standard biventricular pacing. Therefore, by using a protocol that picked the highest of these 4 assessments and then used this measurement to quantify the effect size meant that a positive result could be obtained even if multipoint pacing was no different from biventricular pacing.

Another trial assessing the same question, the multispot trial,[12] avoided this pitfall by prespecifying that researchers were not allowed to choose the "best-of-three" pacing configurations for each patient. Instead, each of the new pacing configurations was compared consistently with the reference of biventricular pacing. This trial showed no advantage of multispot pacing over biventricular pacing.

The 2 trial protocols also differed in other respects. The multipoint pacing trial excluded ventricular ectopics and 2 subsequent beats as well as the first few beats of each pacing configuration. In contrast, the multispot pacing trial[12] focused on the initial period after the transition, because it was argued that the signal was larger in that initial window rather than later, when homeostatic forces had attenuated them, according to combined studies of Doppler and pressure.[13]

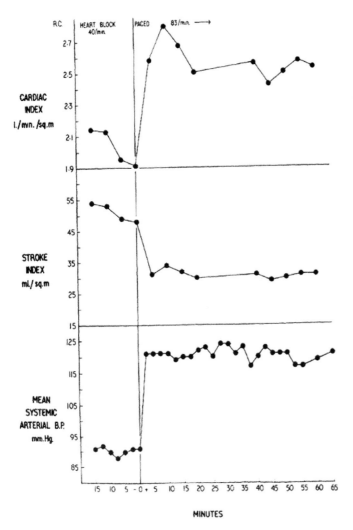

Fig. 1. Hemodynamic benefit of cardiac pacing in complete heart block. Significant hemodynamic benefit of pacing at 83 bpm in a patient with complete heart block secondary to an acute myocardial infarct. Even with the effect of biological variability on the mean systemic arterial blood pressure, the benefit of pacing is so great, in this clinical context, that the hemodynamic benefit is clear despite the variability in the hemodynamic measurements. B.P., blood pressure. (*From* Lassers BW, Anderton JL, George M, Muir AL, Julian DG. Hemodynamic effects of artificial pacing in complete heart block complicating acute myocardial infarction. Circulation. 1968 Aug;38(2):308-23. https://doi.org/10.1161/01.cir.38.2.308. PMID: 5666846; with permission.)

Acquisition Protocol: Features to Maximize Signal-to-Noise Ratio

All hemodynamic markers experience natural spontaneous variability because of numerous unmeasurable and unpredictable intercurrent biological processes. These are not errors of measurement: they are correct measurements of variation in hemodynamics, as can be seen by measuring different hemodynamic markers simultaneously and noticing their fluctuations to be identical.[14] Nevertheless, from the point of view of a researcher assessing the impact of a change in pacing, these fluctuations are an unwanted irritation, and solely for that reason, the authors call them "noise."[15–18]

The hemodynamic benefits of pacing in severe bradycardia and complete heart block are so great that no special effort is needed to distinguish them from noise. However, this noise becomes more of a problem when testing interventions, which are likely to produce smaller hemodynamic improvements. Therefore, special measures are needed to reduce the effects of noise so that the changes occurring owing to the testing pacing configuration can be reliably discerned.

A series of experiments have identified protocol design elements that progressively reduce the impact of noise such that it can now be reduced by 90% to 99%. In the later sections, the authors refer to blood pressure simply because this is readily measurable with high-precision (invasively or noninvasively) calibrated physical units. Many alternative markers are also available. However, regardless of the choice of hemodynamic marker, the considerations discussed later are advisable in protocol design.

Measure values relative to a reference setting

The obvious approach to comparing different pacemaker settings is to measure the blood pressure (or other appropriate marker) in each of the different settings and then compare them. The problem with this is that it will take several minutes at least to complete the acquisition. There are multiple intercurrent processes happening during this time that will be displacing the blood pressure up and down. In general, the longer the time interval between 2 hemodynamic measurements, the greater the variance between the first and second measurement. This is because the various intercurrent biological processes have different periods of oscillation: over longer intervals, slower processes can additionally make an impact, whereas all the faster processes continue to be relevant. The overall pattern is a widening of the spread between blood pressures at different times, which grows approximately in proportion to the square root of the time interval, at least over the interval of seconds to minutes.

The solution to this problem of progressively broadening variation with time is to only measure changes over a few seconds. To allow a wide range of settings to be tested, one can test each setting against a reference setting that is common to all. Therefore, for each tested setting, the authors measure the signed difference in blood pressure produced in that setting compared with the reference setting (**Fig. 2**). For example, if the reference setting is an AV delay of 120 milliseconds, the authors would measure the pressure at 100 milliseconds as "−2.3 mm Hg" and the pressure at 140 milliseconds as "+3.1 mm Hg."[19]

Number of beats to average

The respiratory cycle produces the most dramatic fluctuation in hemodynamics. The authors have found that setting the number of beats to match 1 respiratory cycle gives a good signal-to-noise ratio.[19] If you want to set a protocol that uses a constant number of beats across all patients, the authors suggest a value between 6 and 10 beats, depending on the likely heart rate and respiratory rate of participants during your experiment.[19,20]

Although it can be tempting to extend the number of beats beyond this, to (for example) dozens of seconds or even several minutes, the authors do not recommend this, for 3 reasons. First, it prolongs the acquisition process without corresponding improvements in precision. Second, the signal that the authors are interested in will decay during that time as explained in the next section. Third, the later beats will contain more noise than the earlier beats, for the reasons explained in the previous section.

When to start sampling after a transition?

Some researchers are tempted to wait after a transition for hemodynamics to "stabilize." Unfortunately, this allows 2 undesirable processes to inevitably occur. First, progressively more lower-frequency background physiologic processes will be disturbing the blood pressure. Second, the blood pressure signal itself will be decaying because the increased or decreased pressure is sensed by the body, and the homeostatic response is vasodilatation or vasoconstriction, respectively. This is medically desirable, but experimentally undesirable, because it reduces the pressure increment the authors are trying to measure and therefore makes it more difficult to detect correctly.

The authors' experiments have shown that skipping even just 1 beat after the transition reduces signal-to-noise ratio by about 4%. Skipping 10 beats reduces it by about 40%.[19]

Looking backward from the transition, there is a similar but less severe pattern. Skipping 1 beat before the transition reduces the signal-to-noise ratio by about 3%. Skipping 10 beats reduces it by about 20%.[19]

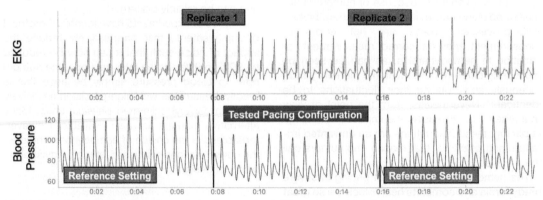

Fig. 2. Sample of a hemodynamic optimization protocol. Extracted sample of a hemodynamic optimization protocol using noninvasive systolic blood pressure measurements. One replicate is a transition between a reference state and a test state. EKG, electrocardiogram.

The authors think that backward skipping has less of an impact because the effect is only through widening of the noise. The forward skipping causes not only widening of the noise but also fading of the signal caused by the physiologic vasodilatation or vasoconstriction described above.

Perform repeated measurements and average
The single most important aspect of the protocol is ensuring that there are adequate replicates. Inadequate replicates make the entire measurement process worse than useless because it will produce misleading results. Averaging of independent repetitions of the same measurement is the single most effective method of increasing precision. It is universally reliable across all fields of science. The number of repetitions required for any degree of precision can now be calculated.[21]

Experiments show the dramatic decline in measurement imprecision with increasing numbers of replicates.[17,20] For example, using 8 replicates with 8 beats per replicate eliminates 90% of the variance seen with a single beat.[20]

Sometimes, the time required to make sufficient measurements is not clinically feasible. In that situation, one should not make the measurements at all.

Pacing at faster heart rates
Pacing at faster rates has dual benefits. First, the impact of changes in pacemaker settings becomes more obvious. This is because the cardiac cycle becomes shorter, and therefore, the distribution of time between the various phases (including the subphases of diastole) becomes more critical to good cardiac function.[22]

Second, at a higher heart rate, the same number of beats is acquired in less time, and therefore (if the protocol has a fixed number of beats), more repetitions can be achieved in the same amount of acquisition time.

Which Hemodynamic Measure?

Many different hemodynamic measures are now possible. The authors group them broadly into "measurements outside the heart" versus "measurements inside the heart."

Measurements outside the heart have the advantage of mutual concordance. Whichever pacing configuration generates the most cardiac output will also generate the highest systolic blood pressure, the highest mean arterial pressure, the widest pulse pressure, the highest pulsatility on a plethysmogram, the highest Doppler flow measured by echocardiography at any systemic artery, and the highest laser Doppler flow in any tissue. These measurements outside the heart can be made invasively or noninvasively. They differ only in their convenience and signal-to-noise ratio. They do *not* differ in which pacemaker configuration is the best.

Measurements inside the heart do not have this desirable feature. One pacemaker setting may generate the loudest heart sounds; another may generate the most positive LV dP/dt_{max}. Another pacemaker setting may generate the most negative dP/dt_{min}, while another may generate the fastest acceleration of an intracardiac structure, such as a pacing lead in a particular chamber, and another may generate the highest or lowest pressure in a particular chamber. There is no reason that (for example) the setting that generates the fastest acceleration of a pacemaker lead with an accelerometer should be the setting that generates the loudest heart sound. Therefore, choosing an intracardiac feature for optimization or measurement of the efficacy of a pacing strategy is necessarily promoting that feature as more important to the patient than all the other intracardiac features.

Outside the heart, however, all the indices are concordant, which is a manifestation that they lie on a final common pathway of cardiac function: the aspect that is detectable by the rest of the body. There is no reason to advocate 1 extracardiac feature as more important than another, because they are always unanimous when measured with adequate precision.

The researcher is free to choose between the extracardiac markers not on importance but on convenience and signal-to-noise ratio. Noninvasive markers are generally more convenient, but if an invasive marker can be easily incorporated into a pacemaker system, then *it* could be more convenient. The key deciding factor is signal-to-noise ratio. For example, simple photoplethysmography at the finger (ie, the signal from a pulse oximeter) gives the same optimum as systemic blood pressure.[14] However, the simple plethysmograph signal is noisier because many time-varying biological features displace it. Therefore, one could choose the plethysmograph, but would need more replicates to achieve the same precision as would be achieved from a blood pressure signal.

Echocardiography provides multiple potential biological markers. When using echocardiography, the authors' preference has been for markers that are universally concordant with the extracardiac measures, that is, Doppler stroke distance through the LV outflow tract (LVOT). When measured with small confidence intervals, this reliably increases and decreases in proportion to cardiac output when the heart rate is fixed, because the size of the LVOT is consistent within a patient. Assessing stroke volume and cardiac output requires assessing the effective cross-sectional area, which cannot be done reliably by echocardiography, not only because of the geometric difficulties but also because the uncertainty of whether all the blood is moving at the same speed. Fortunately, quantifying changes in stroke distance avoids these uncertainties.

With this approach, the authors have shown that when the pacing configuration is improved, cardiac output immediately increases (within a single heartbeat), and this is the cause of the increase in blood pressure. A few seconds later, the increment in blood pressure wanes, and the cardiac output further increases. The authors interpret this as the consequence of systemic vasodilation as a homeostatic response to the increase in blood pressure.

Other studies have used myocardial perfusion index[23,24] as a measure of global ventricular function or stroke volume[25–27] as indirectly calculated from the LVOT velocity time integral. LV dP/dt$_{max}$ can also be calculated with echocardiography using a continuous-wave Doppler trace of mitral regurgitation. With the Bernoulli equation, a pressure gradient can be calculated at times of 1 and 3 meters per second, and the optimal AV delay is that which produces the highest LV dP/dt$_{max}$. This is time-consuming, and clinicians are unlikely to have the patience to do this for the hundreds of beats when blood pressures can be readily acquired by a noninvasive beat-by-beat blood pressure monitor.

Invasive LV dP/dt$_{max}$ is a popular measure because, in general, invasive measurements are considered more reliable than noninvasive. However, because it is an intracardiac measure, maximizing it will necessarily demaximize other intracardiac variables. There is no reason the setting that produces the sharpest instantaneous rate of increase of pressure inside 1 cardiac chamber must also be the one that produces the highest cardiac output. This becomes obvious in hypertrophic obstructive cardiomyopathy, where obstruction of the LVOT causes both an increase in LV pressures and a decline in systemic arterial pressures. Fortunately, experiments indicate that in heart failure, invasive LV dP/dt$_{max}$ does seem to maximize when the systemic circulation is optimized.[17] However, with a catheter inside the LV, a more direct index of systemic circulation might be the peak systolic pressure. One could eliminate the stroke risk by pulling the pressure wire into the aorta distal to the carotids.

In a head-to-head comparison of precision of optimization, invasive systemic arterial blood pressure performed better than both noninvasive beat-by-beat blood pressure and invasive LV dP/dt$_{max}$.[20]

SonR (Livanova) is a heart sound sensor inside the atrial lead. The optimization process is automated and seems to be maximizing the loudness of the first heart sound.[28] When undergoing regular optimizations, there was an improvement in the composite end point of all-cause mortality, heart failure–related hospitalizations, quality of life, and New York Heart Association class.[29]

FUTURE DIRECTIONS

Changing the AV delay has an appreciable effect on hemodynamics, although it is not large. It is a fraction of the effect of switching on a biventricular pacemaker in patients with heart failure and LBBB. There are many methods to choose the best AV delay setting, but most have become accepted into practice without realizing that they have poor test-retest reproducibility under blinded conditions. This is particularly so for echocardiographic optimization with the iterative mitral method. Future studies on optimization methods must begin with assessments of blinded test-retest reproducibility. The authors predict that all methods using measurements outside the heart, when implemented with a reproducible approach (ie, with sufficient replicates for the signal to overwhelm the noise), will indicate the same optimum AV delay in the same patient.

For interventricular delay, the effect of changes is much smaller than that of AV delay, and the hemodynamic optimum is rarely far from 0 milliseconds. Studies that report optima far from 0 milliseconds have usually used noisy methodology that was not much different from selecting a setting at random. Although it could be argued that one should therefore only test "reasonable" VV delays, this argument is incorrect because a method that cannot distinguish an unreasonable from a reasonable VV delay has no chance of finding the best among several reasonable VV delays because the differences will be even smaller.

The greatest utility of hemodynamics will be in identifying favorable pacing configurations, such as lead positions. This may be particularly valuable, as new forms of conduction system pacing are coming to light. The ability to precisely grade the relative hemodynamic merits of different forms of pacing will increase the opportunity to identify useful forms of pacing in general and to personalize the choice for an individual.

The ideal hemodynamic sensor is one that closely accords with all the systemic markers of cardiovascular function, that is, has a monotonic relationship with blood pressure and cardiac output and the other extracardiac variables and can be incorporated into an implantable cardiac device with acceptable energy consumption. Several such sensors are under development.

Regardless of the choice of sensor, it will remain advisable to take the steps the authors described above to minimize the impact of noise.

A final frontier for hemodynamic sensing is its use to assist a defibrillator in deciding whether to deliver therapy when a tachycardia is diagnosed. This is a far more clinically sensitive decision because incorrect choices can lead to obvious and immediate harm, whereas the adverse outcomes from harmful pacing take longer to manifest.[30] There has been some progress in algorithmic development, in learning how to exploit the coupling between the electrical and mechanical signals to maximize the reliability of the automated interpretation. One electromechanical coupling algorithm has been reported to be 100% sensitive and specific at discriminating ventricular fibrillation from T-wave oversensing, noise, and lead fracture.[31] This approach may also prove useful in the more challenging task of making automatic decisions on ventricular tachycardias. Even when the diagnosis is definite, it is not obvious from the electrical data alone whether perfusion is impaired in a patient on a particular occasion. This makes it difficult to determine whether therapy should be delivered or whether it can be delayed to allow more time for spontaneous termination.

CLINICS CARE POINTS

- Although hemodynamic measurements are not routinely performed in clinical practice, they provide us with useful information by quantifying the impact of cardiac pacing on cardiac function.

- This allows us to both compare different pacing modalities and guide optimal programming for each patient.

- It is crucial to use a protocol that reduces the impact of noise to allow for reliable and precise hemodynamic measurements to be made.

FUNDING

This has been funded by the British Heart Foundation (FS/20/11/34750).

REFERENCES

1. Lassers BW, Anderton JL, George M, et al. Hemodynamic effects of artificial pacing in complete heart block complicating acute myocardial infarction. Circulation 1968;38(2):308–23. https://doi.org/10.1161/01.cir.38.2.308.

2. Sowton E. Hemodynamic studies in patients with artificial pacemakers. Br Heart J 1964;26(6):737–46. https://doi.org/10.1136/hrt.26.6.737.

3. Buckingham TA, Janosik DL, Pearson AC. Pacemaker hemodynamics: clinical implications. Prog Cardiovasc Dis 1992;34(5):347–66. https://doi.org/10.1016/0033-0620(92)90039-3.

4. Reiter MJ, Hindman MC. Hemodynamic effects of acute atrioventricular sequential pacing in patients with left ventricular dysfunction. Am J Cardiol 1982;49(4):687–92. https://doi.org/10.1016/0002-9149(82)91947-6.

5. Hartzler GO, Maloney JD, Curtis JJ, et al. Hemodynamic benefits of atrioventricular sequential pacing after cardiac surgery. Am J Cardiol 1977;40(2):232–6. https://doi.org/10.1016/0002-9149(77)90013-3.

6. Cazeau S, Ritter P, Bakdach S, et al. Four chamber pacing in dilated cardiomyopathy. Pacing Clin Electrophysiol 1994;17(11 Pt 2):1974–9. https://doi.org/10.1111/j.1540-8159.1994.tb03783.x.

7. Auricchio A, Stellbrink C, Sack S, et al, Pacing Therapies in Congestive Heart Failure (PATH-CHF) Study Group. Long-term clinical effect of hemodynamically optimized cardiac resynchronization therapy in patients with heart failure and ventricular conduction delay. J Am Coll Cardiol 2002;39(12):2026–33. https://doi.org/10.1016/s0735-1097(02)01895-8.

8. Cleland JG, Daubert JC, Erdmann E, et al. The effect of cardiac resynchronization on morbidity and mortality in heart failure. N Engl J Med 2005;352(15):1539–49. https://doi.org/10.1056/NEJMoa050496.

9. Arnold AD, Shun-Shin MJ, Keene D, et al. His resynchronization versus biventricular pacing in patients with heart failure and left bundle branch block. J Am Coll Cardiol 2018;72(24):3112–22. https://doi.org/10.1016/j.jacc.2018.09.073.

10. Houston BA, Sturdivant JL, Yu Y, et al. Acute biventricular hemodynamic effects of cardiac resynchronization therapy in right bundle branch block. Heart Rhythm 2018. https://doi.org/10.1016/j.hrthm.2018.05.017.

11. Thibault B, Dubuc M, Khairy P, et al. Acute haemodynamic comparison of multisite and biventricular pacing with a quadripolar left ventricular lead. Europace 2013;15(7):984–91. https://doi.org/10.1093/europace/eus435.

12. Sterliński M, Sokal A, Lenarczyk R, et al. In heart failure patients with left bundle branch block single lead MultiSpot left ventricular pacing does not improve acute hemodynamic response to conventional biventricular pacing. A multicenter prospective, interventional, non-randomized study. PLoS One 2016;11(4):e0154024. https://doi.org/10.1371/journal.pone.0154024.

13. Manisty CH, Al-Hussaini A, Unsworth B, et al. The acute effects of changes to AV delay on BP and

stroke volume: potential implications for design of pacemaker optimization protocols. Circ Arrhythm Electrophysiol 2012;5(1):122–30. https://doi.org/10.1161/CIRCEP.111.964205.

14. Kyriacou A, Pabari PA, Whinnett ZI, et al. Fully automatable, reproducible, noninvasive simple plethysmographic optimization: proof of concept and potential for implantability. Pacing Clin Electrophysiol 2012;35(8):948–60. https://doi.org/10.1111/j.1540-8159.2012.03435.x.

15. Pabari PA, Willson K, Stegemann B, et al. When is an optimization not an optimization? Evaluation of clinical implications of information content (signal-to-noise ratio) in optimization of cardiac resynchronization therapy, and how to measure and maximize it. Heart Fail Rev 2011;16(3):277–90. https://doi.org/10.1007/s10741-010-9203-5.

16. Stegemann B, Francis DP. Atrioventricular and interventricular delay optimization and response quantification in biventricular pacing: arrival of reliable clinical algorithms and research protocols, and how to distinguish them from unreliable counterparts. Europace 2012;14(12):1679–83. https://doi.org/10.1093/europace/eus242.

17. Whinnett ZI, Francis DP, Denis A, et al. Comparison of different invasive hemodynamic methods for AV delay optimization in patients with cardiac resynchronization therapy: implications for clinical trial design and clinical practice. Int J Cardiol 2013;168(3):2228–37. https://doi.org/10.1016/j.ijcard.2013.01.216.

18. Whinnett ZI, Davies JE, Willson K, et al. Determination of optimal atrioventricular delay for cardiac resynchronization therapy using acute non-invasive blood pressure. Europace 2006;8(5):358–66. https://doi.org/10.1093/europace/eul017.

19. Whinnett ZI, Nott G, Davies JE, et al. Maximizing efficiency of alternation algorithms for hemodynamic optimization of the AV delay of cardiac resynchronization therapy. Pacing Clin Electrophysiol 2011;34(2):217–25. https://doi.org/10.1111/j.1540-8159.2010.02933.x.

20. Shun-Shin MJ, Miyazawa AA, Keene D, et al. How to deliver personalized cardiac resynchronization therapy through the precise measurement of the acute hemodynamic response: insights from the iSpot trial. J Cardiovasc Electrophysiol 2019;30(9):1610–9. https://doi.org/10.1111/jce.14001.

21. Francis DP. How to reliably deliver narrow individual-patient error bars for optimization of pacemaker AV or VV delay using a "pick-the-highest" strategy with hemodynamic measurements. Int J Cardiol 2013;163(3):221–5. https://doi.org/10.1016/j.ijcard.2012.03.128.

22. Whinnett ZI, Davies JE, Willson K, et al. Hemodynamic effects of changes in atrioventricular and interventricular delay in cardiac resynchronisation therapy show a consistent pattern: analysis of shape, magnitude and relative importance of atrioventricular and interventricular delay. Heart 2006;92(11):1628–34. https://doi.org/10.1136/hrt.2005.080721.

23. Porciani MC, Dondina C, Macioce R, et al. Echocardiographic examination of atrioventricular and interventricular delay optimization in cardiac resynchronization therapy. Am J Cardiol 2005;95(9):1108–10. https://doi.org/10.1016/j.amjcard.2005.01.028.

24. Stockburger M, Fateh-Moghadam S, Nitardy A, et al. Optimization of cardiac resynchronization guided by Doppler echocardiography: hemodynamic improvement and intraindividual variability with different pacing configurations and atrioventricular delays. Europace 2006;8(10):881–6. https://doi.org/10.1093/europace/eul088.

25. Thomas DE, Yousef ZR, Fraser AG. A critical comparison of echocardiographic measurements used for optimizing cardiac resynchronization therapy: stroke distance is best. Eur J Heart Fail 2009;11(8):779–88. https://doi.org/10.1093/eurjhf/hfp086.

26. Gold MR, Niazi I, Giudici M, et al. A prospective comparison of AV delay programming methods for hemodynamic optimization during cardiac resynchronization therapy. J Cardiovasc Electrophysiol 2007;18(5):490–6. https://doi.org/10.1111/j.1540-8167.2007.00770.x.

27. Vanderheyden M, De Backer T, Rivero-Ayerza M, et al. Tailored echocardiographic interventricular delay programming further optimizes left ventricular performance after cardiac resynchronization therapy. Heart Rhythm 2005;2(10):1066–72. https://doi.org/10.1016/j.hrthm.2005.07.016.

28. Cardiocases. Sorin algorithm. In: Cardiocases. Available at: https://www.cardiocases.com/en/pacingdefibrillation/specificities/crt-av-vv-delays-optimization/livanova/sorin-algorithm. October 3, 2021.

29. Delnoy PP, Ritter P, Naegele H, et al. Association between frequent cardiac resynchronization therapy optimization and long-term clinical response: a post hoc analysis of the Clinical Evaluation on Advanced Resynchronization (CLEAR) pilot study. Europace 2013;15(8):1174–81. https://doi.org/10.1093/europace/eut034.

30. Ruschitzka F, Abraham WT, Singh JP, et al. Cardiac-resynchronization therapy in heart failure with a narrow QRS complex. N Engl J Med 2013;369(15):1395–405. https://doi.org/10.1056/NEJMoa1306687.

31. Keene D, Shun-Shin MJ, Arnold AD, et al. Quantification of electromechanical coupling to prevent inappropriate implantable cardioverter-defibrillator shocks. JACC Clin Electrophysiol 2019;5(6):705–15. https://doi.org/10.1016/j.jacep.2019.01.025.

His Bundle Pacing
My Experience, Tricks, and Tips

Francesco Zanon, MD, FESC, FHERA, FHRS*, Lina Marcantoni, MD, Marco Centioni, MD, Gianni Pastore, MD, Enrico Baracca, MD

KEYWORDS

- His bundle pacing • Physiologic pacing • Conduction system pacing

KEY POINTS

- HBP is reliable and effective in preserving the physiologic ventricular synchrony.
- New dedicated tools and customized technologies will continue to improve the implant success rate and system performance.
- Large, randomized trials are needed to definitively prove long-term clinical benefits of HBP.

INTRODUCTION

His bundle pacing (HBP) is a form of physiologic pacing achieved through implantation of a pacing electrode into the His bundle. In patients with narrow QRS, HBP may maintain ventricular synchrony, and in patients with bundle branch block (BBB) HBP may restore ventricular synchrony.[1–3] The complex cardiac anatomy of the atrioventricular node and the His-Purkinje system account for challenging aspects of the HBP procedure.[4–6] The first experiences with HBP were restricted to small single-center series in patients with proximal conduction disturbances mainly due to the scarcity of tools.[7–10] As new tools became available, HBP quickly spread around the world, treating distal conduction disturbances and cardiac resynchronization indications.[11–13] Various technical drawbacks have been solved over time, and it is expected that ongoing research will further simplify HBP.[14–16]

HIS BUNDLE PACING: A 20-YEAR JOURNEY

The idea of HBP came out around the beginning of the pacing era,[17,18] but only in 2000 the first series of patients directly paced at the His bundle were described by Deshmukh and colleagues[19] in 18 patients with history of chronic atrial fibrillation,

narrow QRS, and dilated cardiomyopathy candidate to ablate and pace. The acute implant success rate was 86%, the mean time procedure time was 3.7 ± 1.6 hours, and the mean acute HBP threshold was 2.4 ± 0.9 V. Nevertheless, this pioneering experience really elicited my interest in HBP. Since then, my involvement in HBP has always grown trying to overcome the most challenging aspects of a new pacing technique. At the beginning I tried unsuccessfully to pace the His with standard stylet-driven leads following the technique described by Deshmukh. Some years passed before initial challenges faced at implant were gradually overcome, including high failure rate, electrode dislodgement, high pacing threshold, low R wave sensing. In this journey, the first cornerstone step was the availability of the Select Secure 3830 lead: a 4.1 Fr, lumenless, bipolar, fixed, exposed helix screw, active fixation lead (Medtronic Inc., Minneapolis, MN, USA). This new lead appeared in the market with the specific indication for right septal ventricular pacing. In 2004 we began to use the Medtronic deflectable C304 delivery sheath (Medtronic Inc., Minneapolis, MN, USA) to direct the 3830 lead to the His Bundle region with positive results.[20] Stable HBP was obtained in 92% of patients, the mead lead positioning time was 19 ± 17 min, the mean

Arrhythmia and Electrophysiology Unit, Division of Cardiology, Department of Specialistic Medicine, Santa Maria Della Misericordia General Hospital, Viale Tre Martiri 177, 45100 Rovigo, Italy
* Corresponding author.
E-mail address: franc.zanon@iol.it
Twitter: @ZanonFrancesco (F.Z.); @LinaMarcantoni (L.M.)

Card Electrophysiol Clin 14 (2022) 141–149
https://doi.org/10.1016/j.ccep.2021.12.016

fluoroscopy time 11 ± 8 min, and the mean pacing threshold 2.3 ± 1V.[20] I involved in this pioneering experience various Italian Centers: the result was the successful publication of our first multicenter observational registry demonstrating that the 3830 lead guided by the C304 delivery sheath was helpful in precisely localizing and pacing the His.[21] Sometimes the procedure was complex and often required 2 operators (**Fig. 1**) to manage, at the same time the diagnostic quadripolar catheter preferably introduced from the femoral access aiming to localize the His bundle and the 3830 lead from the superior venous access. At this time the procedure was fluoroscopically centered: the diagnostic catheter located the His bundle, and the operator tried to replicate the same site with the pacing lead and sheath, guided by the fluoroscopic right and left projections.[20] Procedural outcomes gradually become acceptable, and the constant positive clinical results increased my curiosity and the active research on how to pace the conduction system of the heart effectively and feasibly.

Positive results were not unfrequently counterbalanced by challenges also appearing during the follow-up: high pacing thresholds and low R wave sensing were the major pitfalls encountered.[22,23] Those difficulties lengthened the procedure, requiring sometimes several attempts to optimize the final lead location. In selected patients, to overcome electrical parameters, we included an additional apical "backup lead," aiming to ensure optimal sensing and backup pacing in the event of Hisian capture loss.[23] The backup lead ensured ventricular pacing in the case of progression of conduction block below the Hisian pacing site and avoided problems related to an increase of the pacing threshold and low R wave

sensing. Backup stimulation delivered in the event of HBP failure proved to be effective and strengthened the reliability of the pacing system. HBP safety margin could be reduced with total security, allowing a relevant reduction of energy expense with positive impact on device longevity.[24] In a multicenter observational experience, the postimplant increase in threshold was observed in approximately 7% of cases in HBP after a median follow-up of 3 years, probably due to microdislodgment or fibrosis.[22] Loss of capture can occur early after implant or very late. Macrodislodgments are rare but high threshold are not uncommon. Combining macrodislodgment and high threshold as indication for redo procedures, the reintervention rate is between 6% and 8% in larger long-term studies, although in some laboratories it may be up to close to 20%.[22,25,26]

TIMELINE: THE EVOLUTION OF HIS BUNDLE PACING

In our center, after the initial experience started in 2003 to 2004 as depicted in **Fig. 2**, the number of HBP implants increased for the first 4 to 5 years but then decreased later. Limited implantation tools and the contemporary increasing of tools and strong clinical evidence in cardiac resynchronization therapy (CRT) coming from randomized trials[27] probably delayed the HBP evolution.

A renewed interest and significant improvement in HBP implantation outcome were ensured by a series of tridimensional tools equipped with the second orthogonal curve added to the first one. The second curve has made possible to guide the lead perpendicularly to the septum, enabling an easier and efficient lead fixation, allowing better threshold both at implant and during follow-up,

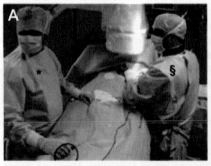 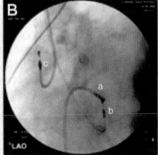 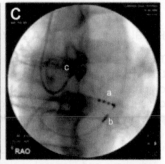

Fig. 1. The initial experience with His bundle pacing (HBP). At the beginning of our experience HBP procedures were "fluoroscopic-centered" and often required 2 operators (*A*). The operator 1 (*) managed the diagnostic quadripolar catheter preferably introduced from the femoral access with the aim to localize the His bundle. The operator 2 (§) managed the 3830 lead from the superior venous access trying to replicate the same site with the pacing lead and sheath, guided by the fluoroscopic left (*B*) and right (*C*) oblique fluoroscopic views. "a": quadripolar diagnostic catheter; "b": 3830 lead; "c": atrial lead.

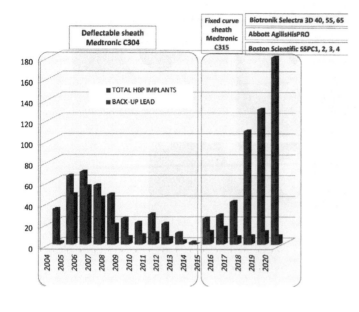

Fig. 2. Evolution of the His bundle pacing (HBP) procedures over time at the Rovigo's Hospital. Blue columns depict the total HBP implant per year. The red columns depict the number of patients who received an additional lead as backup. Our experience started in the period 2003 to 2004. At that time all the implants were performed by the Medtronic C304 deflectable sheath and the Medtronic 3830 bipolar lead. The number of HBP implants increased for the first 4 to 5 years but then decreased later. A renewed interest and significant improvement in HBP implantation outcomes were ensured by a series of new tools equipped with the second orthogonal curve added to the first one, essential to position the lead perpendicularly to the septum. The first tridimensional delivery sheath was the Medtronic C315 fixed curve sheath, still widely used, which was available in Italy since 2015, being the only dedicated tool for 3 to 4 years. In our experience, the fixed curve sheath drastically improved implant success rate and technical performance of the lead during long-term follow-up, thus reducing the number of patients who need the backup leads. During the last few years, the availability of various new tridimensional sheaths furtherly increased the HBP adoption in the daily clinical practice. The use of backup lead still remains in a very low number of cases.

thus reducing the number of reinterventions.[22] The first tridimensional delivery sheath was the C 315 Medtronic fixed curve (Medtronic, Minneapolis, Minnesota, USA), still widely used, which was available in Italy since 2014, being the only dedicated tool for 3 or 4 years. The fixed curve sheath drastically improved implant success rate and technical performance of the lead during long-term follow-up. In our experience, the number of patients who need backup leads has drastically decreased over time.[22]

With the introduction of the new the tridimensional sheath, we standardized our implantation technique, as other centers adopted their own. We usually prefer the 3830-59 cm lead instead of the 3830-69 cm because it is more manageable during screwing even by a single operator. After preparing the sheath and the lead on the surgical table (**Fig. 3** panel A), the sleeve is temporarily removed to gain enough length during the cutting maneuver (see **Fig. 3** panel B). The lead is inserted into the sheath (see **Fig. 3** panel C), and the system assembled is perfused with saline solution (see **Fig. 3** panel D). We usually insert the system (sheath and lead inside) already assembled (see **Fig. 3** panel E) advancing via axillary vein access up to the right atrium, applying small and gentle rotations both clockwise and counterclockwise in sequence.[14]

Since 2019 we rapidly gained experience also with the Selectra 3D introducers. They also have

a 3-dimensional (3D) shape with a primary curve to reach the tricuspid annulus and a second curve to localize the HB region in a perpendicular manner. Three lengths (32, 39, and 42 cm) and 3 different primary curves (40, 55, and 65 cm) are available, allowing to address various anatomies. Today, after more than 100 implants performed with the Selectra 3D, we observed that the 55 cm (M) curve was adequate in most anatomies. The 40 cm (S) curve favors the achievement of more proximal positions, whereas the 65 cm (L) curve leads to more distal sites being especially beneficial in dilated atria.[28]

MOVING FROM FLUOROSCOPIC TO ELECTRICAL APPROACH: THE FLUORO-ZERO TECHNIQUE

The diagnostic mapping catheter was gradually abandoned in favor of the unipolar mapping directly from the tip of the lead. This possibility has allowed to achieve the final His lead position without the use of fluoroscopy, exclusively guided by electrograms. The "fluoro-zero approach" recently was described with positive results in terms of safety, efficacy, and feasibility for HBP.[29] As illustrated in **Fig. 4**, the operator's view is totally focused on electrical signals recorded from the tip of the lead and displayed on the electrophysiology (EP) recording system.

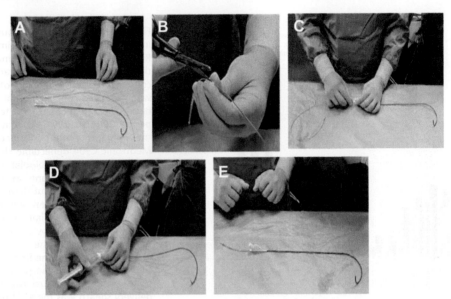

Fig. 3. Lead preparation. In our experience we usually prefer the 3830-59 cm lead instead of the 3830-69 cm because it is more manageable during screwing even by a single operator procedure. After preparing the sheath and the lead on the surgical table (*A*), the sleeve is temporarily removed to gain enough length during the cutting maneuver (*B*). The lead is inserted into the sheath (*C*), and the system assembled is perfused with saline solution (*D*). We usually insert the system (sheath and lead inside) already assembled (*E*) advancing via axillary vein access up to the right atrium, applying small and gentle rotations both clockwise and counterclockwise in sequence.

The lead is connected to the alligator cable in unipolar fashion with the red crocodile on the skin and the black one on the tip of the lead. During the mapping phase the EP recording system is set at a sweep speed of 100 mm/s to clearly visualize the His signal. The x-ray tube is not placed over the surgical field but ready for use. Once the lead is in the atrium and atrial potentials are recorded, the system is advanced. A double atrial and ventricular potential suggests that the lead is facing the septal tricuspid leaflet. In most cases, a further gentle clockwise rotation of the sheath directs the lead superiorly toward the membranous septum, and a prominent ventricular electrogram appears. In a minority of patients, counterclockwise rotation is needed to reach the His area. Our reference to start mapping is usually considered a large ventricular electrogram. The following

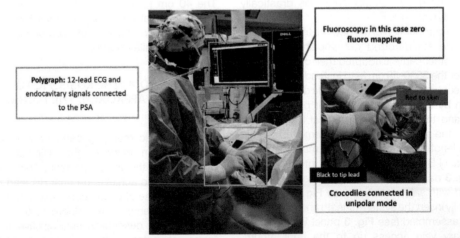

Fig. 4. The "fluoro-zero approach." The operator's view is totally focused on electrical signals recorded in unipolar manner from the tip of the lead and displayed on the EP recording system. The lead is connected with the red crocodile on the skin and the black one on the tip of the lead (*small pink square* and zoom). During the mapping phase the EP recording system is set at a sweep speed of 100 mm/s to clearly visualize the His signal (*small yellow square*). The x-ray tube is not over the surgical field but ready for use (*small red square*). EP, electrophysiology.

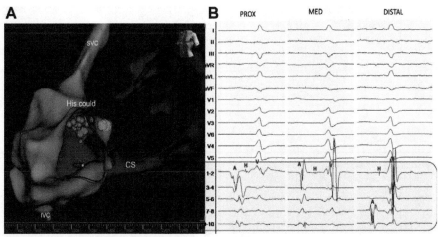

Fig. 5. Three-dimensional (3D) electroanatomic mapping–guided His bundle pacing implant. (*A*) The 3D reconstruction of the right atrium geometry and the His cloud. (*B*) The 12-lead ECG together with the intracardiac signals detected by the decapolar diagnostic catheter in 3 different sites in the His Bundle at a sweep speed 100 mm/s (*red square*). "A" atrial signal; "H" His signal; "V" ventricular signal. The HV duration and the amplitude ratio between atrial signal and ventricular signal differentiate the proximal (longer HV interval) (*B*; "PROX"), intermediate (*B*; "MED"), and distal (shorter HV interval) (*B*; "DISTAL") collected points. Each time the His signal is detected, one tag is drawn on the map following a color code to differentiate the proximal, intermediate, and distal points. ECG, electrocardiogram; CS, coronary sinus; IVC, inferior vena cava; SVC, superior vena cava.

maneuvers are needed to localize and screw properly the lead: the left hand holds with 3 fingers, the sheath moving forward and backward and rotating counterclockwise or vice versa, whereas the right hand continuously and gently pushes and pulls back the lead to assure a contact with the heart and to avoid microentrapment. When a proper His signal is visualized the right hand rapidly screws the lead for 2 to 3 turns, and after verifying satisfactory electrical parameters further 2 to 3 turns are performed to definitively fix the lead. The 12-lead electrocardiogram and the His electrogram are continuously displayed during the procedure to assess selective or nonselective His

bundle capture based on intracardiac recording and paced QRS morphology. Always a few seconds of fluoroscopy were performed while cutting the sheath, to ensure adequate lead slack.

THE LAST FRONTIER: 3-DIMENSIONAL ELECTROANATOMICAL MAPPING–GUIDED IMPLANT
His Cloud

Recently some small experiences showed the safety and feasibility of HBP implant guided by 3D electroanatomic mapping (3D-EAM) systems such as Ensite NavX (Abbott, St. Paul, MN, USA) and CARTO (Biosense Webster, Irvine, CA, USA)

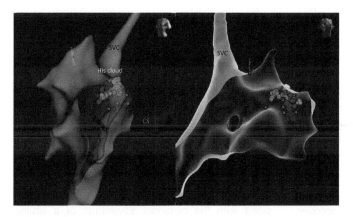

Fig. 6. The 3D electroanatomic mapping could highlight in real time the possible cause of implant failure. The figure depicts a case of HBP implant guided by 3D-EAM showing 2 views. The 3D right atrium geometry has been reconstructed and the His cloud tagged. Proximal, intermediate, and distal His Bundle sites were depicted in yellow, red, and light blue tags, respectively. In this case HBP failed due to inadequate tool: the delivery sheath used and the lead inside were not able to reach the His cloud. The 5 pink tags represent all sites reached with the delivery sheath and the pacing lead inside, far away from the His cloud.

In this case the operator can rapidly decide to change the sheath or change the target in the conduction system without excessive x-ray exposure.

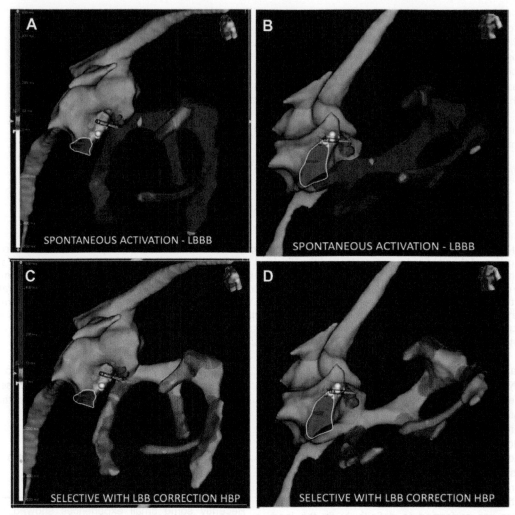

Fig. 7. 3D-EAM shows the recovered left ventricular synchronicity. The figure shows a case report of corrective His bundle pacing (HBP) in patients with left bundle branch block (LBBB) during a 3D electroanatomic mapping–guided implant. After the selective HBP with LBB correction, all the available branches of the coronary sinus were navigated by a Bmw guidewire aiming to compare the global left ventricular activation at baseline and during selective HBP with LBB correction. A color code was used: purple shows delayed and red early left ventricular activation. The map during spontaneous LBBB (*A, B*) confirms delayed activation during LBB particularly evident in the lateral wall of the left ventricle. After turning ON the LBB-corrective HBP pacing, the Bmw guidewire navigating within the CS branches immediately shows homogeneous and normalized left ventricular activation times (*C; D*).

with extremely low fluoroscopic exposure, following the previous demonstration of 3D-EAM in placement of the pacing lead for cardiac resynchronization therapy.[30,31] The first step is the reconstruction of a 3D right atrium geometry; systematically we also map the high interventricular septum to easily shift from HBP to LBBP intraprocedurally, based on electrical parameters. The His cloud is tagged according to the intracardiac signals detection. Each time the His signal is detected, a tag is placed on the map. Moreover, the HV interval is measured for each tag and a color code has been ascribed to differentiate the

proximal (longer HV interval), intermediate, and distal (shorter HV interval) collected points (**Fig. 5**). Interestingly, the resulting picture is a detailed anatomic representation of the His bundle path along the septum contemporarily showing how the electrical signal propagates. Generally, it is possible to recognize a great correspondence with the His cloud tags and the anatomic images of the human conduction system. The lead can then easily direct the pacing lead to the target point with the potential advantage of a limited need for fluoroscopy even in complex cardiac anatomies such as congenital cardiac diseases or enlarged right atria, usually associated with high percentage of implant failure.[32] Furthermore, 3D-EAM could highlight in real-time the possible cause of implant failure: **Fig. 6** depicts a case of implant failure due to inadequate curve of the sheath: the pink tags represent all sites reached with the pacing lead, distant to the His cloud. In this case the operator can rapidly decide to change the sheath or change the target in the conduction system without excessive x-ray exposure.

Validate Synchronicity

3D-EAM allows to validate the recovered ventricular synchronicity in patients with left BBB (LBBB) in whom HBP was used as alternative to standard CRT. **Fig. 7** is a case report of a patient with LBBB paced in the His Bundle in a 3D-EAM–guided approach. After selective HBP with LBB correction, all the available branches of the coronary sinus were navigated with a 0.014-Fr guidewire aiming to analyze the global left ventricular activation. Purple and red color code represents delayed and early left ventricular activation, respectively. Baseline spontaneous LBBB and the selective HBP with LBB correction are compared. The 3D map during spontaneous LBBB (**Fig. 7** panel A and B) confirms delayed activation particularly evident in the lateral wall of the left ventricle. Immediately, after turning ON the LBB-corrective HBP pacing, the guidewire navigating within the CS branches shows homogeneous and normalized left ventricular activation times (see **Fig. 7** panel C and D).

What is Next?

There are still multiple open points that must be addressed to further improve physiologic pacing.

(a) *Clinical indications*: there are no clear indications for HBP. The ideal pacing mode that everyone would like to apply but feels ashamed to ask for. We are waiting for randomized clinical trial indicating HBP as first-line therapy for bradycardia indications.

(b) *Education*: we need to educate physicians to jump into this new modality of pacing. At the same time, we need to educate nurses and technicians on how to assist the HBP implant and manage patients during the follow-up.

(c) *Tools:* important progresses have been made in this technical field, but still further tools are necessary to fill the gaps. Some suggestions may include new deflectable delivery sheaths, with different curves. Leads: shorter dipole, longer helix. Improvement in mapping modalities.

Unmet features:

- *Devices*: algorithms for His electrograms detection, selective or nonselective, battery capacity, device diagnostics.
- *Imaging*: easy localization of His/left bundle.
- *Follow-up*: easy way for diagnostic and programming.
- *Remote monitoring*: easy way to diagnose different threshold (ie, selective vs nonselective vs septal capture only).

Electrocardiogram recording for better follow-up.

SUMMARY

The HBP is increasingly proving to be a viable alternative to traditional right ventricle pacing, being able to avoid pacing-induced cardiomyopathy. HBP is reliable and effective in preserving the physiologic ventricular synchrony with clinical benefits particularly evident when a high percentage of pacing is required. New tools specifically designed for selective site pacing currently allow reliable HBP in routine clinical practice, increase procedural success rate, and reduce both fluoroscopy time and total procedural time. New customized technologies will continue to improve the implant success rate and system performance. Large, randomized trials can definitively prove long-term clinical benefits of HBP and will bolster HBP to be considered as a first approach in patients who need a pacemaker.

CLINICS CARE POINTS

- Apical ventricular pacing is detrimental for left ventricular function, conduction system pacing is a physiologic mode of pacing that mantain the natural mechanics of the heart.

DISCLOSURE

F. Zanon reports speaker fees (modest) from Abbott, Biotronik, Boston Scientific, Medtronic, and Microport. Other authors report no disclosure.

REFERENCES

1. Arnold AD, Whinnett ZI, Vijayaraman P. His-purkinje conduction system pacing: State of the Art in 2020. Arrhythm Electrophysiol Rev 2020;9(3):136–45.

2. Sharma PS, Vijayaraman P, Ellenbogen KA. Permanent His bundle pacing: shaping the future of

physiological ventricular pacing. Nat Rev Cardiol 2020;17(1):22–36.

3. Vijayaraman P, Chung MK, Dandamudi G, et al. His bundle pacing. J Am Coll Cardiol 2018;72(8): 927–47.

4. Padala SK, Cabrera JA, Ellenbogen KA. Anatomy of the cardiac conduction system. Pacing Clin Electrophysiol 2021;44(1):15–25.

5. Nagarajan VD, Ho SY, Ernst S. Anatomical considerations for his bundle pacing. Circ Arrhythm Electrophysiol 2019;12(7):e006897.

6. Cabrera JA, Porta-Sánchez A, Tung R, et al. Tracking down the anatomy of the left bundle branch to optimize left bundle branch pacing. JACC Case Rep 2020;2(5):750–5.

7. Occhetta E, Bortnik M, Marino P. Permanent parahisian pacing. Indian Pacing Electrophysiol J 2007; 7(2):110–25.

8. Catanzariti D, Maines M, Cemin C, et al. Permanent direct his bundle pacing does not induce ventricular dyssynchrony unlike conventional right ventricular apical pacing. An intrapatient acute comparison study. J Interv Card Electrophysiol 2006;16(2): 81–92.

9. Zanon F, Bacchiega E, Rampin L, et al. Direct His bundle pacing preserves coronary perfusion compared with right ventricular apical pacing: a prospective, cross-over mid-term study. Europace 2008;10(5):580–7.

10. Kronborg MB, Poulsen SH, Mortensen PT, et al. Left ventricular performance during para-His pacing in patients with high-grade atrioventricular block: an acute study. Europace 2012;14(6):841–6.

11. Sharma PS, Dandamudi G, Naperkowski A, et al. Permanent His-bundle pacing is feasible, safe, and superior to right ventricular pacing in routine clinical practice. Heart Rhythm 2015;12(2):305–12.

12. Ajijola OA, Upadhyay GA, Macias C, et al. Permanent His-bundle pacing for cardiac resynchronization therapy: initial feasibility study in lieu of left ventricular lead. Heart Rhythm 2017;14(9): 1353–61.

13. Lustgarten DL, Crespo EM, Arkhipova-Jenkins I, et al. His-bundle pacing versus biventricular pacing in cardiac resynchronization therapy patients: a crossover design comparison. Heart Rhythm 2015; 12(7):1548–57.

14. Marcantoni L, Zuin M, Baracca E, et al. Implantation technique of His bundle pacing. Herzschrittmacherther Elektrophysiol 2020;31(2):111–6.

15. Lustgarten DL, Sharma PS, Vijayaraman P. Troubleshooting and programming considerations for His bundle pacing. Heart Rhythm 2019;16(5):654–62.

16. Zanon F, Ellenbogen KA, Dandamudi G, et al. Permanent His-bundle pacing: a systematic literature review and meta-analysis. Europace 2018;20(11): 1819–26.

17. Scherlag BJ, Kosowsky BD, Damato AN. A technique for ventricular pacing from the His bundle of the intact heart. J Appl Phys 1967;22(3): 584–7.

18. Narula OS, Scherlag BJ, Samet P. Pervenous pacing of the specialized conducting system in man. His bundle and A-V nodal stimulation. Circulation 1970;41(1):77–87.

19. Deshmukh P, Casavant DA, Romanyshyn M, et al. Permanent, direct His-bundle pacing: a novel approach to cardiac pacing in patients with normal His-Purkinje activation. Circulation 2000;101(8): 869–77.

20. Zanon F, Baracca E, Aggio S, et al. A feasible approach for direct his-bundle pacing using a new steerable catheter to facilitate precise lead placement. J Cardiovasc Electrophysiol 2006;17(1): 29–33.

21. Zanon F, Svetlich C, Occhetta E, et al. Safety and performance of a system specifically designed for selective site pacing. Pacing Clin Electrophysiol 2011;34(3):339–47.

22. Zanon F, Abdelrahman M, Marcantoni L, et al. Long term performance and safety of His bundle pacing: a multicenter experience. J Cardiovasc Electrophysiol 2019;30(9):1594–601.

23. Zanon F, Marcantoni L, Pastore G, Baracca E, Picariello C, Lanza D, Giatti S, Aggio S, Conte L, D'Elia K, Roncon L, Rinuncini M, Galasso M. Hisian pacing with apical back-up on demandi s safe and effective (abstract). Article presented at: Annual congress of the European Heart Rhythm Association, Barcelona, Spain, March 18, 2018; Abstract RF 43.

24. F Zanon, L Marcantoni, G Pastore, et al. The energy cost of His bundle pacing can be curtailed. Article presented at: ESC Congress 2019 together with World Congress of Cardiology. 31 August-4,September 2019, Paris-France. P6547. European Heart Journal, Volume 40, Issue Supplement_1, October 2019.

25. Subzposh FA, Vijayaraman P. Long-term results of his bundle pacing. Card Electrophysiol Clin 2018; 10(3):537–42.

26. Bhatt AG, Musat DL, Milstein N, et al. The efficacy of his bundle pacing: lessons learned from implementation for the first time at an experienced Electrophysiology center. JACC Clin Electrophysiol 2018; 4(11):1397–406.

27. Vardas PE, Auricchio A, Blanc JJ, et al. Guidelines for cardiac pacing and cardiac resynchronization therapy: the Task Force for cardiac pacing and cardiac resynchronization therapy of the European Society of Cardiology. Developed in collaboration with the European Heart Rhythm Association. Eur Heart J 2007;28:2256–95.

28. Marcantoni L, Pastore G, Baracca E, Andreaggi S, Pellegrini N, Galuppi E, Bartolomei M, Centioni M,

Rigatelli G, Roncon L, Zanon F. Selectra 3D- guided conduction system pacing: single-center experience. European Heart Journal, Volume 42, Issue Supplement_1, October 2021, ehab724.0683. Abstract presented at: ESC Congress 2021-The Digital Experience. 27-30 August 2021.

29. Zanon F, Marcantoni L, Zuin M, et al. Electrogram-only guided approach to His bundle pacing with minimal fluoroscopy: a single-center experience. J Cardiovasc Electrophysiol 2020;31(4):805–12.

30. Richter S, Ebert M, Bertagnolli L, et al. Impact of electroanatomical mapping-guided lead implantation on procedural outcome of His bundle pacing. Europace 2021;23(3):409–20.

31. Orlov MV, Koulouridis I, Monin AJ, et al. Direct Visualization of the his bundle pacing lead placement by 3-Dimensional electroanatomic mapping: technique, anatomy, and practical considerations. Circ Arrhythm Electrophysiol 2019;12(2):e006801.

32. Marcantoni L, Pastore G, Baracca E, Pellegrini N, Andreaggi S, Bartolomei M, Centioni M, Rigatelli G, Galuppi E, Roncon L, Zanon F. 3D electro-anatomical mapping to guide conduction system pacing in complex cardiac anatomies. European Heart Journal, Volume 42, Issue Supplement_1, October 2021, ehab724.0684. Abstract presented at: ESC Congress 2021-The Digital Experience. 27-30 August 2021.

Physiologic Differentiation Between Selective His Bundle, Nonselective His Bundle and Septal Pacing

Marek Jastrzębski, MD, PhD

KEYWORDS

• His bundle pacing • Conduction system pacing • Programmed stimulation • V6 R- wave peak time
• Capture diagnosis

KEY POINTS

- During His bundle (HB) pacing 3 distinct capture types are possible: selective-HB capture when only HB is activated, nonselective (ns) HB capture when there is simultaneous activation of the adjacent right ventricular septal (RVS) myocardium, and selective RVS capture, when only septal myocardium is activated.
- The electrocardiogram-based diagnosis of ns-HB capture is sometimes challenging because there is substantial overlap between QRS morphologies of ns-HB and RVS capture, and loss of HB capture might be masked by the still maintained RVS capture.
- The electrocardiographic hallmark of physiologic pacing is the preservation or restoration of physiologic depolarization sequence and physiologic activation times in the left ventricle, and this forms the basis for electrocardiographic differentiation between ns-HB capture and selective RVS capture.
- Diagnostically most useful QRS morphology criteria include notch/slur/plateau in left ventricular leads and V6 R-wave peak time.
- Dynamic diagnostic maneuvers include decremental output pacing, programmed stimulation, and burst/incremental pacing.

INTRODUCTION

His bundle (HB) pacing is an increasingly popular method of physiologic ventricular pacing. The electrocardiographic (ECG) hallmark of physiologic pacing is the preservation or restoration of physiologic activation times in the left ventricle (**Fig. 1**)—a principle of paramount diagnostic importance.[1,2]

The current review focuses on the differentiation between 3 possible capture types when the pacing lead is placed in the HB region: selective (s-) HB capture when only HB is activated, nonselective (ns-) HB capture when there is simultaneous activation of the adjacent right ventricular septal (RVS) myocardium, and selective RVS capture, when HB is not activated at all but only septal myocardium.

The ECG-based diagnosis of ns-HB capture is sometimes challenging because there is substantial overlap between QRS morphologies of ns-HB and RVS capture, and loss of HB capture might be masked by the still maintained RVS capture. Within this context it is particularly important to

First Department of Cardiology, Interventional Electrocardiology and Hypertension, Jagiellonian University Medical College, Jagiellonian University in Krakow, Ul. Jakubowskiego 2, Kraków 30-669, Poland
E-mail address: mcjastrz@cyf-kr.edu.pl

Card Electrophysiol Clin 14 (2022) 151–163
https://doi.org/10.1016/j.ccep.2021.12.009
1877-9182/22/© 2021 Elsevier Inc. All rights reserved.

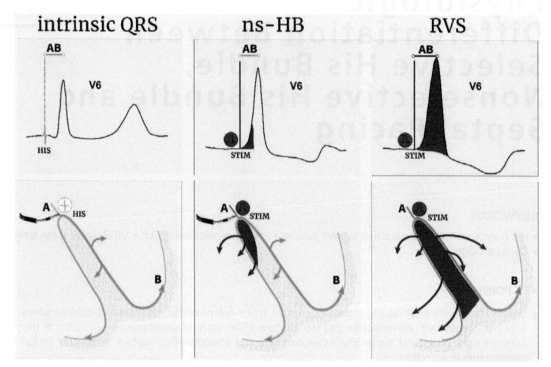

Fig. 1. The principle of preservation of physiologic activation times in the left ventricle during His bundle (HB) pacing. During intrinsic activation, the time from the His bundle potential (HIS) to the activation of the lateral wall of the left ventricle equals the time from the pacing stimulus (STIM) to the activation of the lateral wall of the left ventricle during nonselective (ns-) HB pacing. During right ventricular septal (RVS) capture, the corresponding interval is longer by the time it takes for the depolarization wavefront to cross the interventricular septum and engage the conduction system of the left ventricle. (*Adapted from* Jastrzebski M, Moskal P, Kukla P et al. Novel approach to diagnosis of His bundle capture using individualized left ventricular lateral wall activation time as reference. J Cardiovasc Electrophysiol 2021. doi.org/10.1111/jce.15233; with permission.)

develop accurate criteria for the ECG diagnosis of HB capture/loss of HB capture during follow-up.

SELECTIVE HIS BUNDLE CAPTURE

The presence of a latency interval between the pacing spike and QRS that corresponds to the His-ventricle (HV) interval in endocardial recording is nearly pathognomonic for this type of capture, especially when the paced QRS morphology is either nearly identical as supraventricular QRS morphology or conforms to the criteria for normal supraventricular QRS. In endocardial tracing this is accompanied by discrete ventricular potential, in contrast to ns-HB and RVS capture when the local potential follows immediately the stimulus, and is, therefore, fused with it (**Fig. 2**). Consequently, the diagnosis of s-HB capture is very straightforward. For this reason, the rest of this review discusses only methods for differentiation between ns-HB capture and RVS capture (more precisely, selective para-Hisian myocardial capture).

HIS BUNDLE CAPTURE DIAGNOSIS BASED ON PACED QRS MORPHOLOGIC CRITERIA

HB pacing results in fast and homogenous depolarization of the LV, rather than prolonged and sequential as during RVS capture. Moreover, during HB pacing depolarization of the LV does not require slow myocardial spread of activation from the right side to the left side of the interventricular septum but commences simultaneously with QRS onset. The impact of these phenomena on QRS morphology was exploited in the first validated ECG algorithm for the differentiation between HB versus RVS pacing (**Fig. 3**).[3]

QRS Notching and Slurring

The development of a mid-QRS notch/slur/plateau in left ventricular leads (I, V4–V6), and V1, which appears immediately with the loss of HB capture, provides an easy to assess and reliable morphologic diagnostic criterion (see **Fig. 3**).[3] This morphologic feature has similar cause as the QRS notch/slur seen during left bundle branch

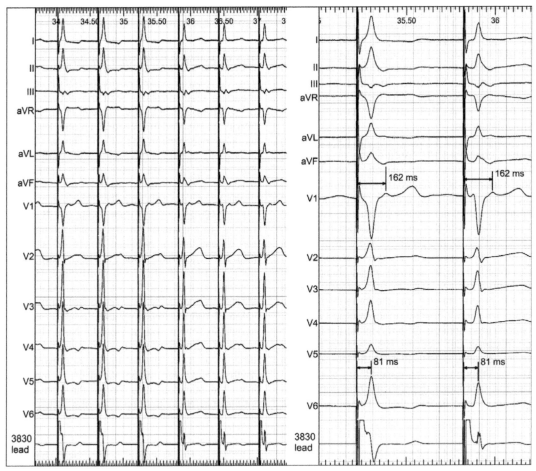

Fig. 2. Transition from nonselective to selective His bundle pacing. Typical features of selective capture can be appreciated: after the pacing stimulus instead of pseudo-delta, which was present during nonselective capture, the latency interval appears, and also the discrete potential on the endocardial channel (3830 lead) becomes evident. In the right panel it can be appreciated that despite QRS morphology transition the activation time in the left ventricle remains unchanged (as evidenced by stable time to R-wave peak in V6 of 81 ms), similarly the retrograde conduction time remains unchanged (as evidenced by stable VA interval of 162 ms). (*Left panel*) Sweep speed 25 mm/s; (*right panel*) sweep speed 67 mm/s.

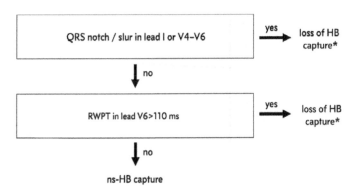

Fig. 3. Algorithm for the electrocardiographic diagnosis of loss of nonselective His bundle capture (ns-HB). RWPT, R-wave peak time. (*) lack/loss of left intraventricular conduction disturbance correction should also be considered. (*From* Jastrzebski M, Moskal P, Curila K et al. Electrocardiographic characterization of non-selective His-bundle pacing: validation of novel diagnostic criteria. Europace 2019; 21:1857–1864; with permission.)

block (LBBB). It is most likely caused by slow cell-to-cell conduction through the interventricular septum and the delayed activation of the lateral wall of the LV. Loss of HB capture parallels the situation seen with loss of conduction in the left bundle branch. Similarly, the use of a QRS notch/slur to recognize loss of HB capture parallels the use of a QRS notch/slur as criterion for LBBB diagnosis.

Occasionally, a QRS notch/slur can be seen despite confirmed HB capture; this likely results from a noncorrected intra-Hisian or intra-left ventricular conduction disturbance. A noncorrected intra-Hisian conduction problem results in a long HV interval and leads to a substantial contribution of the direct septal myocardial depolarization to the fused QRS morphology. Note that HV of 60 ms or more gives the direct septal depolarization enough time to activate whole thickness of the interventricular septum and already invade the LV before the left bundle branch starts to depolarize the LV. During noncorrected LBBB (or noncorrected nonspecific intraventricular conduction disturbance) despite HB capture there is continued delay in activation of the lateral wall of the LV. Although in such cases there is HB capture, the ventricular depolarization is nonphysiologic, more akin to RVS than HB pacing and for

clinical purposes could be categorized as equivalent to loss/lack of HB capture.

The V_6 R-Wave Peak Time Criterion

The V_6 R-wave peak time (V_6RWPT) is an ECG measure that correlates with the activation time of the lateral wall of the LV. The velocity of conduction in the His-Purkinje system is higher than in the working myocardium, resulting in shorter V_6RWPT during HB capture than during RVS capture (see **Fig. 1**; **Fig. 4**).[3] With loss of HB capture the V_6RWPT prolongs by at least 20 ms.[2] The ROC curve–based analysis of V_6RWPT values observed during HB capture and during loss of HB capture pointed to a value of 106 ms as an optimal cutoff for differentiation between these 2 situations (**Fig. 5**).[2] The area under the ROC curve, sensitivity, and specificity of the fixed cutoff V_6RWPT criterion in that study were 97.8%, 90.2%, and 95.7%, respectively. For practical purposes a value of 100 ms (more specific) or 110 ms (more sensitive) might be adopted. Note that the V_6RWPT corresponds to the intrinsicoid deflection time in lead V_6 during native supraventricular rhythm. However, when V_6RWPT is measured from the stimulus, it is longer than physiologic intrinsicoid deflection time by the value of HV

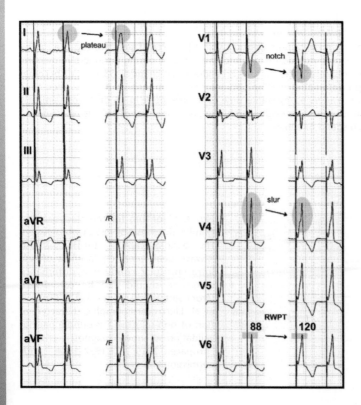

Fig. 4. Typical beat-to-beat changes in QRS morphology related to loss of His bundle capture. In lead I the pointy peak changes into a slur/plateau, in leads V1 and V3 a notch appears, and in leads V4 and V5 a slur develops. The R-wave peak time (RWPT) in lead V6 prolongs from 88 ms to 120 ms. (*From* Jastrzebski M, Moskal P, Curila K et al. Electrocardiographic characterization of non-selective His-bundle pacing: validation of novel diagnostic criteria. Europace 2019; 21:1857-1864; with permission.)

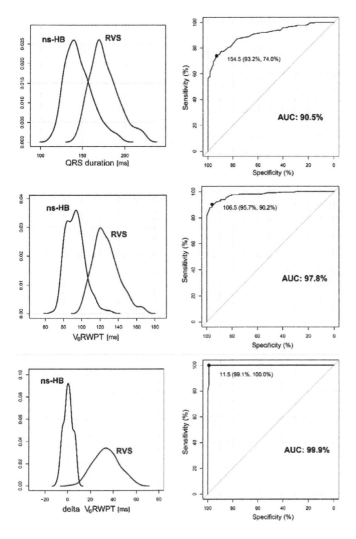

Fig. 5. Density plots and receiver operating characteristics curves for the QRS duration, R-wave peak time in lead V_6 (V_6RWPT) and delta V_6RWPT during nonselective His bundle capture (ns-HB) and right ventricular septal (RVS) capture. Delta V_6RWPT criterion offers perfect separation of values without any overlap between ns-HB and RVS capture and best diagnostic performance (area under the curve [AUC]). (*From* Jastrzebski M, Moskal P, Kukla P et al. Novel approach to diagnosis of His bundle capture using individualized left ventricular lateral wall activation time as reference. J Cardiovasc Electrophysiol 2021. doi.org/10.1111/jce.15233; with permission.)

latency interval, which is "filled" with the pseudo-delta wave during nonselective capture. Because the upper normal value for intrinsicoid deflection time in lead V_6 is 50 ms and the upper normal value of HV interval is 55 ms, then by adding them we obtain the recommended cutoff value of 100 to 110 ms for HB capture diagnosis provided earlier.

Global QRS Duration

The QRS duration measured from the pacing stimulus to the QRS offset using all 12 standard ECG leads can also be used for differentiation between ns-HB capture and RVS capture. However, as we have shown (see **Fig. 5**), there is a considerable overlap of values between the ns-HB QRS and the RVS QRS duration.[2] In patients with normal HV interval, the paced QRS duration during ns-HB capture equals the sum of the HV interval

and the baseline intrinsic QRS duration. Because the upper normal values of HV interval and QRS complex are 55 ms and 110 ms, respectively, then an ns-HB paced QRS can be as wide as 165 ms. A diagnostically optimal differentiating cutoff for QRS duration determined by ROC curve analysis was found to be 154 ms, whereas values less than 120 to 130 ms are 100% specific for ns-HB capture (but not sensitive).[2] It is important to ensure that the analyzed QRS is a fully paced QRS and not a QRS fused with native conduction.

The V_6RWPT should be preferred over global QRS duration for capture diagnosis. Apart from smaller overlap of values between ns-HB capture and RVS capture, the R-wave peak offers a very distinct point for precise measurements, whereas QRS offset has a low amplitude and transitions smoothly into ST-T complex, making QRS duration measurements less precise.

USING NATIVE QRS AND NATIVE CONDUCTION INTERVALS AS PHYSIOLOGIC REFERENCE

The fixed cutoff criteria for V6RWPT and QRS duration described earlier are limited by the substantial variability in HV interval and native QRS duration, both showing show typical bell curve distribution (see **Fig. 5**); this leads to overlap of values during RVS capture and ns-HB capture. Therefore, any fixed cutoff duration criteria for diagnosis of HB capture would be limited by a trade-off between the sensitivity and specificity.

This problem can be approached on the grounds of the paradigm of physiologic pacing, stating that proximal conduction system capture is characterized by equal LV lateral wall activation times during pacing and during native conduction.[1,2] During ns-HB pacing, the physiologic activation of the LV remains largely unaffected (see **Fig. 1**), despite direct nonphysiologic septal activation that leads to pseudo-delta formation and QRS prolongation that characterizes ns-HB pacing; this is because the velocity of conduction in the His-Purkinje system is much higher than in the septal myocardium, and the lateral wall of LV is depolarized purely via the His-Purkinje conduction system. Consequently, during ns-HB pacing, the time from the pacing stimulus (that corresponds to HB recording/depolarization during supraventricular rhythm) to the activation of the lateral wall of the LV is not influenced by the direct septal capture and should be equal to the corresponding time during native supraventricular conduction (that is HB-V6RWPT should equal stimulus-V6RWPT) (**Fig. 6**).

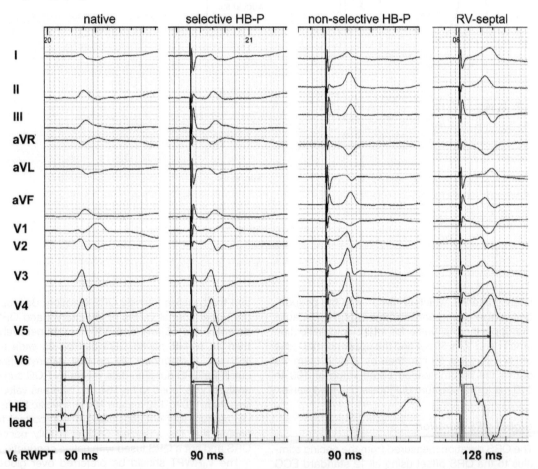

Fig. 6. Activation time of the lateral wall of the left ventricle, as indicated by the time to the R-wave peak in lead V6 (V6RWPT), remained constant during native conduction and His bundle pacing (HB-P). Loss of HB capture, that is right ventricular (RV) septal-only capture, resulted in prolongation of the paced V6RWPT by 38 ms (90 ms–128 ms). In contrast to the LV lateral wall activation time, the global ventricular activation could not serve in this case as a reference, as RV septal QRS was narrower than the HB potential to QRS offset interval during native conduction (178 ms vs 206 ms, respectively). (*From* Jastrzebski M, Moskal P, Kukla P et al. Novel approach to diagnosis of His bundle capture using individualized left ventricular lateral wall activation time as reference. J Cardiovasc Electrophysiol 2021. doi.org/10.1111/jce.15233; with permission.)

Therefore, using native LV lateral wall activation time (HB-V$_6$RWPT) as reference instead of fixed cutoffs allows individualization of duration criteria. Such an approach was already validated both for HB pacing and for the diagnosis of left bundle branch capture during deep septal pacing.[1,2] We found that if the paced V$_6$RWPT (measured from stimulus) and native V$_6$RWPT (measured from HB potential) differ by more than 12 ms then HB capture was not obtained. This individualized V$_6$RWPT criterion resulted in diagnostic accuracy of 99.7%

that surpassed the fixed V$_6$RWPT cutoff criterion and QRS duration–based criteria.[2]

Attempts were made to use native global QRS duration as reference.[2,4] However, although this works well for narrow QRS with normal HV interval, it is inaccurate for cases with right bundle branch morphology (see **Fig. 6**) or LBBB.[2]

Comparison of paced and native V$_6$RWPT offers fast and simple alternative for the determination of HB capture in cases where the threshold determination fails as a diagnostic test. It might also be

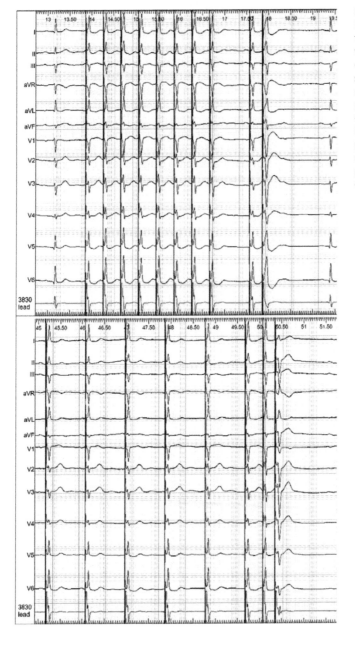

Fig. 7. In the same patient both selective His bundle (HB) response and right ventricular septal (RVS) myocardial response were obtained. (*Upper panel*) Fast basic drive train (S1) with long coupling of S2 shortens refractory period of RVS myocardium and prolongs refractory period of HB, and consequently, S3 finds only RVS myocardium excitable. Slow basic drive train with short-coupled S2 prolongs refractoriness of the RVS myocardium and shortens the refractory period of HB, and consequently, S3 finds only HB excitable.

useful for ECG follow-up of patients with HB pacing devices to determine if HB capture is still maintained. For this it would be necessary to routinely include in the implantation procedure report the final HB-V$_6$RWPT (or paced V$_6$RWPT) value, along with the capture thresholds, sensitivity values, and other relevant data.

QRS TRANSITION DURING CAPTURE THRESHOLD TEST

During the implantation procedure and device follow-up, the most common method to determine HB capture is a standard threshold test.[5] This method exploits differences in capture threshold between HB and adjacent septal myocardium. It is important to perform the test in the unipolar pacing mode from the lead tip to avoid pseudo-transition due to loss of anodal capture. When the pacing output slowly decreases it is possible to observe a sudden change in QRS morphology (**Figs. 2** and **4**). When HB or RVS capture is lost, a transition to the RVS QRS or selective (s)-HB QRS, respectively, is observed. The type of transition (ns-HB → RVS or ns-HB → s-HB) depends on which tissue has the lower capture threshold. It is pertinent to define when a change in QRS morphology can be considered a diagnostic transition. Transition to s-HB capture is diagnosed by the appearance of a latency interval after the pacing stimulus (see **Fig. 2**) and QRS morphology usually identical to the native supraventricular QRS, whereas transition to RVS capture is diagnosed by QRS prolongation, appearance of a notch/slur/plateau in the left ventricular leads, and sudden prolongation in the V$_6$RWPT by 20 ms or more (see **Fig. 4**).[2,3] In patients with an undamaged distal conduction system, the V$_6$RWPT on average prolongs by 33 ms with loss of HB capture. Prolongation by less than 20 ms might result from noncorrected conduction disturbance that leads to a long V$_6$RWPT already during ns-HB capture. Ambiguous threshold test result and equal HB and RVS capture thresholds seen in 6% to 10% of cases require other maneuvers to determine HB capture (see later discussion).

In patients with bundle branch blocks, it is possible to observe more QRS morphology transitions, as additionally correction/loss of correction of LBBB or RBBB often occurs.[6] In essence, any obvious transition is diagnostic of conduction system capture, as during RVS pacing the QRS

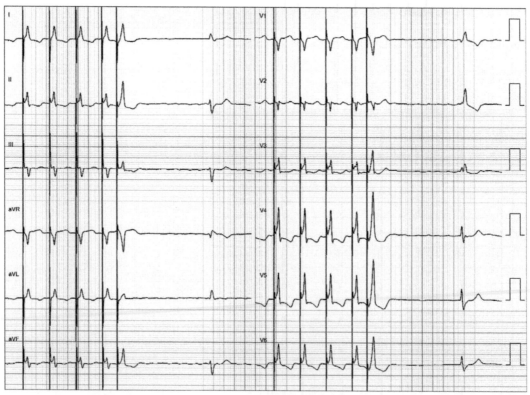

Fig. 8. A single extrastimulus delivered at the coupling rate of 290 ms results in sudden change of paced QRS morphology (myocardial response); this was because at 290 ms His bundle was refractory, whereas septal myocardium was still excitable.

morphology remains constant till complete loss of capture.

PROGRAMMED HIS BUNDLE STIMULATION

When the capture thresholds of the HB and the RVS myocardium are equal, the method of output-dependent QRS transition does not work. To address this problem, the technique of programmed conduction system stimulation was developed.[7] This method rests on the physiologic differences between conduction system and working myocardium with regard to the refractoriness. The idea is simple: when an appropriately timed extrastimulus is delivered during absolute refractory period of HB or RVS, there will be loss of capture of the refractory tissue, and an evident transition of the extrastimulus QRS morphology must ensue. Depending on the type of QRS transition obtained we classified the responses to programmed stimulation as "selective response" (ns-HB → s-HB) or "myocardial response" (ns-HB → RVS).

Although the average absolute refractory period of HB is 80 ms shorter than RVS absolute refractory period (when assessed with an 8-beat basic drive train of 600 ms; 271.1 ± 34 ms vs 353.1 ± 30 ms), thus facilitating myocardial response,[7] both type of responses can be obtained most of the patients when dedicated pacing protocols are used. These are based on the physiology described by Denker and colleagues: refractoriness of the myocardium is mainly influenced by the several preceding cycles (S1 basic drive train), whereas refractoriness of the conduction system is manly influenced by the last, immediately preceding RR cycle (**Fig. 7**).[8,9]

To obtain myocardial response it is enough to perform an 8-beat drive (S1) with a 600-m cycle + S2 starting from 400 to 450 ms and

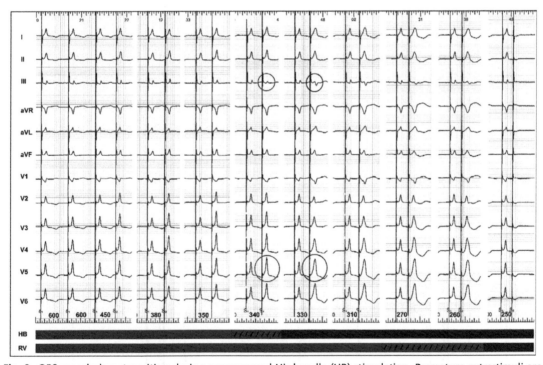

Fig. 9. QRS morphology transition during programmed His bundle (HB) stimulation. Premature extrastimuli are delivered after a drive train of 600 ms at progressively shorter coupling intervals. At coupling intervals of 450 to 350 ms, the S2 morphology (nonselective HB QRS, HB blue bar, excitable period) is stable. At coupling interval of 330 ms evident transition occurs; this corresponds with encroachment with S2 on the absolute refractory period of HB (HB brown bar). At coupling intervals of 330 to 260 ms, only right ventricular (RV) septal myocardial QRS morphology is present. During relative refractory period of the HB (340–330 ms; HB dashed blue bar), there is already some QRS prolongation due to decrement in HB conduction and hence bigger contribution of RV myocardial depolarization wavefront to the fused ns-HB QRS complex. During the relative refractory period of the RV myocardium (270–250 ms, RV dashed blue bar), some QRS widening can also be observed albeit gradual and without sudden increase in V6 R-wave peak time. (*From* Jastrzebski M, Moskal P, Bednarek A, Kielbasa G, Vijayaraman P, Czarnecka D. Programmed His Bundle Pacing: A Novel Maneuver for the Diagnosis of His Bundle Capture. Circ Arrhythm Electrophysiol 2019; 12:e007052; with permission.)

decreasing at 10-ms steps; this will provide a diagnostic response in nearly 100% of cases (**Fig. 8**). With progressively shorter coupling intervals, a sudden evident change in the QRS morphology of S2 occurs, usually around a coupling interval of 380 to 320 ms. With further shortening of the coupling interval some additional, gradual QRS prolongation might be present, when RVS relative refractory period is encroached on (**Fig. 9**); this must not be mistaken as myocardial response in RVS cases; to avoid this, the last 4 coupling intervals should be considered as nondiagnostic or sudden V_6RWPT increase greater than 20 ms should be considered as obligatory.

To obtain a s-HB response, single or double extrastimuli on intrinsic rhythm or slow basic drive train protocols are necessary (see **Fig. 7**; **Fig. 10**). An extrastimulus delivered during intrinsic rhythm is more likely to produce s-HB capture because the local timing of the HB and para-Hisian myocardial depolarization during supraventricular rhythm is different (more time for the HB to recover and

less time for the myocardium to recover (**Fig. 11**).[7] Note that the programmed HB stimulation method is thus capable of visualizing s-HB QRS morphology in cases with obligatory nonselective pacing (the RVS threshold is lower than the HB threshold), providing a very rewarding and unquestionable proof of HB capture.

Programmed stimulation can be easily used during implantation, when a programmable external pacemaker/electrophysiologic system is used, but also during follow-up using a noninvasive programmed stimulation function implemented in most pacemakers. When these options are not available asynchronous slow pacing mode can be used, as it also results in scanning of the diastole with stimuli.

Apart from programmed stimulation, differences in refractoriness can be also exploited using burst pacing[10] or incremental pacing. Burst pacing was investigated systematically by Liang and colleagues and found to be useful in cases where threshold test failed to provide diagnosis.[10]

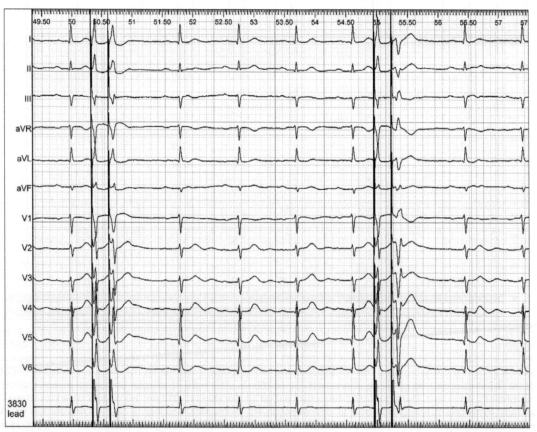

Fig. 10. Double extrastimuli delivered during intrinsic sinus rhythm. At coupling interval of 290 ms the S2 morphology is nonselective His bundle capture, albeit different than S1 due to decremental conduction in His bundle. At the coupling interval of 280 ms S2 morphology transitions to selective HB capture. Note discrete potential on the endocardial channel "3830 lead" and dramatic change of QRS morphology in all 12 leads.

Incremental pacing deserves more attention than burst, as this maneuver should always be performed to assess distal His-Purkinje system conduction anyway. In my experience burst pacing predominantly results in myocardial response, whereas with incremental pacing selective response can be observed more frequently (**Fig. 12**). Occasionally, incremental pacing will even provide selective response that was not obtainable with programmed stimulation (https://twitter.com/Marek_Jastrz_EP/status/1108810446214254592?s = 20.).

MISCELLANEOUS METHODS
Ventriculoatrial Interval

Analysis of ventriculoatrial (VA) interval for diagnosis of HB capture is based on the seminal observation by Jackman and colleagues that formed the basis of the para-Hisian pacing maneuver for the diagnosis of concealed accessory pathway.[11]

For the presently discussed use, this method is limited to patients without atrial fibrillation and with preserved retrograde conduction, that is, a relatively small percentage of patients with

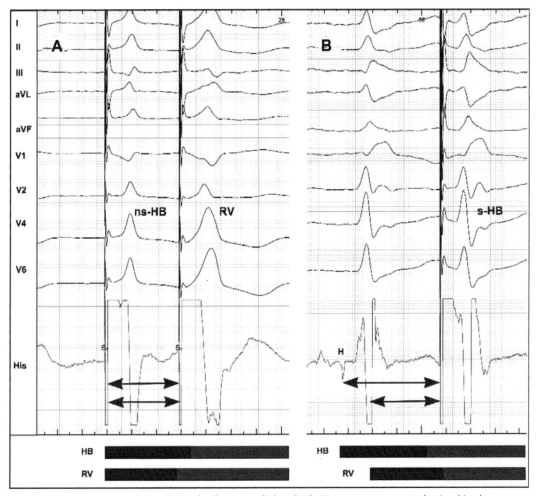

Fig. 11. During programmed stimulation both myocardial and selective responses were obtained in the same patient. (*A*) After a drive train an extrastimulus is delivered at a coupling interval of 300 ms; this resulted in right ventricular (RV) septal myocardial capture. (*B*) An extrastimulus is delivered also at a coupling interval of 300 ms, albeit, during native conduction; this resulted in a selective His bundle (s-HB) capture. Divergent responses can be explained by a different activation sequence in the para-Hisian region with the drive train and native conduction. During native conduction HB is excitable (*blue bar*), whereas RV myocardium is not, because HB is activated 100 ms before the adjacent ventricular myocardium, resulting in HB coupling interval of 400 ms (*arrow*). In contrast, during the drive train both the HB and the adjacent RV myocardium are depolarized simultaneously. HB, His bundle; s-HB, selective HB; ns-HB, non-selective HB; His, endocardial signals from the screwed-in HB pacing lead; H, HB potential; RV, right ventricle. (*From* Jastrzebski M, Moskal P, Bednarek A, Kielbasa G, Vijayaraman P, Czarnecka D. Programmed His Bundle Pacing: A Novel Maneuver for the Diagnosis of His Bundle Capture. Circ Arrhythm Electrophysiol 2019; 12:e007052; with permission.)

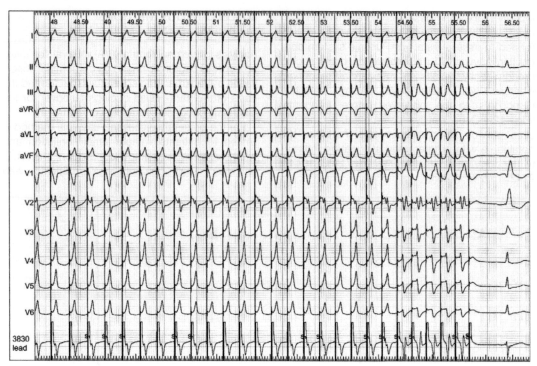

Fig. 12. During incremental pacing nonselective His bundle pacing transitions into selective HB capture (last 5 beats).

indication for permanent pacing. Moreover, a major practical limitation comes from fact that VA interval prolongation is nearly always accompanied by diagnostic QRS morphology transition that is easier to rely on than retrograde P wave analysis. However, occasionally VA interval prolongation might support the presence of transition when this is unequivocal or when ECG is limited to a single lead tracing.

Device Electrograms

Device electrogram (EGM) analysis can also be useful for the differentiation of the 3 types of capture during HB pacing.[12] The following criteria were analyzed in the study by Saini and colleagues: far-field EGM QRS duration, near-field EGM time-to-peak, and near-field EGM polarity. The device EGM transition correlated well with QRS morphology transition on 12-lead ECG. The near-field EGM time-to-peak was found to be a device-based equivalent of the presence/absence of discrete local potential on the endocardial channel during implantation, whereas the far-field EGM QRS duration was the equivalent of global QRS duration in the surface ECG. As could be expected, the far-field EGM QRS duration was shorter during ns-HB capture than during RVS capture (103 vs 145 ms), and transition to RVS

capture was always accompanied by prolongation of the far-field EGM QRS duration by at least 40 ms. The device marker channel data can provide additional valuable information, as sudden increase in VA interval (mean delta VA of 70 ms), which indicates loss of HB capture, can be easily ascertained. The EGM-based methods might be useful for follow-up when 12-lead is ECG is not feasible or for automated analysis or device-based HB capture monitoring.

DISCLOSURE

The author has nothing to disclose.

REFERENCES

1. Jastrzebski M, Kielbasa G, Curila K, et al. Physiology-based electrocardiographic criteria for left bundle branch capture. Heart Rhythm 2021;18: 935–43.
2. Jastrzebski M, Moskal P, Kukla P, et al. Novel approach to diagnosis of His bundle capture using individualized left ventricular lateral wall activation time as reference. J Cardiovasc Electrophysiol 2021. https://doi.org/10.1111/jce.15233.
3. Jastrzebski M, Moskal P, Curila K, et al. Electrocardiographic characterization of non-selective His-

bundle pacing: validation of novel diagnostic criteria. Europace 2019;21:1857–64.

4. Liang Y, Wang N, Yu H, et al. A simple and practical criterion for determining a failed His-bundle pacing. Europace 2020;22:ii61–6.

5. Vijayaraman P, Dandamudi G, Zanon F, et al. Permanent His bundle pacing: Recommendations from a Multicenter His bundle pacing Collaborative working Group for standardization of definitions, implant measurements, and follow-up. Heart Rhythm 2018; 15:460–8.

6. Burri H, Jastrzebski M, Vijayaraman P. Electrocardiographic analysis for His bundle pacing at implantation and follow-up. JACC Clin Electrophysiol 2020; 6:883–900.

7. Jastrzebski M, Moskal P, Bednarek A, et al. Programmed His bundle pacing: a novel maneuver for the diagnosis of His bundle capture. Circ Arrhythm Electrophysiol 2019;12:e007052.

8. Denker S, Lehmann MH, Mahmud R, et al. Divergence between refractoriness of His-Purkinje system and ventricular muscle with abrupt changes in cycle length. Circulation 1983;68:1212–21.

9. Jastrzebski M. Permanent left bundle branch pacing: what is the mechanism of divergent responses during programmed stimulation? J Cardiovasc Electrophysiol 2020;31:1222–5.

10. Liang Y, Yu H, Wang N, et al. Cycle length criteria for His-bundle capture are capable of determining pacing types misclassified by output criteria. Heart Rhythm 2019;16:1629–35.

11. Jackman WM, Beckman KJ, McClelland J, et al. Para-Hisian RV pacing site for differentiating retrograde conduction over septal accessory pathway and AV node. Abstract. Jackman WM, Beckman KJ, McClelland J et al. Pacing Clin Electrophysiol 1991;670.

12. Saini A, Serafini NJ, Campbell S, et al. Novel method for Assessment of His bundle pacing morphology using near field and far field device Electrograms. Circ Arrhythm Electrophysiol 2019;12:e006878.

Left Bundle Branch Pacing
How I Do It?

Lan Su, MD[a,b], Kenneth A. Ellenbogen, MD[c], Weijian Huang, MD[a,b],*

KEYWORDS

- Left bundle branch pacing (LBBP) • His bundle branch pacing (HBP) • Conduction system capture
- Cardiac resynchronization therapy • Implantation technology

KEY POINTS

- Definition, classification of left bundle branch pacing (LBBP), and the electrophysiological characteristics of left bundle branch capture are reviewed.
- Describe the process of LBBP to improve implant success rate using the "Wenzhou experience."
- Techniques to avoid the intraoperative and postoperative complications of LBBP.
- Discuss the more advanced solutions for challenging cases.

Of vital*, major#, and minor• importance:

  * LBB captures criteria and standardized testing methods.

  * How to distinguish LBBP from left ventricular septal pacing.

  * Preoperative evaluation including arrhythmia, etiology, and anatomic abnormalities.

  * Preparation including implant tools and setting of electrophysiology recording systems.

  * The basic technique and key steps of LBBP, including the optimization of initial position on the right ventricular septum, lead fixation, and estimation of the depth under the LV septum.

  # Assist in lead positioning by various methods including the utility of His bundle location.

  # The value of LBB potential.

  # Prevention of complications and preventive measures of ventricular septal perforation.

  # The postoperative follow-up

- Special tips for challenging cases.
- Fusion technique to eliminate RBB delay.

INTRODUCTION

The first case of permanent left bundle branch pacing(LBBP)was reported in 2017, which was achieved using the 3830 lead (SelectSecure; Medtronic Inc., Minneapolis, MN) delivered through a fixed curve sheath (C315HIS; Medtronic) via a transvenous approach to capture the left conduction system.[1] Since then, LBBP has rapidly evolved into clinical practice because it is a simpler and more reliable procedure with a high success rate, and satisfactory pacing/sensing parameters compared with His bundle pacing (HBP).[2–4] In recent years, several researchers have described various implant techniques and new methods to facilitate LBBP-.[5] In this article, we describe the standard procedural work-flow, basic technique, key steps, and the Wenzhou experience.

BASIC CONCEPTS AND TECHNIQUES
Anatomic and Electrophysiology Basis of Left Bundle Branch Pacing

LBBP is relatively easy to perform because the left bundle and its branches are a wide conduction network along the subendocardial aspect of the left interventricular septum in a fan-like shape.[6,7] Theoretically, if the pacing lead is screwed deep into the LV septum, the LBB can be captured with synchronized left ventricular activation. The paced QRS morphology mainly depends on the

a Department of Cardiology, The First Affiliated Hospital of Wenzhou Medical University, Wenzhou, China;
b The Key Lab of Cardiovascular Disease of Wenzhou, Wenzhou, China; c Virginia Commonwealth University/Pauley Heart Center, Richmond, VA, USA
* Corresponding author. Department of Cardiology, The First Affiliated Hospital of Wenzhou Medical University, Nanbaixiang, Wenzhou 325000, P.R. China.
E-mail address: weijianhuang69@126.com

Card Electrophysiol Clin 14 (2022) 165–179
https://doi.org/10.1016/j.ccep.2022.01.003
1877-9182/22/© 2022 Elsevier Inc. All rights reserved.

following factors: (1) the pacing site and the site of block; (2) distal conduction system disease; (3) retrograde conduction to the His and right bundle; (4) local myocardia capture (unipolar or bipolar). The lead position and the anatomic distribution of the LBB are shown in **Fig. 1**.

Definition and Classification of Left Bundle Branch Pacing

LBBP is defined as direct capture of the left bundle branch and surrounding myocardium, while left ventricular septal pacing (LVSP) is defined as the capture of the left ventricular septal myocardium only without direct capture of the LBB. Left bundle branch area pacing (LBBAP) includes LVSP and LBBP with or without direct evidence of LBB capture.[8,9]

Electrophysiological Characteristics and Standardized Testing Methods

During LBBP lead implantation, the following electrophysiological characteristics are tested:

1. Selective and nonselective LBBP: During threshold testing, a transition from nonselective to selective LBBP (loss of septal myocardial capture with short isoelectric interval) or nonselective to LVSP can be observed[10,11]
2. Paced QRS morphology and duration[8]: Paced QRS duration is defined as stimulus to the

end of QRS, measured by the electrophysiology (EP) recording system and reflects the fusion of LV and right ventricular (RV) electrical activation. The LBB paced QRS duration was longer in patients with LBBB or RBBB compared with those with narrow QRS, possibly due to absent retrograde conduction to the RBB. Bipolar pacing with anodal capture during LBBP could eliminate or attenuate the paced RBBB pattern and shorten the QRS duration; however, this may not be always feasible because of the high anodal capture threshold. These observations indicate that using the paced QRS duration as one of the criteria for LBB capture is not accurate.[8]

3. The stimulus to LV activation time (Stim-LVAT): The Stim-LVAT is assessed by measuring the stimulus to the peak of the R wave in leads V4–V6.[10,11]
4. LBB potential: In patients with non-LBBB during intrinsic rhythm, LBB potentials should always be recorded on the intracardiac electrogram (IEGM) from the LBBP lead, with the potential to a ventricular interval of 20 to 35 ms to help confirm the lead position and the level of conduction block.[12] However, in patients with LBBB, LBB potentials can only be recorded during the restoration of left bundle conduction by means of HBP or during premature ventricular contractions (PVCs) from the LBB region). LBB potentials can also be visualized in the LBB

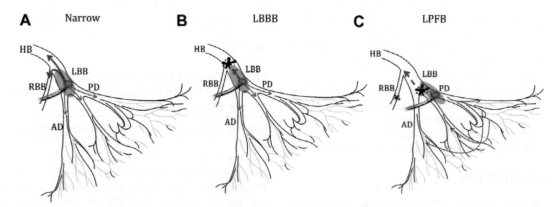

Fig. 1. The anatomic distribution and lead position of the LBB. Left bundle branch is a wide conduction network along the left subendocardial part of the interventricular septum in a fan shape. Optimization principle for LBB pacing site selection: 1. pacing beyond the site of conduction block; 2. pacing close to the proximal left bundle branch to achieve the optimal left ventricular synchronization. (A) Normal retrograde and anterograde conduction: Stimulus can conduct to the left bundle branch and right bundle branch through retrograde and anterograde conduction to achieve left ventricular and interventricular synchronization when pacing at the trunk of the left bundle branch. (B) Pacing beyond the site of block to capture proximal LBB and ensure the left ventricular synchronization when the block site is located at proximal LBB. (C) When the block site is at distal LBB including the left anterior branch (LAF) and left posterior branch (LPF), pacing should be more performed distally. In this position, the stimulus first anterogradely conducts from the branch of LPF to the distal conduction bundle and then retrogradely conducted to LAF to achieve left ventricular activation. The conduction delay in the left anterior branch area shows the QRS morphology of LAF block and the left deviation of the electrical axis.

pacing lead during conducted beats with narrow QRS or during RBBB morphology escape rhythm from the LBB fascicles.

5. Premature ventricular contractions (PVCs)[12,13]: PVCs with an RBBB morphology induced during lead implantation, are a marker that indicates that the LBB area is already reached and lead rotations should be immediately stopped to prevent perforation.

6. Pacing parameters: Including pacing thresholds (unipolar and bipolar pacing thresholds), R-wave amplitudes, and unipolar impedances. The unipolar LBB capture thresholds should be less than 1 V/0.5 ms and unipolar pacing impedance should be around 600 Ω at implant. The average sensed R-wave amplitude is usually more than 10 mv.[14]

Standard testing methods during LBBP implantation is recommended:

1. During LBBP lead implantation, low- and high-output pacing is performed early and repeatedly to confirm direct LBB capture (illustrated in **Fig. 2**) during the following scenario: (1) when the tip of the LBBP lead is in the interventricular septum to a depth of approximately 6 to 8 mm (confirmed by the fulcrum sign or during contrast injection); (2) when the paced QRS morphology demonstrates an RBBB pattern; (3) if premature ventricular beats with an

RBBB morphology are observed; (4) if LBB potential is observed;

2. Distinguish LBB and myocardial capture thresholds: Repeated testing should be performed after implanting the LBB lead and during the waiting period. If the LBB capture threshold is similar to the LVS myocardial threshold, we attempt to differentiate the 2 thresholds by changing pacing outputs, pulse width, pacing rate, or by using programmed stimulation[8,15,16] (illustrated in **Fig. 3**). The response to the above maneuvers can prove that direct capture of LBB was achieved and that the lack of QRS morphology change with lowering of the pacing output was related to identical capture thresholds of both myocardium and LBB, which is not uncommon.

The Practical Criteria for LBB Pacing

Flowchart for the diagnosis of LBB capture from Wenzhou experience is shown in **Fig. 4**.[8] When the pacing lead is implanted close to the LBB area, the following electrophysiologic characteristics can be used for confirming LBB capture.

1. Paced QRS morphology of RBBB: Paced RBBB pattern was necessary but not sufficient to confirm LBB capture because a higher proportion of patients during pacing from the LVS will have a RBBB morphology.

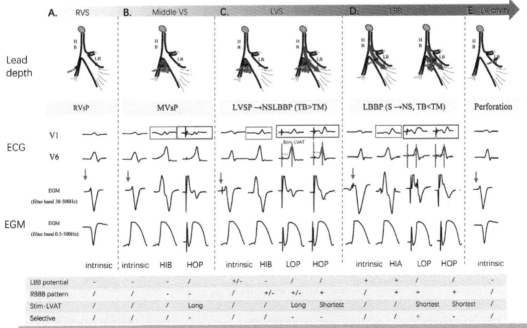

	RVS	Middle VS	LVS	LBB	LV cavity
	RVsP	MVsP	LVSP →NSLBBP (TB>TM)	LBBP (S →NS, TB<TM)	Perforation
	intrinsic	intrinsic HIB HOP	intrinsic HIB LOP HOP	intrinsic HIA LOP HOP	intrinsic
LBB potential	-	- - /	+/- - / /	+ + / /	-
RBBB pattern	/	/ - -	/ +/- +/- +	/ + + +	/
Stim-LVAT	/	/ / Long	/ / Long Shortest	/ / Shortest Shortest	/
Selective	/	/ / -	/ / - -	/ / + -	/

- Test earlier and more times with low and high output (width) at different depth, time to confirm LBB capture and avoid perforation
- The lead depth can be determined by contrast injection, hinge point, echocardiogram, CT

Fig. 2. Relationship between lead depth, pacing parameters, ECG, and EGM characteristics.

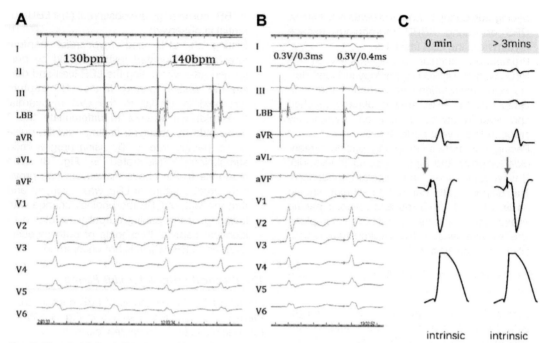

Fig. 3. Threshold discrimination and lead stability testing. (*A–C*): to distinguish myocardial and LBB capture when they were similar by changing the pacing rate (*A*), pulse width (*B*); (*C*): lead stability testing by monitoring LBB potential, fluoroscopy image, and assessing pacing parameters when the sheath is pulled back to the atrium. (*From* Jastrzębski M. Permanent left bundle branch pacing: What is the mechanism of divergent responses during programmed stimulation?. *J Cardiovasc Electrophysiol.* 2020;31(5):1222–1225; with permission).

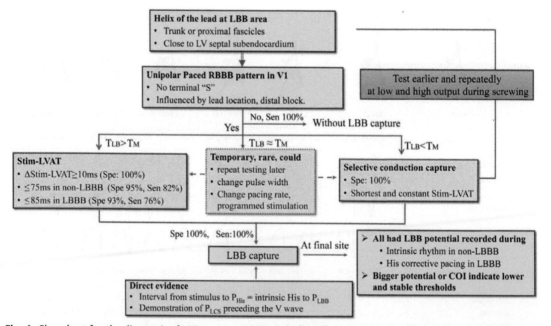

Fig. 4. Flowchart for the diagnosis of LBB capture. RBBB: right bundle branch block; LBB: left bundle branch; LVAT: left ventricular activation time; COI: current of injury. (*From* Wu S, Chen X, Wang S, et al. Evaluation of the Criteria to Distinguish Left Bundle Branch Pacing From Left Ventricular Septal Pacing. aged 8 and older 3. *JACC Clin Electrophysiol.* 2021;7(9):1166–1177; with permission).

2. LBB potential and current of injury (COI): LBB potential should be noted in all patients with normal LBB activation successfully undergoing LBB pacing and is a good marker that the lead is located around the LBB; however, LBB capture cannot be established based only on this finding. A larger LBB potential or COI indicates that the lead is associated with a lower threshold.

3. Stim-LVAT:From LVSP to NS-LBBP or from NS-LBBP to LVSP, an abrupt change in Stim-LVAT of > 10 ms was observed in all cases with a specificity of 100% for confirming LBB capture (shown in **Fig. 2**). LBBP results in the shortest and constant Stim-LVAT in the same patient regardless of increasing pacing output. The native QRS can serve as a reference for the diagnosis of LBB capture in the same patient because LBBP results in the physiologic depolarization of the LV.

4. Selective LBBP: Selective LBBP is characterized by a discrete isoelectric period between the stimulus artifact and onset of ventricular activation recorded on the EGM from the LBBP lead with a specificity of 100% for the confirmation of LBB capture in 90% of patients, in a small series of successful LBBP (27 of 30 patients).[8]

Electrophysiology Recording System Settings for Left Bundle Branch Pacing Implantation

EP recording system is required to record surface ECG and IEGM to assess paced QRS morphology, conduction system potential, and current of injury (COI) of left bundle branch and local myocardium to guide LBBP implantation. When routinely configured with a bandpass filter of 30 ~ 500 Hz for collecting high-frequency signals, His bundle potential can be recorded. While setting the bandpass filter at 0.5 ~ 500 Hz specially for the detection and visualization of low-frequency signals, the COI of both LBB and myocardium can be documented. A pacing system analyzer (PSA) can sometimes be used to record the His bundle potential when the amplitude is > 0.3 mV. Experienced operators can perform LBBP implantation only under the guidance of routine ECG monitor and PSA.

PREOPERATIVE PREPARATION AND EVALUATION
Patient Assessment

In addition to the routine preoperative preparation and evaluation (ECG, cardiac function, and blood test) for pacemaker implantation, special considerations for the LBBP implantation are highlighted in **Table 1**. These techniques increase the success rate of LBBP and reduce the risk of complications[17]:

(1) types of conduction disturbances: LBBB; (2) assessment of the thickness and scar burden of basal segment of the interventricular septum; (3) patients with anatomic abnormalities including persistent left superior vena cava (PLSVC), Ebstein anomaly, aneurysm of aortic sinus, and so forth; (4) patients with postvalve surgery (illustrated in **Fig. 5**)[18,19]; (5) selection of venous access.

Tools for Left Bundle Branch Pacing Implantation

LBBP Implantation tools include pacing lead, delivery sheath, PSA, and EP recording system. The Medtronic 3830 active fixation lead delivered via C315HIS delivery sheath is the most widely used lead for LBBP in clinical practice at present because the lead has a conductive helix electrode that is nonretractable. Over the last several years, a growing number of newly developed implantation tools and equipment from a variety of device manufacturers have been released, including dedicated sheaths for right-sided venous access, to deliver conventional leads, novel active fixation leads, and for anatomic variations and can even be used for 3D mapping. Other tools include the bridle cable for continuous recording of IEGM and anti-interference technology.

ROUTINE PROCEDURE FOR LEFT BUNDLE BRANCH PACING IMPLANTATION

The general operation for LBBP is shown in **Fig. 6**.

Choice of Venous Access and Placement of the Delivery Sheath

A left transvenous approach is preferably recommended since the most used preshaped delivery sheaths (C315His) are designed primarily for left-sided access. Additional advantages of left-sided approach include: (1) when the CS delivery sheath is used as a "sheath in sheath" technology for optimal support; (2) when conduction system pacing fails and one need to switch to biventricular pacing; (3) when ICD therapy is considered. Compared with subclavian puncture, axillary vein access has a lower risk of pneumothorax and subclavian crush. It is appropriate to consider right-sided access when the distance from the left venous puncture to the pacing site is too long.

The delivery sheath is advanced gently over the guidewire to decrease the risk of bending and damage from the blood vessels and heart on the pacing lead. Once the His bundle is identified approximately by locating the atrioventricular groove and tricuspid valve annulus under

Table 1
Preoperative preparation and evaluation.

	Preoperational Assessment and Preparation	Special Considerations
Conduction disturbances	The level of atrioventricular block (AVB)	Pacing beyond the site of block
	LBBB	Temporary ventricular pacing for a backup
	Nonspecific intraventricular conduction delay (IVCD)	LOT-CRT might be considered
Basal segment interventricular septum	Ventricular septal thickness	Change the initial site for LBBP Strong support of the deliver sheath required
	Fibrotic scar burden	
Anatomical abnormalities	Persistent left superior vena cava (PLSVC)	Special skills is needed in these challenging conditions
	Transposition of great arteries	
	Ebstein's anomaly	
	Ventricular of septal aneurysm	
	Aneurysm of aortic sinus	
Surgical operation	Transcatheter Aortic Valve Replacement (TAVR)	Pacing distal to the site of surgical injury
	Ventricular septal defect reparation	
	Ventricular septum ablation or resection of Hypertrophic cardiomyopathy (HCM)	
Selection of venous access	Left axillary vein preferred	Specialized delivery sheath or reshaped technique required or right access
EP recording system	Bandpass filter setting	Setting band filter of 30–500 Hz for recording the conduction bundle potential
		Setting band filter of 0.5–500 Hz for recording currents of injury

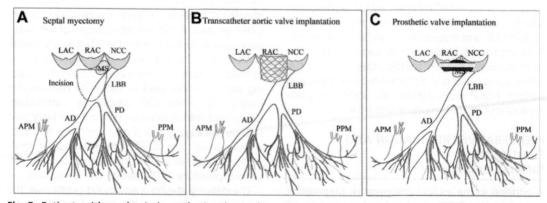

Fig. 5. Patients with mechanical prosthetic valve replacement or posttranscatheter aortic valve implantation. (*A*) Patient with septal myectomy; (*B*) patient with transcatheter aortic valve implantation; (*C*) patient with prosthetic valve implantation.*(From* Zheng R, Dong Y, Wu S, et al. Conduction system pacing following septal myectomy: Insights into site of conduction block [published online ahead of print, 2022 Jan 13]. J Cardiovasc Electrophysiol. 2022;10.1111/jce.15362; with permission).

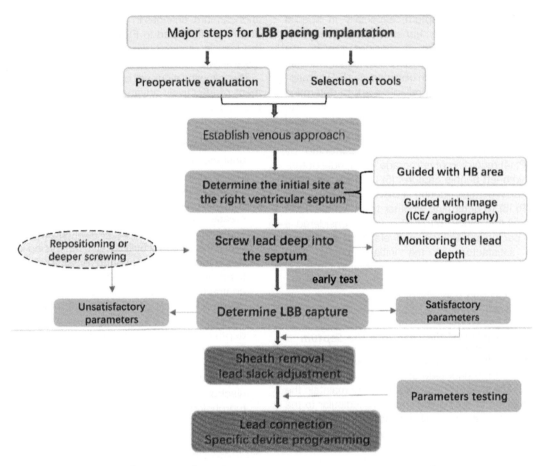

Fig. 6. Routine procedure for LBBP implantation.

fluoroscopy, then gently advance the tip of the pacing lead out of the sheath for further mapping.

Determination of Initial Site of Right Side of Interventricular Septum for Left Bundle Branch Pacing

Except for routine fluoroscopic imaging and intracardiac echocardiography (ICE), other methods including the Nine-Partition method,[20] dual-lead technique and subtricuspid valve angiography[21] can also help locate the position of His bundle and left bundle branch. His bundle mapping initially may help identify the anatomic distribution of the proximal trunk of the LBB. Usually, experienced operators can achieve His bundle mapping within a few minutes under fluoroscopy. His bundle mapping combined with image assist in determining the position of the proximal LBB after screwing the lead

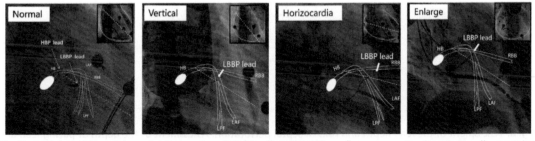

Fig. 7. Initial position and conduction system (His bundle/RBB/LBB) on fluoroscopy Precise His Bundle mapping (pacing or his potential mapping) to locate His bundle as a marker for distal his bundle or proximal LBBP, is especially valuable in those with abnormal anatomy, such as horizontal or vertically rotated heart, large right atrium, and to avoid RBB injury.

in the ventricular septum, especially in special cases including cardiac transposition and anatomic variation (shown in **Fig. 7**). Besides, precise His bundle mapping offers more additional benefits including: (1) HB position obtained via HBP or mapping can be used as a reliable mark to determine the proximal LBB especially for patients with anatomic abnormality; (2) confirmation of the level of AV block; (3) to determine whether the wide QRS (LBBB or RBBB) ikcan be corrected by HBP; (4) recording of retrograde His bundle potential with left bundle capture; (5) LBB potential can be documented during LBBB correction with HBP; (6) to determine whether there is multi-level conduction block; (7) HBP can be considered if the pacing parameters and electrical synchrony are satisfactory at the initial attempt. His-optimized cardiac resynchronization therapy (HOT-CRT) is an alternative option for patients with IVCD and consists of pacing the His bundle and the left ventricle (via the coronary sinus).

Deep Fixation of the Lead into the Septum

After the delivery sheath reaches the initial site for LBBP on the right side of the ventricular septum, rotate the sheath counterclockwise to maintain the orientation of the pacing lead perpendicular to the ventricular septum and get adequate support to screw the lead into the interventricular septum. Furthermore, we should turn the pacing lead clockwise rapidly to penetrate the RV endocardium of the ventricular septum. When the pacing lead is screwed approximately 7 mm deep into the septum, or fixation beat-like RBBB pattern occurs, or paced QRS morphology with an RBBB pattern, we recommend to measure pacing parameters. As the pacing lead is gradually screwed deeper into the ventricular

endocardium, changes in QRS morphology can be observed (illustrated in **Fig. 2**). If deep fixation of the lead is required, we have to rotate the lead more slowly to avoid septal perforation.

The following signs will be helpful for the assessment of effectively advancing the lead deep into the ventricular septum:

1. The notch on the paced QRS in lead V1 will move from the nadir up to the end of the QRS until the latter part of the R′ wave appears (ie, paced morphology changes from an LBBB pattern to an RBBB pattern).
2. Unipolar pacing impedance will gradually increase and then gradually decrease with the final impedance being more than 500 Ω;
3. When the sheath is pulled back, the pacing lead inside the ventricular septum remains relatively fixed, while the rest of the lead wobbles with the contraction of heart which we call the "fulcrum sign" on fluoroscopy. The different movements between these 2 parts can help assess the depth of the lead into the ventricular septum.
4. Deep septal fixation/template beats can be observed as the pacing lead is screwed into the ventricular septum. The approximate depth of electrode tip can be evaluated by the morphology of PVCs or paced QRS morphology.

Methods for the Evaluation of Depth of the Pacing Lead in the Septum

A variety of methods including echocardiographic measurements, angiography via the lead delivery sheath, pacing parameters from both tip and ring of the lead, and IEGM characteristics on LBB pacing lead can be used to evaluate the depth of

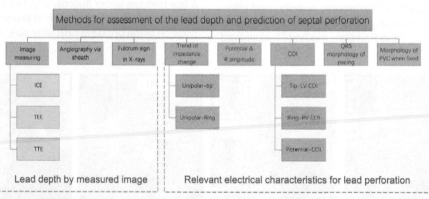

Fig. 8. Assessment of the lead depth and risks of septal perforation. Assessment of the depth of pacing lead and septal perforation: (1) image evidence includes echocardiography, angiography via delivery sheath, "fulcrum sign" in X-rays; (2) relevant electrophysiological characteristics includes: the trend of impedance change; R-wave amplitude; V-COI at the tip and ring of the pacing lead; morphology of paced QRS and PVCs during lead fixation.

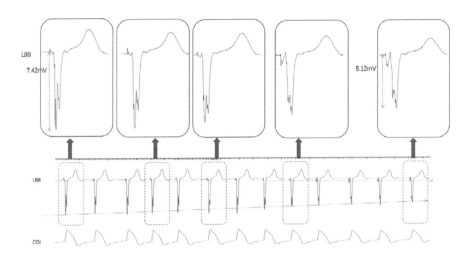

Fig. 9. Continuous recording of LBB and COI on intracardiac electrocardiogram continuous recording of intracardiac electrocardiogram. During screwing in, the amplitude of LBB potential gradually increased and was accompanied by an occurrence of LBB COI, suggesting that the lead electrode was getting deeper and closer to LBB. At the same time, monitoring the downtrend of the R wave and local V-COI amplitude can be used to avoid septal perforation.

pacing lead in the ventricular septum during the procedure (shown in **Fig. 8**).

Special Considerations as Indirect Evidence for the Identification of Successful Left Bundle Branch Pacing

Acceptable LBBP is usually identified based on threshold testing. LBB potential with COI of the the left bundle (shown in **Fig. 9**) indicates that the pacing lead tip meets the left bundle, and, in this scenario, there will be a low and stable LBB capture threshold.[16]

When the morphology of the PVC observed during lead fixation is similar to the selective LBBP morphology (typical RBBB pattern with short peak LVAT), it is thought to originate from the left bundle's fascicles. Monitoring the morphology of the PVC within the interventricular septum can predict whether the lead has reached the final desired position[13](shown in **Fig. 10**).

Special Consideration as Signs for High Risk of Septal Perforation During Procedure

We should continuously monitor the changes in the depth of the lead, pacing parameters, paced QRS morphology, and IEGM characteristics to avoid perforation into the LV cavity during the procedure. (1) The thickness of the ventricular septum by echocardiography or other imaging as a reference for the depth of the lead to be screwed into the ventricular septum. (2) The amplitude of ventricular myocardium injury current (V-COI) is usually more than 5mv. If the amplitude declines to less than 3mv, it indicates that the lead is very close to the left ventricular subendocardium, especially with a change in COI contour (illustrated in **Fig. 11**). Once there is a loss of V-COI, it means there is ventricular septal perforation.

Sheath Removal

It is important to not pull the lead when slitting the sheath. Before removal, the sheath should be withdrawn to the right atrium and adjusted to achieve appropriate lead slack. In addition, it is important to compare pacing parameters and LBB potential before and after sheath removal and assess the slack of pacing lead with deep inspiration.

Adequate Slack of the Pacing Lead

Appropriate lead slack is important during conduction system pacing which may ensure stable pacing parameters and avoid septal perforation postoperatively. During the procedure, it is necessary to observe the overall lead tension via fluoroscopy, and firmly fix the pacing lead in the pocket, so as to avoid lead dislodgement caused by device movement postoperatively. The amplitude of intracardiac potentials remains constant means that the lead is properly fixed. Examples of low and adequate lead slacks are shown in **Fig. 12**.

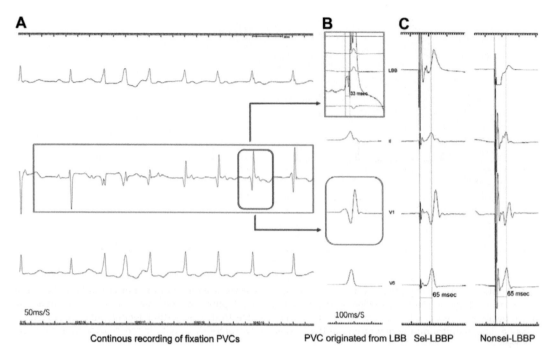

Fig. 10. Recording of continuous PVCs which indicates the depth of pacing lead. (*A*) When the electrode tip is screwed deeply to LBB in the ventricular septum, the surface ECG continuously records the premature ventricular complexes (PVCs), and the QRS morphology changes from right ventricular origin to left ventricular septum origin. (*B*)The morphology of this PVC is consistent with the morphology of selective LBBP which indicates that the PVC originated from LBB and the electrode tip is close to the conduction bundle. The depth of pacing lead can also be assessed by the morphology of PVCs. (*C*) Selective and nonselective LBBP.

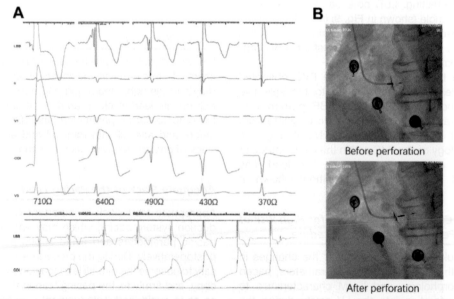

Fig. 11. Tracing of EGM during lead fixation, septal perforation, and following retraction of the lead. (*A*) Case: Monitor the unipolar V-COI during deep screwing of the pacing lead. The morphology of V-COI gradually changed and decreased from spike shape to hump shape. Once ventricular septum was perforated, V-COI disappeared accompanied by a decrease in pacing impedance to less than 400 Ω. (*B*) Intracardiac angiography shows that the pacing lead perforated through the left ventricular septal endocardium.

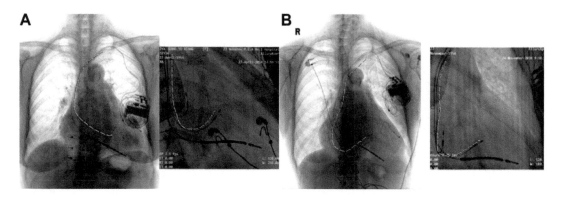

Low slack   Appropriate slack

Fig. 12. Different slacks of pacing lead Case: Patient with cardiomyopathy and complete LBBB. (*A*) The lead slack was normal during the procedure while it decreased postprocedure associated with an increase in LBBB correction threshold to 3.75 V/1.0 ms. (*B*)The lead tension was adjusted to an appropriate state after lead repositioning, and the pacing threshold was stable.

ADDITIONAL CONSIDERATIONS AND CHALLENGING CASES

It is difficult to perform LBB pacing in the following conditions including ventricular septal hypertrophy, heavy septal scar burden and complex congenital heart disease. The basal interventricular septum is assessed preprocedure.[11] The selection of an adequate delivery sheath can strengthen support and increase the success of lead fixation with short fluoroscopy and procedural duration.

1. How to manage difficulty in pacing lead fixation: The pacing lead may rebound counterclockwise immediately after each clockwise rotation when it is difficult to screw the lead in deeply, indicating that the tip of pacing lead is stuck in the tissue. The implanter must adjust the support to keep the sheath perpendicular and

repeatedly confirm that there is no advancement of the lead and then pay attention to eliminate the possible causes: deformation of the sheath results in difficulty screwing the pacing lead and inadequate support of the delivery sheath. It is also possible that the lead may be screwed on the tricuspid annulus or septal leaflet of the valve, and so forth. The solution is as follows:
(1) Change the screwing site on the RV surface of the ventricular septum under the guidance of His bundle mapping to avoid the septal leaflet of the tricuspid valve;
(2) Replace the implantation tools: It is recommended to replace the implantation tools as early as possible including the use of a deflectable delivery sheath to assist in strengthening and improving the support for screwing or use "sheath in sheath"

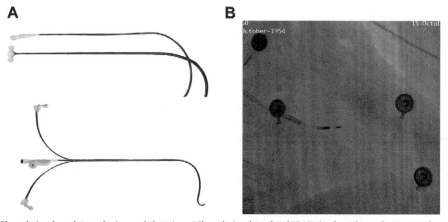

Fig. 13. "Sheath in sheath" technique. (*A*) Using "Sheath in sheath" (C315His sheath as the inner sheath and CS sheath as the outer sheath) technique can facilitate the lead fixation with better support. (*B*) "Sheath in sheath" demonstrated on fluoroscopy.

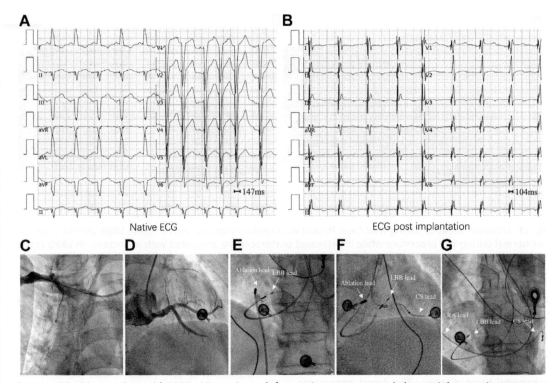

Fig. 14. LBBAP in a patient with LBBB, AF, persistent left superior vena cava and absent right superior vena cava. (*A*) Native ECG showed AF and LBBB with QRS duration of 147 ms; (*B*) ECG shows LBBAP postatrioventricular nodal ablation with QRS duration of 104 ms, Stim-LVAT of 80 ms and RBBB morphology; (*C*) angiography revealed absent right superior vena cava; (*D*) coronary venography; (*E*) the LBBAP lead was 11 mm deep determined by the contrast injection through the reshaped C315 His sheath; (*F*) the ablation catheter, LBB pacing lead and CS lead in the right anterior oblique 30° view; (*G*) the LBBP lead, CS lead, and RA lead. LBBAP, left bundle branch area pacing; LBBB, left bundle branch block; AF, atrial fibrillation; CS, coronary sinus; RA, right atrium.

technique (C315His sheath as the inner sheath and CS sheath as the outer sheath) to help deliver the sheaths to the proper position as in patients with huge right atrium or severe tricuspid regurgitation (shown in **Fig. 13**). C315 His sheath plus CS delivery sheath (peelable or slit) is recommended to be used for LBBP.

2. Challenging cases/anatomy: An example of a patient with PLSVC case is described in **Fig. 14**. An 80-year-old man with hypertension was admitted with recurrent chest tightness and dyspnea. ECG demonstrated atrial fibrillation with a rapid ventricular rate and left bundle branch block (LBBB) with a QRS duration of 147 ms. The left ventricular ejection fraction (LVEF) was 31%. Atrioventricular nodal ablation combined with LBBP was performed in March 2019. During the procedure, the transaxillary angiography showed persistent left superior vena cave with absent right superior vena cava. HBP failed to correct the LBBB and finally left LBBAP fused with coronary sinus lead pacing was achieved. The acute threshold of LBBAP was 0.5 V @0.5 ms and unipolar impedance was 430 Ω. The symptoms were significantly relieved and LVEF improved to 51% at 2-year follow-up. The pacing parameters remained stable and no lead-related complication was observed during the follow-up.

3. Atrial septal pacing: Use of 3830 lead via sheath implantation for atrial septal pacing can be seen in "Dual-lead method."[22] The implanter should pay attention to whether the two 3830 leads are intertwined (especially during the slitting of the second sheath). The unipolar impedance of atrial septal pacing is typically greater than 600 Ω with significant atrial COI (illustrated in **Fig. 15**).

LEFT BUNDLE BRANCH PACING COMPLICATIONS AND MANAGEMENT STRATEGIES
Intraoperative Complications

1. Bundle branch injury: The incidence of right bundle branch injury is higher in LBBP than HBP because the pacing lead needs to bypass

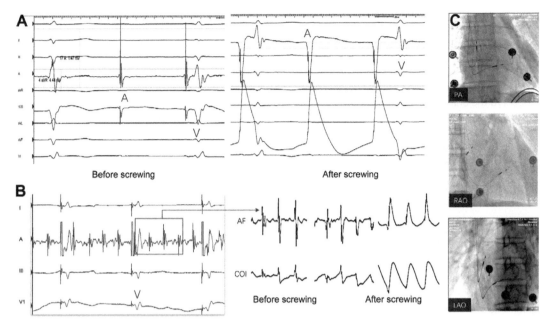

Fig. 15. Atrial septal lead fixation. (*A*) Case 1, sinus rhythm with complete AV block. After 3830 lead is fixed in the high position of atrial septum with 780 Ω unipolar impedance, A. giant atrial COI in the intracardiac electrocardiogram. (*B*) Case 2, atrial fibrillation with complete AV block. 3830 lead is fixed in the atrial septum, COI with fibrillation wave was recorded in intracardiac electrocardiogram. Unipolar impedance was more than 600 Ω. (*C*) Posteroanterior (PA), right (RAO), and left anterior oblique (LAO) fluoroscopic views of the atrial lead are shown.

the tricuspid valve during LBBP. The implanter should gently manipulate the sheath and the lead, as the lead crosses the tricuspid annulus and maintain the lead tip inside the sheath and below the level of His bundle to avoid RBB injury. The subvalvular potential recorded from the conducting tissue below the tricuspid annulus is typically the RBB potential. If the RBB is injured or RBBB occurs during lead advancement into the septum, avoid further fixation, and most transient injuries will recover. Temporary backup ventricular pacing is needed in patients with LBBB because of the possibility of complete heart block with lead manipulation or fixation.

2. Lead dislodgement and septal perforation: Closely monitoring the depth of the lead tip into the interventricular septum and the impedance changes during the procedure may help reduce the risk of dislodgement or perforation.[17,23] As the lead is screwed into the septum, perforation risks need to be evaluated when the impedance starts to drop or when the unipolar impedance is < 500 Ω. The decrease of amplitude of V-COI on intracardiac electrocardiogram is a sensitive indicator for perforation. If perforation occurs, simply withdrawing the lead is not recommended. The lead should be repositioned at a different location.

3. Other possible complications: Complications such as interventricular septal injury, pacing lead damage, coronary artery injury, coronary vein injury, electrode mistakenly entering the noncoronary aortic cusp, and pacing lead wrapping the tricuspid leaflet have been reported in rare cases. Although only sporadic cases of septal hematoma have been reported[24], particular attention to the presence of chest pain during surgery, ST-T changes in the electrocardiogram, and postoperative echocardiography may help. Repeatedly screwing the lead into and out of the septum at the same site should be avoided as this may lead to the development of a small ventricular septal defect. When the lead is stuck in the septum or valve, pull the lead back within the sheath with proper tension while rotating the entire system counterclockwise to release the lead to avoid septal myocardial disruption or damage to the tricuspid valve leaflet.

Postoperative Complications

The incidence of conduction system pacing threshold increase was less than 1% (LBB capture threshold >3 V/0.5 ms) in our center.[14] This is a rare phenomenon but may occur for the following reasons: (1) the pacing site does not bypass the site of block; (2) conduction disease progression; (3) electrode dislodgement, and so forth. The following are recommended: (1) estimate whether the pacing site bypasses the site of conduction block; (2) adjust the lead to maintain proper slack with adequate lead anchoring to pectoral muscle tissue; (3) observe the change in amplitude of the LBB potential and COI and whether capture threshold increases after fixation, before and after sheath removal. If perforation or micro-dislodgement occurs, reposition should be considered.

CLINICS CARE POINTS

The term left bundle branch pacing implies demonstrating evidence for direct left bundle branch capture.

Dual lead technique improves the success rate of Left bundle branch pacing in patients with left bundle branch block.

Monitoring for lead-depth during implantation with special attention to myocardial current of injury is necessary to prevent perforation into left ventricular cavity.

ACKNOWLEDGMENTS

This work was supported by the Key Research and Development Program of Zhejiang (grant no. 2019C03012), and Major Project of the Health Commission of Zhejiang Province (grant no. 2021KY787).

DISCLOSURE

The authors have nothing to disclose.

REFERENCES

1. Huang W, Su L, Wu S, et al. A novel pacing strategy with low and stable output: pacing the left bundle branch immediately beyond the conduction block. The Can J Cardiol 2017;3(12):1736.e1–3.
2. Wu S, Su L, Vijayaraman P, et al. Left bundle branch pacing for cardiac resynchronization therapy: non-randomized on-treatment comparison with his bundle pacing and biventricular pacing. Can J Cardiol 2021;37(2):319–28.
3. Sharma PS, Patel NR, Ravi V, et al. Clinical outcomes of left bundle branch area pacing compared to right ventricular pacing: results from the geisinger-rush conduction system pacing registry. Heart Rhythm 2022;19:3–11. S1547-5271(21)02102-0. 5.
4. Liu X, Niu HX, Gu M, et al. Contrast-enhanced image-guided lead deployment for left bundle branch pacing. Heart Rhythm 2021;18(8):1318–25.
5. Zhang J, Sun Y, Zhang Z, et al. Intracardiac ultrasound-guided left bundle branch pacing in a bradycardia patient. Clin Case Rep 2020;8(6):1030–3.
6. Massing GK, James TN. Anatomical configuration of the his bundle and bundle branches in the human heart. Circulation 1976;53(4):609–21.
7. Anderson RH, Yanni J, Boyett MR, et al. The anatomy of the cardiac conduction system. Clin Anat 2009;22(1):99–113.
8. Wu S, Chen X, Wang S, et al. Evaluation of the criteria to distinguish left bundle branch pacing from left ventricular septal pacing. JACC Clin Electrophysiol 2021;7(9):1166–77.
9. Wu S, Sharma PS, Huang W. Novel left ventricular cardiac synchronization: left ventricular septal pacing or left bundle branch pacing? Europace 2020;22(Suppl_2):ii10–8.
10. Chen X, Wu S, Su L, et al. The characteristics of the electrocardiogram and the intracardiac electrogram in left bundle branch pacing. J Cardiovasc Electrophysiol 2019;30(7):1096–101.
11. Huang W, Chen X, Su L, et al. A beginner's guide to permanent left bundle branch pacing. Heart Rhythm 2019;16(12):1791–6.
12. Vijayaraman P, Subzposh FA, Naperkowski A, et al. Prospective evaluation of feasibility and electrophysiologic and echocardiographic characteristics of left bundle branch area pacing. Heart Rhythm 2019;16:1774–82.
13. Jastrzębski M, Kiełbasa G, Moskal P, et al. Fixation beats: a novel marker for reaching the left bundle branch area during deep septal lead implantation. Heart Rhythm 2021;18(4):562–9.
14. Su L, Wang S, Wu S, et al. Long-term safety and feasibility of left bundle branch pacing in a large single-center study. Circ Arrhythm Electrophysiol 2021;14(2):e009261.
15. Jastrzębski M. Permanent left bundle branch pacing: what is the mechanism of divergent responses during programmed stimulation? J Cardiovasc Electrophysiol 2020;31(5):1222–5.
16. Su L, Xu T, Cai M, et al. Electrophysiological characteristics and clinical values of left bundle branch current of injury in left bundle branch pacing. J Cardiovasc Electrophysiol 2020;31(4):834–42.
17. Chen X, Wei L, Bai J, et al. Procedure-related complications of left bundle branch pacing: a single-center experience. Front Cardiovasc Med 2021;8:645947.
18. Zheng R, Wu S, Wang S, et al. Case report: interventricular septal hematoma complicating left bundle branch pacing lead implantation. Front Cardiovasc Med 2021.

19. Zheng R, Dong Y, Wu S, et al. Conduction system pacing following septal myectomy: Insights into site of conduction block [published online ahead of print, 2022 Jan 13]. J Cardiovasc Electrophysiol. 2022;10.1111/jce.15362. doi:10.1111/jce.15362.

20. Zhang J, Wang Z, Zu L. Simplifying physiological left bundle branch area pacing using a new nine-partition method. Can J Cardiol 2021;329–38.

21. Hu Y, Gu M, Hua W, et al. Left bundle branch pacing from distal His-bundle region by tricuspid valve annulus angiography. J Cardiovasc Electrophysiol 2019;2550–3.

22. Su L, Wu S, Wang S, et al. Pacing parameters and success rates of permanent His-bundle pacing in patients with narrow QRS: a single-centre experience,. Europace 2019;21(5):763–70.

23. Guo J, Li L, Meng F, et al. Short-term and intermediate-term performance and safety of left bundle branch pacing. J Cardiovasc Electrophysiol 2020; 31(6):1472–81.

24. De Pooter Jan, Calle Simon, Demulier Laurent, et al. Septal Coronary Artery Fistula Following Left Bundle Branch Area Pacing. JACC Clin Electrophysiol 2020; 6:1337–8.

Physiology of Left Ventricular Septal Pacing and Left Bundle Branch Pacing

Jesse Rijks, MD[a], Justin Luermans, MD, PhD[a,b], Luuk Heckman, MD[c],
Antonius M.W. van Stipdonk, MD, PhD[a], Frits Prinzen, PhD[c],
Joost Lumens, PhD[d], Kevin Vernooy, MD, PhD[a,b],*

KEYWORDS

- Left ventricular septal pacing • Left bundle branch pacing • Bradycardia pacing
- Cardiac resynchronization therapy • Physiologic pacing

KEY POINTS

- Electrical activation of the left ventricle starts in the left bundle branch followed by three endocardial areas at the left side of the interventricular septum.
- Right ventricular pacing is associated with adverse effects such as heart failure and atrial fibrillation.
- Left ventricular septal pacing results in (near) physiologic activation of the left ventricle and shows promising results in cardiac resynchronization therapy.
- Left bundle branch pacing proves to maintain or restore (in LBBB) left ventricular electrical and mechanical synchrony with promising results in cardiac resynchronization therapy.
- Implantation techniques for LVSP and LBBP are similar, although more advanced electrophysiological knowledge and equipment is needed to verify left bundle branch capture.
- Theoretically left bundle branch pacing leads to a more synchronous activation of the left ventricle due to capture of the specialized conduction system.

INTRODUCTION

For decades in cardiac pacing, the right ventricular (RV) apex has been the preferred site for ventricular stimulation.[1] The RV apex has proved to be an easily accessible and stable site for lead fixation. However, RV pacing (RVP) causes electrical and mechanical dyssynchrony of the heart, frequently leading to a reduced systolic left ventricular function.[2,3] This, so-called, pacing-induced cardiomyopathy has been associated with an increased risk for heart failure (HF) hospitalization, atrial fibrillation (AF), and cardiovascular death.[4,5] Following the recognition of these adverse effects of RVP, new pacing strategies to maintain or restore interventricular and intraventricular synchrony have been developed. These techniques include biventricular pacing (BVP) and His bundle pacing (HBP). BVP is applied by implantation of 2 ventricular pacing leads. One lead is positioned in the RV, and the other lead is placed on the left ventricular free wall via the coronary sinus. Simultaneous stimulation of the leads aims to restore the ventricular electrical synchrony. Despite the more

[a] Department of Cardiology, Cardiovascular Research Institute Maastricht (CARIM), Maastricht University Medical Centre (MUMC+), the Netherlands; [b] Department of Cardiology, Radboud University Medical Centre (RadboudUMC), Nijmegen, the Netherlands; [c] Department of Physiology, Cardiovascular Research Institute Maastricht (CARIM), Maastricht University, the Netherlands; [d] Department of Biomedical Engineering, Cardiovascular Research Institute Maastricht (CARIM), Maastricht University, the Netherlands
* Corresponding author. Cardiovascular Research Institute Maastricht, Maastricht University Medical Center, PO BOX 5800, Maastricht 6202 AZ, the Netherlands.
E-mail address: Kevin.vernooy@mumc.nl

Card Electrophysiol Clin 14 (2022) 181–189
https://doi.org/10.1016/j.ccep.2021.12.010

synchronous electrical activation, biventricular pacing still results in a nonphysiologic activation.

The most physiologic form of pacing is provided by HBP, as there is complete recruitment of the conduction system to both ventricles. HBP remains challenging due to several factors. First, implantation is challenging with a narrow anatomic target zone, resulting in moderate success rates varying from 81% to 87% after ~40 procedures.[6,7] Furthermore, HBP has been associated with high pacing thresholds and low R wave amplitudes, possibly resulting in atrial oversensing and ventricular undersensing.[8] Another downside of HBP is the possible failure of recruitment of conduction in distal conduction disorders.[7,9] More recently, left ventricular septal pacing (LVSP) and left bundle branch pacing (LBBP) were introduced.

In this review the authors elaborate on the physiology and potential beneficial effects of LVSP and LBBP.

PHYSIOLOGIC ACTIVATION OF THE LEFT VENTRICLE
Electrical Activation

In 1970, Durrer and colleagues[10] described the physiologic electrical activation of the left ventricle in 7 isolated human hearts. During sinus rhythm (SR) with normal ventricular activation through the His-Purkinje system, the activation of the left ventricle starts in the left bundle branch(LBB). The investigators found that, subsequently, 3 endocardial areas are activated first. These areas are located high on the anterior paraseptal wall just below the attachment of the mitral valve, central on the left-sided surface of the interventricular septum (IVS), and on the posterior paraseptal wall about one-third of the distance from apex to base.[10]

In the IVS electrical activation starts on the left septal surface in the middle third part anteriorly and at the lower third part at the junction of septum and posterior wall.[10] The activation then proceeds from the left to the right septum and in apico-basal direction.[10]

It has been demonstrated that endocardial conduction is much faster than endocardium-to-epicardium conduction.[11] One of the reasons for this difference in conduction speed is the more uniform geometric alignment of myocardial fibers in the subendocardium when compared with the epicardium[11]; this facilitates a preferential flow current and more rapid conduction parallel to the aligned myocardial fibers in the endocardium.[12] Another study showed that myocardial fiber arrangement rotates between endocardial and epicardial surfaces,[13] possibly contributing to a

nonaligned area slowing endocardium-to-epicardium conduction. Furthermore, most of the endocardium contains a layer of Purkinje tissue, electrically parallel with the myocardium, contributing to the faster spreading of the endocardial activation front.[14]

Mechanical Activation

The electrical activation or action potential triggers calcium influx, which initiates calcium-induced calcium release. This released calcium binds to the myofibrils, resulting in contraction of the cardiac muscle cells.[15] Various studies in canine hearts showed the close relation between electrical activation and subsequent mechanical activation.[16–18] This tight coupling in a normal synchronous activated left ventricle leads to a synchronous LV contraction.[19]

ADVERSE EFFECTS OF RIGHT VENTRICULAR PACING
Pathophysiology of Right Ventricular Pacing

Different ventricular activation sequences, induced by artificial electrical stimulation (pacing), have been described to influence cardiac pump function.[20] In RVP, electrical activation mainly depends on slow conduction through the myocardial cells (from the right side of the IVS to left side of the IVS and subsequently the left ventricle) instead of using the fast-conducting Purkinje fibers, leading to a dyssynchronous electrical activation. This dyssynchronous activation can lead to a depressed systolic and diastolic LV function.[3] However, the overall dyssynchronous activation does not fully explain the occurrence of pacing-induced LV dysfunction, as total ventricular activation time on the surface electrocardiogram (ECG) (QRS duration) correlates poorly to the occurrence of LV dysfunction.[3] When focusing on electromechanical coupling in RVP, it has been shown that not only the shift of activation in time contributes to a depression of LV function. Strain imaging, used to display electromechanical coupling in RVP, shows a completely different morphology of shortening patterns, indicating discoordination of contraction. This discoordination is characterized by early systolic shortening in early activated regions and systolic prestretch in late-activated regions. Later in systole the opposite phenomenon is observed. Late-activated regions show pronounced shortening, whereas early activated regions may be stretched.[21–23] In considerable dyssynchrony, for instance in RVP, this results in the external work (calculated as the area of the fiber stress-fiber length loop) in early activated regions to be close to zero or even negative and double the normal values in late activated regions, leading to an inefficient contraction.[23]

Clinical Outcomes of Right Ventricular Pacing

The possible adverse effects of RVP first became clinically apparent in patients in the Mode Selection (MOST) trial, a randomized trial comparing DDD pacing versus VVI pacing in patients with a pacing indication due to bradycardia. In 1339 patients with narrow QRS and preserved LV ejection fraction at baseline, it was shown that the percentage of ventricular pacing is a strong predictor for development of AF and HF hospitalization.[4] Later, the Dual Chamber and VVI Implantable Defibrillator (DAVID) trial showed similar results. Patients with an indication for ICD implantation and reduced LV ejection fraction, but without bradycardia, were randomized to dual chamber pacing (DDDR-70) and ventricular back-up pacing (VVI-40). The ventricular pacing percentage was markedly higher in the dual-chamber pacing group compared with the ventricular back-up pacing group, 60% versus 1%, respectively. Dual-chamber pacing showed no clinical benefit over ventricular back-up pacing and even showed a worse outcome regarding the composite end point of death and HF hospitalization.[5] The fact that not every individual treated with RVP will develop pacing-induced cardiomyopathy indicates that more factors contribute to this. It is shown that the presence of structural heart disease, that is, hypertrophy and diastolic dysfunction, contribute to prolonged paced QRS duration and therefore electrical dyssynchrony, independent of the pacing site (RV apex vs RV outflow tract).[24] Furthermore, a lower preimplantation LV ejection fraction, higher ventricular pacing rates, and second- or third-degree atrioventricular block as indication for pacing are associated with higher percentages of pacing-induced cardiomyopathy.[25]

LEFT VENTRICULAR SEPTAL PACING
Acute Effects of Left Ventricular Septal Pacing

After the recognition of the potential adverse effects of RVP, the search for more physiologic forms of pacing gained interest. As described in the first paragraph, during normal SR with normal ventricular activation through the His-Purkinje system, the electrical impulse first exits the Purkinje system at sites on the LV endocardial surface of the IVS. It was therefore hypothesized that pacing near these exit sites will result in a more physiologic activation of the LV. In a canine experiment in 1982, Little and colleagues[26] showed that pacing on the left side of the IVS resulted in the following similar findings as during SR: the IVS was activated from left to right, preejection LV pressure exceeded RV pressure, and IVS motion was the same in LVSP and normal SR.[26] Moreover, invasively measured LV stroke volume and contractility (expressed by LV dP/dTmax) were found to be better during LVSP when compared with RVP in a study in 7 anesthetized open-chest dogs with healthy hearts, despite longer QRS duration in LVSP as compared with RVP[27]; this supports the earlier hypothesis that LV function is dependent not only on QRS duration but more importantly on the sequence of activation.

A subsequent study, comparing different sites of LV pacing, RVP, and normal SR in anesthetized, open-chest dogs, showed that LV function measured in terms of LV dP/dT max and LV stroke work (calculated as the loop area in the pressure-volume loop) was indeed maintained during LVSP to a level comparable with normal SR (Fig. 1).[28]

Long-Term Effects of Left Ventricular Septal pacing

The aforementioned studies showed the beneficial acute hemodynamic effects of LVSP but did not

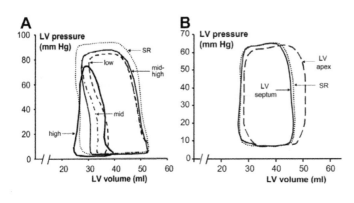

Fig. 1. (A) Pressure volume loops during sinus rhythm (SR) with normal intrinsic ventricular activation and during pacing at the low, mid, mid-high, and high right ventricular (RV) septum. Note that the loop area in the RV-paced loops is smaller than during SR, indicating lower LV stroke work. (B) Pressure volume loops during SR and during pacing the left ventricular septum (LVSP) and left ventricular apex. Note that the pressure volume loop during LVSP is comparable with SR. (Modified from Peschar M, de Swart H, Michels KJ, Reneman RS, Prinzen FW. Left ventricular septal and apex pacing for optimal pump function in canine hearts. J Am Coll Cardiol. 2003;41(7):1218-1226. https://doi.org/10.1016/s0735-1097(0300091-3; with permission.)

investigate the long-term effects of LVSP. The longer term effects of LVSP were studied in canine hearts after 16 weeks of pacing and were compared with RVP and normal SR.[29] First, it was demonstrated that LVSP led to a rapid activation of the LV endocardium, resulting in a pattern that, of all tested pacing sites, most closely resembled the pattern during normal SR, albeit that the RV free wall was slightly delayed. MRI tagging was used to determine strain patterns. During 16 weeks of RVP, circumferential strain was significantly lower in the IVS and higher in the LV free wall. Furthermore, dP/dTmax was significantly lower during RVP compared with baseline, both at implantation and after 16 weeks of pacing. Such differences were not observed during LVSP. The contraction pattern in LVSP was very similar to normal SR. The pattern for regional time to peak shortening (time to peak shortening [ms] of the septal, anterior, lateral, and posterior segments relative to the earliest activated region) were identical for LVSP and normal SR. Besides this, external efficiency (ratio of stroke work, calculated as the loop area in the pressure-volume loop, and oxygen consumption) was decreased by 30% to 40% during RVP, when compared with normal SR, whereas there was no decrease in efficiency during LVSP.[29]

Left Ventricular Septal Pacing in the Human Heart

After preclinical studies successfully demonstrated the advantages of LVSP over RVP and even showed that electrical and mechanical activation and their subsequent hemodynamic effects were comparable with normal SR, clinical studies were needed. The first study of LVSP in patients was conducted in 10 patients with structurally normal hearts with mainly a pacing indication because of sick sinus syndrome.[30] Acute hemodynamic measurements showed that in LVSP values of LV dP/dtmax were maintained to levels comparable with baseline atrial pacing with normal ventricular conduction.[30] Furthermore, the acute hemodynamic benefits of LVSP over RVP were consistently observed in all patients. Not only were favorable hemodynamic effects observed, but QRS duration was shorter during LVSP (144 ms ± 20 ms) than during RV septal pacing (165 ms ± 17 ms).[30] This large difference in QRS duration and the differences in hemodynamic effect between LVSP and RV septal pacing, although pacing sites are only ~1 cm apart, might be due to a significant delay in transseptal conduction during RV septal pacing. This causes delayed LV electrical and mechanical activation with even

more pronounced delayed contraction of the LV lateral wall, causing both interventricular and intraventricular dyssynchrony.[31] On the other hand, it is imaginable that LVSP causes significant delay in RV electrical and mechanical activation, inducing interventricular dyssynchrony. Although LVSP maintains physiologic septal and LV activation, a delayed electrical activation of the right RV free wall is observed in LVSP. Data on the hemodynamic effects of delayed RV activation during LVSP are not available yet.

Left Ventricular Septal Pacing in Cardiac Resynchronization Therapy

Subsequently to showing that LVSP leads to an electrical and mechanical activation of the left ventricle comparable with normal SR, LVSP was explored as alternative pacing strategy for cardiac resynchronization therapy (CRT) for dyssynchronous HF.

In patients with HF induced by LBBB it makes sense to create the most physiologic sequence of activation by pacing at the earliest activated site in the left ventricle with fast endocardial spread of activation. Also, in LBBB the use of the LVSP site seems favorable because a considerable part of the total dyssynchrony in LBBB originates from the delay in conduction across the IVS.[32] Rademakers and colleagues[33] explored LVSP in CRT in both ischemic and nonischemic canine LBBB hearts. LVSP, in combination with RVP, resulted in electrical (measured as QRS duration and total activation time) and acute hemodynamic (measured as LVdP/dT max and stroke work) benefits similar to conventional BVP (generally applied as CRT pacing strategy), when compared with baseline LBBB.[33] An acute hemodynamic pacing study, comparing LVSP with BVP in 12 patients with HF with an indication for CRT, confirmed these results.[33] More recently, an extensive acute electrical and hemodynamic study was performed, comparing LBBB with LVSP, LVSP in combination with RVP (LVSP + RVP), BVP, and HBP, in patients undergoing CRT implantation. QRS duration, QRS area determined by vectorcardiography, and standard deviation of activation time (SDAT) obtained with the ECG belt were measured as indicators of electrical dyssynchrony. LV function was determined by measuring the LV dP/dT max. LVSP resulted in a larger reduction in electrical dyssynchrony than BVP and LVSP + RVP compared with baseline AAI pacing with LBBB, while being similar to HBP. Regarding LV function, improvement in LV dP/dtmax was similar in LVSP, BVP, and HBP with an increase of ~17% compared with baseline

LBBB (**Fig. 2**).[34] These results indicate that LVSP provides short-term hemodynamic improvement and electrical resynchronization comparable with BVP and even HBP in patients undergoing CRT.

LEFT BUNDLE BRANCH PACING

In normal ventricular conduction via the His-Purkinje system, electrical activation of the endocardium on the left-sided IVS is preceded by activation of the His bundle and subsequently the LBB.

Pacing the LBB has recently been introduced as an alternative method of physiologic pacing to maintain left ventricular synchrony.[35] The LBB arises from the branching portion of the His bundle. The proximal left bundle spreads out beneath the LV subendocardium, forming a wider target for pacing when compared with the narrow His bundle.[7] Zhang and colleagues[36] analyzed ECG parameters in 23 consecutive patients undergoing LBBP. At baseline QRS duration in the LBBP group was 130 ms ± 43.3 ms, whereas after LBBP implantation QRS duration shortened to 112 ms ± 12 ms. Echocardiographic strain imaging in LBBP showed similar global longitudinal strain rates when compared with baseline normal SR.[37] When comparing mechanical synchrony between LBBP and conventional RVP using 2-dimensional echocardiographic strain imaging, there was a significantly shorter maximal time difference to peak strain in LBBP (66 ms in LBBP vs 149 ms in RVP),[38] indicating a more synchronous

left ventricular activation in LBBP. Another study evaluated BNP and diastolic echocardiographic parameters measured before and 7 days after permanent LBBP or RVP.[39] BNP levels were significantly lower in the LBBP group compared with RVP. Peak E-wave velocity and E/e' decreased and e' increased significantly after 7 days compared with preimplantation in the LBBP group, whereas there were no significant changes in the RVP group.[39]

When comparing LBBP with HBP, looking at mechanical synchrony using phase analysis of single-photon emission computed tomography myocardial perfusion imaging, no differences regarding left ventricular mechanical synchrony between LBBP and HBP were found in 56 pacemaker-indicated patients with normal cardiac function.[40]

Left Bundle Branch Pacing in Cardiac Resynchronization Therapy

LBBP has also been performed in CRT candidates as an alternative for BVP. LBBP showed a significant shortening of QRS duration from 168 ms ± 38 ms to 119 ms ± 12 ms, when compared with baseline LBBB.[36]

The positive effects of LBBP in LBBB are probably due to pacing beyond the site of conduction block in the left bundle.[37] The correction of LBBB during LBBP indicates its usefulness in CRT. Huang and colleagues[41] performed LBBP in 63 patients with nonischemic cardiomyopathy,

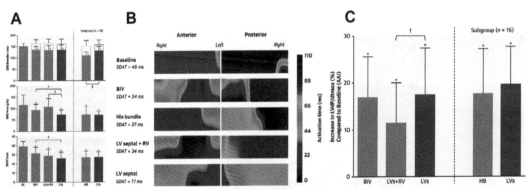

Fig. 2. (*A*) QRS duration as time between onset QRS to end QRS (*closed bars*) and as time between pacing stimulus to end QRS (*open bars*) (*upper panel*), QRS area determined by vectorcardiography (*middle panel*) and SDAT obtained with ECG belt (lower panel), during baseline LBBB(BL), biventricular pacing (BiV), LVSP + RVP, LVSP alone, and during HBP and LVSP. Results are presented as mean ± SD. *P < .05 versus BL; †P < .05 BVP versus LVSP; ‡P < .05 LVSP + RV versus LVSP; §P < .05 HB versus LVSP. (*B*) Isochronal maps together with corresponding SDAT during baseline LBBB, BVP, HBP, LVSP + RVP, and LVSP alone. (*C*) Acute hemodynamic effects measured as percentual increase in LV dP/dtmax compared with baseline LBBB during BVP, LVSP + RVP, and LVSP alone and in a subgroup during HBP and LVSP. Results are presented as mean ± SD. *P < .05 versus BL; †P < .05 LVSP + RV versus LVSP. (*Modified from* Salden FCWM, Luermans JGLM, Westra SW, et al. Short-Term Hemodynamic and Electrophysiological Effects of Cardiac Resynchronization by Left Ventricular Septal Pacing. J Am Coll Cardiol. 2020;75(4):347-359. https://doi.org/10.1016/j.jacc.2019.11.040; with permission)

LBBB, and an indication for CRT. There was significant shortening of QRS duration and within 75% of included patients improvement of LVEF greater than 50% at 1-year follow-up.[41] A large retrospective multicenter study regarding LBBP in CRT showed clinical response (improvement in NYHA class ≥1 without HF hospitalization) and echocardiographic response (≥5% improvement in LVEF) in 72% and 73% of patients, respectively.[42]

LEFT VENTRICULAR SEPTAL PACING OR LEFT BUNDLE BRANCH PACING?

Although implantation techniques do not differ that much, in LBBP (as opposed to LVSP) more advanced electrophysiological knowledge and equipment is needed to verify LBB capture. Recording of a 12-lead ECG for assessment of QRS morphology and measurement of left ventricular activation time (LVAT), measured from the pacing spike to the peak of the R wave in lead V5 or V6, is usually performed. Furthermore, intracardiac electrograms from the tip of the lead are used for searching the His potential as a reference point and recording of the LBB potential to identify the LBB region. Moreover, electrophysiological knowledge on the response of ventricular pacing maneuvers is helpful to confirm LBB capture.[7] The LVSP implantation method is more straightforward, as it is not necessary to identify LBB capture. The paced QRS morphology, visible on 12-lead ECG, is used to validate the right position on the right side of the IVS. Advancement of the lead through the IVS is monitored by QRS morphology, either via continuous pacing[43] or via evaluating fixation beats (ectopic ventricular beats caused by lead fixation).[44] A qR morphology in V1 indicates deep left-sided septal deployment. Deep septal deployment can also be evaluated by septal contrast angiography. **Fig. 3** shows the location of the left ventricular septal lead in LVSP and LBBP.

The difference between LVSP and LBBP is capture of the LBB in LBBP and only myocardial capture in LVSP. In LBBP, theoretically a more synchronous electrical activation of the left ventricle is obtained by capturing the specialized conduction system.[45] While attempting LBBP, actual LBB capture rates differ in literature, with capture rates varying from 60% to 90%[46–48]; this means that a considerable amount of patients intendedly being treated with LBBP are in fact treated with LVSP. A recent study compares LV electrical synchrony between LBBP and LVSP by determining QRS area and LVAT (both markers of electrical synchrony).[46] LBB capture was defined by the presence of (1) paced (pseudo) RBBB morphology, (2) recording of an LBB potential during intrinsic rhythm, (3) constant left ventricular activation time during high- and low-output pacing, and (4) demonstration of transition from nonselective LBBP to selective LBBP or nonselective LBBP to LVSP. The study showed that, compared with conventional RV pacing, the largest reduction in QRS area and LVAT are achieved at the first steps penetrating the IVS and that a reasonably acceptable level of ventricular synchrony is achieved when an R′ becomes apparent in lead V1 (evidence of pacing at the

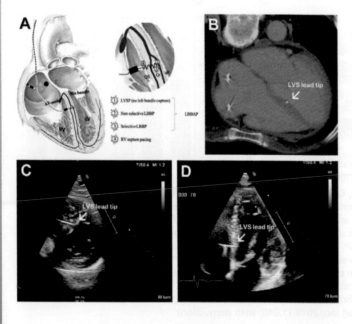

Fig. 3. Location of the LVSP/LBBP lead. (A)The heart and conduction system. It is illustrated where the lead is positioned in the interventricular septum. The different definitions of capture are shown and which QRS morphologies are typically seen. (B) Cardiac CT image showing the LVSP/LBBP lead tip deployed deep in the interventricular septum (IVS). (C) Parasternal short axis transthoracic echo (TTE) view showing the LVSP/LBBP lead tip in the IVS. (D) Apical 4 chamber TTE view showing the LVSP/LBBP lead tip in the IVS. (Panel A modified from Heckman LIB, Luermans JGLM, Curila K, Van Stipdonk AMW, Westra S, Smisek R, Prinzen FW, Vernooy K. Comparing Ventricular Synchrony in Left Bundle Branch and Left Ventricular Septal Pacing in Pacemaker Patients. Journal of Clinical Medicine. 2021; 10(4):822. https://doi.org/10.3390/jcm10040822.)

left side of the IVS).[46] Comparing LVSP and LBBP using ultrahigh-frequency ECG indicates that although LV lateral wall depolarization is accelerated in LBBP compared with LVSP, LBBP results in greater interventricular dyssynchrony, because the RV is activated relatively later.[45] This difference in interventricular synchrony is most likely due to immediate left-to-right transseptal depolarization in LVSP and delayed left-to-right transseptal depolarization in (selective) LBBP, resulting in a more balanced ventricular depolarization in LVSP, compared with (selective) LBBP.[45,49] Most of the aforementioned studies focus on the acute or short-term effect of LVSP and LBBP. Data on long-term effects are lacking and needed. Furthermore, the differences and similarities between LVSP and LBBP need to be explored beyond the current knowledge.

SUMMARY

LVSP and LBBP are emerging forms of ventricular pacing, due to their more physiologic pattern of electrical activation of the left ventricle and probably better feasibility than HBP. Both animal and patient studies have demonstrated their (near) physiologic electrical and mechanical activation of the left ventricle. Although data in large randomized trials regarding long-term effects are lacking, these new pacing strategies form a promising alternative to conventional RVP in bradycardia pacing. Studies regarding CRT show promising results for both LVSP and LBBP.

CLINICS CARE POINTS

- LVSP and LBBP result in (near) physiologic electrical and mechanical activation of the left ventricle.
- Studies regarding CRT show promising results for both LVSP and LBBP.
- More studies regarding long-term effects of LVSP and LBBP are needed.
- More studies comparing LVSP and LBBP are needed to further evaluate and compare both pacing strategies.

CONFLICT OF INTEREST

F. Prinzen: research grants from Medtronic, Abbott, MicroPort CRM, and Biotronik. K. Vernooy: consultancy agreement with Medtronic, Abbott, and Philips. J. Luermans: Consultancy agreement with Medtronic.

REFERENCES

1. Burri H, Starck C, Auricchio A, et al. EHRA expert consensus statement and practical guide on optimal implantation technique for conventional pacemakers and implantable cardioverter-defibrillators: endorsed by the Heart Rhythm Society (HRS), the Asia Pacific Heart Rhythm Society (APHRS), and the Latin-American Heart Rhythm Society (LAHRS). Europace 2021;23(7):983–1008.
2. Nielsen JC, Kristensen L, Andersen HR, et al. A randomized comparison of atrial and dual-chamber pacing in 177 consecutive patients with sick sinus syndrome: echocardiographic and clinical outcome. J Am Coll Cardiol 2003;42(4): 614–23.
3. Prinzen FW, Peschar M. Relation between the pacing induced sequence of activation and left ventricular pump function in animals. Pacing Clin Electrophysiol 2002;25(4 Pt 1):484–98.
4. Sweeney MO, Hellkamp AS, Ellenbogen KA, et al. Adverse effect of ventricular pacing on heart failure and atrial fibrillation among patients with normal baseline QRS duration in a clinical trial of pacemaker therapy for sinus node dysfunction. Circulation 2003;107(23):2932–7.
5. Wilkoff BL, Cook JR, Epstein AE, et al. Dual-chamber pacing or ventricular backup pacing in patients with an implantable defibrillator: the Dual Chamber and VVI Implantable Defibrillator (DAVID) Trial. JAMA 2002;288(24):3115–23.
6. Keene D, Arnold AD, Jastrzebski M, et al. His bundle pacing, learning curve, procedure characteristics, safety, and feasibility: Insights from a large international observational study. J Cardiovasc Electrophysiol 2019;30(10):1984–93.
7. Ponnusamy SS, Arora V, Namboodiri N, et al. Left bundle branch pacing: a comprehensive review. J Cardiovasc Electrophysiol 2020;31(9):2462–73.
8. Vijayaraman P, Dandamudi G. How to perform permanent his bundle pacing: tips and tricks. Pacing Clin Electrophysiol 2016;39(12):1298–304.
9. Vijayaraman P, Naperkowski A, Ellenbogen KA, et al. Electrophysiologic Insights into site of atrioventricular block: Lessons from permanent His bundle pacing. JACC Clin Electrophysiol 2015;1(6):571–81.
10. Durrer D, van Dam RT, Freud GE, et al. Total excitation of the isolated human heart. Circulation 1970; 41(6):899–912.
11. Myerburg RJ, Gelband H, Nilsson K, et al. The role of canine superficial ventricular muscle fibers in endocardial impulse distribution. Circ Res 1978; 42(1):27–35.
12. Roberts DE, Hersh LT, Scher AM. Influence of cardiac fiber orientation on wavefront voltage, conduction velocity, and tissue resistivity in the dog. Circ Res 1979;44(5):701–12.

13. Streeter DD Jr, Spotnitz HM, Patel DP, et al. Fiber orientation in the canine left ventricle during diastole and systole. Circ Res 1969;24(3):339–47.

14. Spach MS, Huang SN, Ayers CR. Electrical and anatomic study of the Purkinje system of the canine heart. Am Heart J 1963;65:664–73.

15. Eisner DA, Caldwell JL, Kistamas K, et al. Calcium and excitation-contraction coupling in the heart. Circ Res 2017;121(2):181–95.

16. Prinzen FW, Augustijn CH, Allessie MA, et al. The time sequence of electrical and mechanical activation during spontaneous beating and ectopic stimulation. Eur Heart J 1992;13(4):535–43.

17. Badke FR, Boinay P, Covell JW. Effects of ventricular pacing on regional left ventricular performance in the dog. Am J Phys 1980;238(6):H858–67.

18. Wyman BT, Hunter WC, Prinzen FW, et al. Mapping propagation of mechanical activation in the paced heart with MRI tagging. Am J Phys 1999;276(3): H881–91.

19. Sengupta PP, Tondato F, Khandheria BK, et al. Electromechanical activation sequence in normal heart. Heart Failure Clin 2008;4(3):303–14.

20. CJ W. The muscular reactions of the mammalian ventricles to artificial surface stimuli. Am J Phys 1925;73:346–78.

21. Prinzen FW, Augustijn CH, Arts T, et al. Redistribution of myocardial fiber strain and blood flow by asynchronous activation. Am J Phys 1990;259(2 Pt 2):H300–8.

22. Delhaas T, Arts T, Prinzen FW, et al. Regional fibre stress-fibre strain area as an estimate of regional blood flow and oxygen demand in the canine heart. J Physiol 1994;477(Pt 3):481–96.

23. Prinzen FW, Hunter WC, Wyman BT, et al. Mapping of regional myocardial strain and work during ventricular pacing: experimental study using magnetic resonance imaging tagging. J Am Coll Cardiol 1999;33(6):1735–42.

24. Ogano M, Tsuboi I, Iwasaki YK, et al. Structural heart disease, not the right ventricular pacing site, determines the QRS duration during right ventricular pacing. Heart Vessels 2021;36(12):1870–8.

25. Safak E, Ince H, Gkouvatsou L, et al. Pacing-induced cardiomyopathy in chronic right ventricular apical pacing: a midterm follow-up study. Eur J Med Res 2019;24(1):23.

26. Little WC, Reeves RC, Arciniegas J, et al. Mechanism of abnormal interventricular septal motion during delayed left ventricular activation. Circulation 1982;65(7):1486–91.

27. Prinzen FW, Van Oosterhout MF, Vanagt WY, et al. Optimization of ventricular function by improving the activation sequence during ventricular pacing. Pacing Clin Electrophysiol 1998;21(11 Pt 2):2256–60.

28. Peschar M, de Swart H, Michels KJ, et al. Left ventricular septal and apex pacing for optimal pump function in canine hearts. J Am Coll Cardiol 2003; 41(7):1218–26.

29. Mills RW, Cornelussen RN, Mulligan LJ, et al. Left ventricular septal and left ventricular apical pacing chronically maintain cardiac contractile coordination, pump function and efficiency. Circ Arrhythm Electrophysiol 2009;2(5):571–9.

30. Mafi-Rad M, Luermans JG, Blaauw Y, et al. Feasibility and acute hemodynamic effect of left ventricular septal pacing by Transvenous Approach through the interventricular septum. Circ Arrhythm Electrophysiol 2016;9(3):e003344.

31. Strik M, van Deursen CJ, van Middendorp LB, et al. Transseptal conduction as an important determinant for cardiac resynchronization therapy, as revealed by extensive electrical mapping in the dyssynchronous canine heart. Circ Arrhythm Electrophysiol 2013;6(4):682–9.

32. Prinzen FW, Auricchio A. Is echocardiographic assessment of dyssynchrony useful to select candidates for cardiac resynchronization therapy? Echocardiography is not useful before cardiac resynchronization therapy if QRS duration is available. Circ Cardiovasc Imaging 2008;1(1):70–7.

33. Rademakers LM, van Hunnik A, Kuiper M, et al. A possible role for pacing the left ventricular septum in cardiac resynchronization therapy. JACC Clin Electrophysiol 2016;2(4):413–22.

34. Salden F, Luermans J, Westra SW, et al. Short-term hemodynamic and electrophysiological effects of cardiac resynchronization by left ventricular septal pacing. J Am Coll Cardiol 2020;75(4):347–59.

35. Huang W, Su L, Wu S, et al. A novel pacing strategy with low and stable output: pacing the left bundle branch immediately beyond the conduction block. Can J Cardiol 2017;33(12):1736 e1731–3.

36. Zhang J, Wang Z, Cheng L, et al. Immediate clinical outcomes of left bundle branch area pacing vs conventional right ventricular pacing. Clin Cardiol 2019; 42(8):768–73.

37. Li X, Li H, Ma W, et al. Permanent left bundle branch area pacing for atrioventricular block: feasibility, safety, and acute effect. Heart Rhythm 2019; 16(12):1766–73.

38. Sun Z, Di B, Gao H, et al. Assessment of ventricular mechanical synchronization after left bundle branch pacing using 2-D speckle tracking echocardiography. Clin Cardiol 2020;43(12):1562–72.

39. Liu Q, Yang J, Bolun Z, et al. Comparison of cardiac function between left bundle branch pacing and right ventricular outflow tract septal pacing in the short-term: a registered controlled clinical trial. Int J Cardiol 2021;322:70–6.

40. Hou X, Qian Z, Wang Y, et al. Feasibility and cardiac synchrony of permanent left bundle branch pacing through the interventricular septum. Europace 2019;21(11):1694–702.

41. Huang W, Wu S, Vijayaraman P, et al. Cardiac re-synchronization therapy in patients with Nonischemic cardiomyopathy using left bundle branch pacing. JACC Clin Electrophysiol 2020;6(7):849–58.

42. Vijayaraman P, Ponnusamy S, Cano O, et al. Left bundle branch area pacing for cardiac resynchronization therapy: results from the international LBBAP Collaborative study group. JACC Clin Electrophysiol 2021;7(2):135–47.

43. Jastrzebski M, Moskal P. Reaching the left bundle branch pacing area within 36 heartbeats. Kardiol Pol 2021;79(5):587–8.

44. Jastrzebski M, Kielbasa G, Moskal P, et al. Fixation beats - a novel marker for reaching the left bundle branch area during deep septal lead implantation. Heart Rhythm 2020;18(4):562–9.

45. Curila K, Jurak P, Jastrzebski M, et al. The left bundle branch pacing compared to left ventricular septal myocardial pacing increases interventricular dyssynchrony but accelerates left ventricular lateral wall depolarization. Heart Rhythm 2021;18(8):1281–9.

46. Heckman LIB, Luermans J, Curila K, et al. Comparing ventricular synchrony in left bundle branch and left ventricular septal pacing in pacemaker patients. J Clin Med 2021;10(4).

47. Jastrzebski M, Kielbasa G, Curila K, et al. Physiology-based electrocardiographic Criteria for left bundle branch capture. Heart Rhythm 2021;18(6):935–43.

48. Heckman L, Vijayaraman P, Luermans J, et al. Novel bradycardia pacing strategies. Heart 2020;106(24):1883–9.

49. Jastrzebski M, Burri H, Kielbasa G, et al. The V6-V1 interpeak interval: a novel criterion for the diagnosis of left bundle branch capture. Europace 2021;24(1):40–7.

Evaluation of Criteria for Left Bundle Branch Capture

Shunmuga Sundaram Ponnusamy, MD[a], Pugazhendhi Vijayaraman, MD[b],*

KEYWORDS

- Left bundle branch pacing • Left ventricular activation time • R-wave peak time
- Left bundle branch potential • Conduction system capture

KEY POINTS

- Left bundle branch pacing (LBBP) provides electrical and mechanical synchrony at low and stable pacing output and effectively corrects distal conduction system disease.
- The criteria for differentiating LBBP from LV septal pacing has not been validated in large trials.
- There are several electrocardiography based and intracardiac electrogram based criteria to confirm LBB capture.
- It is essential to confirm conduction system capture for synchronized activation of the ventricle.

INTRODUCTION

Cardiac pacing is the definitive therapy for patients with symptomatic bradycardia. The right ventricular apex has been the standard pacing site over years, as it is a safe, time-tested procedure supported by plenty of clinical data. But there are clinical concerns, as chronic RV apical pacing produces electrical and mechanical dyssynchrony resulting in ventricular dysfunction, atrial arrhythmias, and recurrent heart failure.[1,2] The alternative pacing sites including RV septum and RV outflow tract were tried with limited success.[3] The role of biventricular devices in improving heart failure has been restricted to small group of patients with wide QRS on the surface electrocardiography.

Deshmukh and colleagues[4] first demonstrated the clinical feasibility of permanent His bundle pacing (HBP) in 12 patients with atrial fibrillation. Left ventricular ejection fraction (LVEF) improved from 20% to 31% with reduction in LV end-diastolic diameter. Subsequently conduction system as an alternative site of pacing was explored

extensively, supported by multiple nonrandomized observational studies. With the widespread adoption of HBP, the limitations were soon recognized. Higher capture thresholds, need for lead revisions, R-wave undersensing, premature battery depletion, and inability to correct distal conduction system disease are the major concerns that prevent HBP from being a workhorse pacing strategy.[5]

LEFT BUNDLE BRANCH PACING

Huang and colleagues[6] suggested direct capture of left bundle branch (LBB) by placing the lead deep inside the proximal interventricular septum. In view of high HBP correction threshold for left bundle branch block (LBBB), LBBP was performed by placing the lead deep in the septum, 15 mm apical to distal His signals. LVEF improved from 32% to 62% at 1-year follow-up with reduction in end-diastolic diameter from 76 mm to 42 mm. A prospective study by Vijayaraman and colleagues[7] showed 93% success rate for LBBP

Funding: None.
[a] Department of Cardiology, Velammal Medical College hospital and research institute, Airport Ring road, Madurai -625009, Tamilnadu, India; [b] Cardiac Electrophysiology, Geisinger Heart Institute, Geisinger Commonwealth School of Medicine, MC 36-10, 1000 E Mountain Blvd, Wilkes-Barre, PA 18711, USA
* Corresponding author.
E-mail addresses: pvijayaraman1@geisinger.edu; pvijayaraman@gmail.com

(93 out of 100 patients) with paced QRS duration of 136 ± 17 ms. The pacing parameters remained stable at median follow-up of 3 months. Anatomically, LBB is a wide target with broad fan of fibers on the left subendocardial aspect of the interventricular septum as opposed to narrow band of His bundle. LBBP is defined as direct capture of the proximal left bundle or one of its fascicles along with septal myocardium at a low threshold.[8] LBBP provides electrical and mechanical synchrony at low and stable pacing output and effectively corrects distal conduction system disease.

WHY TO CONFIRM LEFT BUNDLE BRANCH CAPTURE?

The criteria for selective and nonselective capture of His bundle have been described and validated in several studies.[5] Similar criteria for LBBP are lacking. It is essential to differentiate the LBBP from left ventricular septal pacing (LVSP) as the latter would also produce relatively narrow QRS with similar morphology. LVSP results in delayed left ventricular lateral wall depolarization, as the myocytes are activated first before engaging the left conduction system.[9] Conduction system capture is essential to have synchronized ventricular activation and to avoid pacing-related complications. Currently the term LBB area pacing includes both LBBP, where there is clear evidence of direct LBB capture, and those with LVSP, where only LV septal myocardial capture without evidence for direct LBB capture. In this section, the authors review these criteria (**Table 1**) and their overall accuracy.

LEFT BUNDLE BRANCH CAPTURE CONFIRMATION CRITERIA
Paced QRS Morphology in Lead V1

Pacing the LBB would produce early activation of the left ventricle with right bundle branch (RBB) delay in the surface ECG. A paced QRS morphology of RBB delay pattern (qR/rSR) in lead V1 (**Fig. 1**) is seen in nearly 100% of patients with LBB capture.[8] But RBB delay pattern is also seen in 23.4% to 44.4% of patients with LV septal only capture (LVSP).[10] R' wave was seen in 100% of patients with LBB capture as opposed to 23.4% of patients with LVSP (*P* < .001). A terminal S wave is absent in lead V1 in LBBP and is seen in 60% of LVSP (*P* < .001). Large R wave amplitude (0.78–0.82 mV) and broad R wave duration (46–58 ms) are noted during LBBP as compared with LVSP (0.18 mV and 35 ms, respectively).[10] Hence, a paced QRS morphology of RBB delay pattern is sensitive but not specific for LBBP.

Demonstration of Left Bundle Branch Potential

In patients with normal LBB activation during sinus rhythm, sharp high-frequency potential with amplitude of 0.3 ± 0.13 mV can be recorded (**Fig. 2**A) and confirms the lead to be in the vicinity of the LBB area although it does not prove direct LBB capture.[10] Su and colleagues[11] showed in patients with sinus node dysfunction and atrioventricular block (QRS duration <120 ms) that LBB potentials can be recorded in 98.3% (115/117) of patients. In patients with complete LBBB, potentials may be concealed toward the terminal part of the ventricular electrogram. His corrective pacing could unmask the potential (**Fig. 2**C) by restoration of LBB conduction[12] in these patients by dual lead pacing technique. LBB current of injury (COI) often predicts a lower and stable threshold. Among 115 patients studied, Su and colleagues demonstrated LBB-COI in 67% of patients. Based on the morphology, 3 distinct patterns were noted using the electrophysiology system with filter setting of 30 to 500 Hz. In type 1, high-frequency potential is followed by a horizontal PV segment elevation, which returned to baseline at the end of the procedure. In type 2, the potential is concealed inside the PV segment (**Fig. 2**B). With gradual resolution in the COI, the potential resurges as a sharp high-frequency deflection and evolve into type I. In type 3, the potential is associated with a deep negative PV segment deflection, which gradually tapers off to isoelectric level.

Demonstration of Abrupt Decrease in Stim-LVAT Greater than or Equal to 10 ms with Short and Constant Peak Left Ventricular Activation Time

The peak left ventricular activation time or R-wave peak time (RWPT) is measured in the lateral ECG leads (V5 or V6) from the onset of the pacing spike to the peak of R wave to measure the lateral myocardial depolarization.[8,10] It indicates the rapidity of LV free wall activation. LVSP usually results in prolonged pLVAT, as the wavefront activates the free wall through myocardium. Huang and colleagues[10] showed a mean value of 90.2 ± 15.2 ms in 21 patients with LVSP. Once LBB is captured with further advancement of the lead inside the septum rapid LV activation occurs through conduction system. There will be abrupt shortening pLVAT and remains constant irrespective of the pacing output (**Fig. 3**A). An abrupt shortening in stim-LVAT of greater than or equal to 10 ms occurs during transition from LVSP to LBB capture.[10] As the conduction system is engaged by increasing the pacing output, there will be a

Table 1
Electrocardiogram- and electrogram-based left bundle branch capture confirmation criteria

Electrocardiography based	Electrogram based
Paced QRS morphology-RBB delay pattern	Demonstration of LBB potential
Abrupt shortening of LVAT ≥ 10 ms with short and constant LVAT	Demonstration of retrograde His or antegrade left conduction system potential
RWPT between corrective HBP and LBBP	Nonselective to selective or nonselective to septal capture transition
V6-V1 interpeak interval	Programmed deep septal stimulation
Template or fixation beat	Physiology-based criteria a. QRS onset to RWPT ≤native RWPT (+10 ms) b. Stim to RWPT ≤LBB potential to V6 RWPT (+10 ms) c. Stim to V6 RWPT +10 ms < (IDT-TCT)

rapid activation of the left ventricular, resulting in reduction in LVAT by greater than or equal to 10 ms. Huang and colleagues suggested that stim-LVAT was at least 5 ms more than native LBB potential to LVAT in 50% of the patients due to variation in initial sequence of LV activation during LBBP.[10] An abrupt shortening of stim-LVAT of greater than or equal to 10 ms has 100% specificity in confirming LBB capture. Although pLVAT helps in predicting the required depth of the lead

inside the septum, the absolute value less than which conduction system capture could be confirmed is still not known. A pilot study[13] using SPECT MPI to assess LV mechanical synchrony showed that patients with LVAT less than 76 ms had better mechanical synchrony with sensitivity of 88.9% and specificity of 87.5%. Huang and colleagues[10] showed that pLVAT of 75 ms in patients with non-LBBB has sensitivity of 82% and specificity of 95% for confirming LBB capture. Similarly,

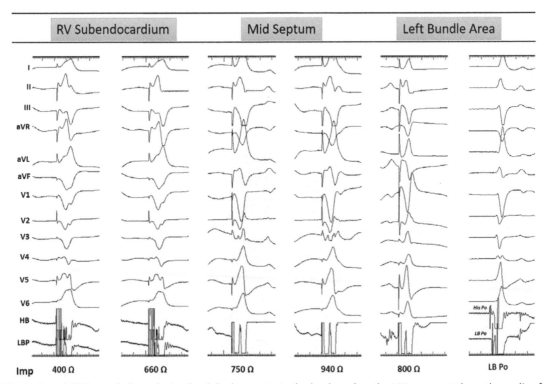

Fig. 1. Paced QRS morphology during lead deployment. As the lead reaches the LBB area, notch on the nadir of the QS will gradually ascend up to form qR pattern in lead V1 along with LBB potential on the lead electrogram.

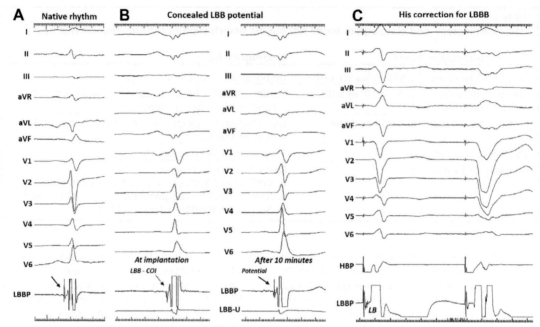

Fig. 2. Demonstration of LBB potential (*black arrow*) during native rhythm with baseline narrow QRS duration (*A*) and during His corrective pacing with baseline LBBB morphology (*B*) Concealed LBB potential (*C*) due to current of injury (*dotted arrow*) immediately with resurgence of potential 10 minutes after implantation.

for patients with baseline LBBB, a value of 85 ms has sensitivity of 76% and specificity of 93%. In patients with cardiomyopathy with significant scar pLVAT may be prolonged. Vijayaraman and colleagues in their retrospective study used less than 90 ms as an arbitrary cutoff for pLVAT to account for delay in conduction due to cardiomyopathy.[14]

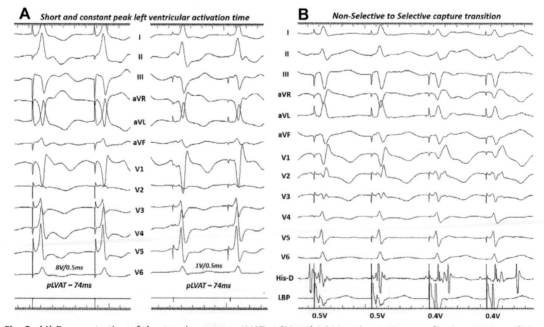

Fig. 3. (*A*) Demonstration of short and constant pLVAT at 8V and 1.0 V pacing output confirming capture of LBB. (*B*) Nonselective to selective capture transition with lead electrogram showing distinct isoelectric interval as the output is reduced from 0.5 V to 0.4 V.

Demonstration of Nonselective to Selective or Nonselective to Septal Capture Transition

Decremental unipolar pacing while checking the threshold will show transition in nonselective to selective capture of LBB at near-threshold value. Nonselective capture of LBB and septal myocardium is characterized by RBB delay pattern in ECG, short RWPT in lateral ECG leads with pacing lead not demonstrating a discrete ventricular electrogram after the pacing spike (**Fig. 3**B). Selective capture is characterized by change in QRS morphology from qR to rSR' in lead V1, increase in S wave duration in lead V6 with pacing lead showing discrete ventricular electrogram from the pacing artifact (**Fig. 4**).[10] The duration of the isoelectric interval between pacing artifact and local ventricular electrogram corresponds to the interval between LBB potential to the onset of QRS. The distinct feature of selective LBB capture "M" pattern or rsR' pattern and wide R' with a notch in lead V1 had a specificity of 100% for confirmation of LBB capture.[15] Selective capture of LBBP could be demonstrated in 39.6% to 90% of study population.[10–12] In a large single-center study by Su and colleagues,[16] 75.4% (460/618) patients were noted to have selective LBB capture. The threshold of local septal myocardium and LBB could vary at different time intervals. Hence repeated testing after a waiting period for the COI to settle, programmed deep septal stimulation, and different pacing rate and pulse width could help in demonstration of selective LBB capture in higher percentage of patients. During this transition, the pLVAT remains constant.

Nonselective to septal myocardial capture transition is characterized by sudden prolongation of pLVAT by more than 10 ms when the pacing output is reduced gradually. Huang and colleagues[10] demonstrated absolute change of stim-RWPT by 10 to 30 ms during transition from nonselective LBB capture to myocardial capture among 30 patients who underwent LBBP. Nonselective to septal capture transition occurs due to (1) higher LBB threshold as compared with myocardial threshold and (2) pacing lead anatomically away from the LBB area with conduction system capture occurring only at high output; this can be differentiated by differential pacing at high and low output where the stim-RWPT will be constant in the former group and shortening of stim-RWPT at high output is noted in the latter group. It is important to differentiate this, as further rotations are required in the latter group to reach the LBB area.

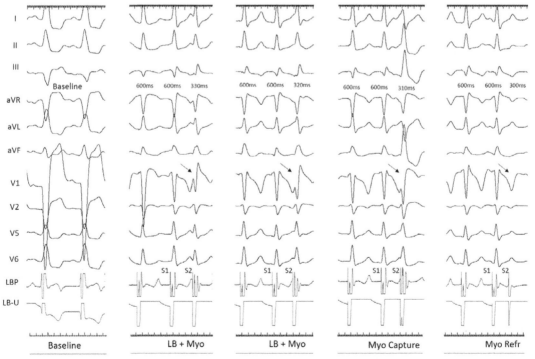

Fig. 4. Programmed deep septal stimulation showing change in QRS morphology with loss of R in lead V1 and duration as LBB lose its capture. (*From* Ponnusamy SS, Arora V, Namboodiri N, Kumar V, Kapoor A, Vijayaraman P. Left bundle branch pacing: A comprehensive review. J Cardiovasc Electrophysiol. 2020;31(9):2462-2473. https://doi.org/10.1111/jce.14681; with permission.)

Programmed Deep Septal Stimulation

Once the pacing lead is deployed in the deep intra-septal location, programmed deep septal pacing can be performed to confirm the LBB capture (see **Fig. 4**).[17] The concept is based on the difference in effective refractory period (ERP) of LBB and septal myocardium; this can be done by using either electrophysiology system or pacing system analyzer. Pacing output must be kept at 2 times the capture threshold in unipolar configuration. Premature beats are introduced after 8-beat basic drive of 600 milliseconds and after during intrinsic sinus rhythm at a sweep speed of 50 to 100 mm/s. The coupling interval is decreased gradually in 10 ms step until complete loss of capture. Three different responses can be seen based on change in QRS morphology.

(a) Diagnostic response type 1 ("myocardial"): as the coupling interval is gradually reduced less than 300 ms, there will be a loss of conduction system capture, resulting in selective myocardial capture and change in paced QRS morphology(**Fig. 5**). This response will be seen in patients with conduction system ERP higher than myocardial ERP. The changes that can be observed include rightward axis shift, higher amplitudes in precordial leads (V2–V5), loss/decrease in amplitude of "R" wave in lead V1, prolonged global QRS duration, and notched or slurred R wave peak; this can be challenging at times to differentiate the changes in QRS morphology due to the myocardial conduction delay during shorter premature stimulus versus actual differences in refractory periods.

(b) Diagnostic response type 2 ("selective LBB"): paced QRS of RBB delay pattern with an isoelectric interval preceding it indicates selective capture of LBB. Selective response will be seen more frequently when the extrastimuli are delivered during intrinsic rhythm rather than after 8-beat basic drive, as the conduction system will always be depolarized earlier and easily excitable than the adjacent myocardium. Selective response to programmed stimulation is observed in only one-third of the patients, as the difference in local activation times between LBB and septal myocardium is relatively small.

(c) Nondiagnostic response: progressive minor change in QRS morphology and duration not suggestive of type 1 or type 2 may be seen in 20% of the patients.[17] It is possible that in some cases change in QRS morphology may not be recognized due to nearly similar ERP of myocardium and LBB or fast engagement of conduction system from myocardial capture.

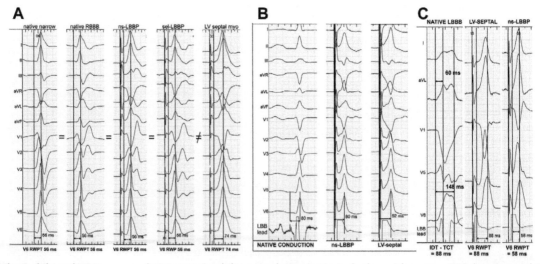

Fig. 5. (*A*) Lead V6 R-wave peak time remained the same during intrinsic rhythm with narrow QRS duration, right bundle branch block, and nonselective LBBP and selective LBBP. LVSP resulted in prolongation of V6-RWPT to 74 ms. (*B*) LBB potential to R-wave peak in lead V6 equaled the pacing stimulus to R wave peak in lead V6 during nonselective LBB capture as compared with a longer interval during LVSP. (*C*) During native LBBB rhythm, LBB capture would show stim to RWPT in lead V6 shorter than (IDT-TCT) as opposed to a longer interval during LVSP capture. (*From* Jastrzębski M, Kiełbasa G, Curila K, et al. Physiology-based electrocardiographic criteria for left bundle branch capture. Heart Rhythm. 2021;18(6):935-943. https://doi.org/10.1016/j.hrthm.2021.02.021; with permission.)

Marek and colleagues[17] showed diagnostic response (type 1 and type 2) in 79.7% of patients. Selective LBB response was noted more often when premature beats were introduced during intrinsic rhythm rather than after basic drive train (30.1% vs 1.4%). Myocardial response on the other hand was seen more often after basic drive train rather than during intrinsic rhythm (72.7% vs 23.1%). Programmed deep septal stimulation will help in confirming conduction system capture when other criteria are not fulfilled.

Physiology-Based Electrocardiography Criteria

These ECG criteria are based on the concept that LBB capture results in restoration of normal physiologic activation of lateral wall of the left ventricle. Marek and colleagues[18] proposed that (1) QRS onset to RWPT equals the RWPT during native non-LBBB rhythm in lead V6; (2) stim to RWPT equals the LBB potential to RWPT in lead V6 during non-LBBB rhythm; and (3) stim to RWPT in lead V6 will be less than the difference between intrinsicoid deflection time (IDT) and transeptal conduction time (TCT) during baseline LBBB rhythm. A 10 ms difference is allowed for some imprecision in measurement between native conduction interval and the corresponding interval during pacing. Because of notched/slurred QRS the intrinsicoid deflection time is measured in patients with baseline LBBB rhythm rather than RWPT. The IDT is measured from the earliest onset of QRS in any lead to the beginning of final rapid downslope in lead V6. TCT is measured from the onset of QRS to the beginning of the first notch in the lateral leads, preferably I and aVL.

They analyzed a total of 357 ECGs: 118 with native rhythm, 124 with nonselective LBB capture, 69 with selective LBB capture, and 45 with LV septal capture. The first criterion: QRS onset to RWPT less than or equal to native V6 RWPT (+10 ms) in non-LBBB rhythm has a sensitivity of 98% and specificity of 85.7% for diagnosing LBB capture (see **Fig. 5**A). The second criterion: stim to RWPT less than or equal to LBB potential to V6 RWPT (+10 ms) has a sensitivity of 88.2% and specificity of 95.4% for diagnosing LBB capture (see **Fig. 5**B). There should not be any difference in stim-RWPT or QRS onset to V6 RWPT between nonselective and selective LBB capture. In patients with baseline LBBB, stim to V6 RWPT will be shorter by greater than 10 ms than the difference between IDT-TCT, whereas in LV septal pacing it will be less than 10 ms or even longer (see **Fig. 5**C). The third criterion: stim to V6 RWPT +10 ms < (IDT-TCT) has a sensitivity of

77.8% and specificity of 100%. The optimal V6-RWPT to differentiate LBB capture from LV septal capture during non-LBB rhythm is 83 ms (sensitivity 84.7%; specificity 96.3%). A V6 RWPT of less than 74 ms has a specificity of 100% for LBB capture confirmation. Similarly, in patients with baseline LBBB rhythm, the optimal V6-RWPT for differentiating LBB capture from LV septal capture is 101 ms (sensitivity 90.4%; specificity 78.9%). A V6 RWPT of less than or equal to 80 ms has a specificity of 100% for confirming LBB capture in patients with LBBB.

Retrograde His Bundle Potential and Anterograde Left Conduction System Potential

Pacing from the LBB area would result in retrograde activation of His bundle and/or antegrade activation of left conduction system (LCS). His bundle potential or LCS potential could be recorded by the pacing lead (HB) or a multielectrode catheter (LCS during LBB stimulation). Capture of LBB could be confirmed by (1) demonstrating stimulus to His potential = intrinsic His potential to LBB potential and (2) demonstration of left conduction system potential preceding the local ventricular electrogram recorded on the multielectrode catheter (**Fig. 6**). Both these findings could provide direct evidence for confirmation of LBB capture. Huang and colleagues[10] demonstrated stim-HB potential duration of 21±5 ms and intrinsic HB potential to LBB potential duration of 21±6 ms in 21 patients with baseline non-LBBB morphology. Also, the stim-HB potential duration was similar during selective LBBP and nonselective LBBP at low and high output. LCS potential could be obtained by His corrective pacing or by direct LBB pacing in patients with baseline LBBB.

ΔRWPT Between Corrective HBP and LBBP in LBBB

LBB potentials are not usually recorded in patients with LBBB. However, if LBBB is corrected with HBP, the PRWT during corrective HBP can be used to confirm LBB capture during LBBP. For a successful LBBP, delineation of distal His bundle signal is essential. Hence mapping of distal His bundle with a diagnostic quadripolar catheter or pacing lead is a routine practice prior of LBBP lead implantation. As the pacing site is distal in LBBP as compared with HBP, RWPT have to be shorter due to earlier activation of LV (**Fig. 7**). An absolute value of 8 ms for ΔRWPT during LBBP and HBP provides 100% sensitivity and 93% specificity and greater than 10 ms has 100% specificity and 81% sensitivity in patients with LBBB.[19]

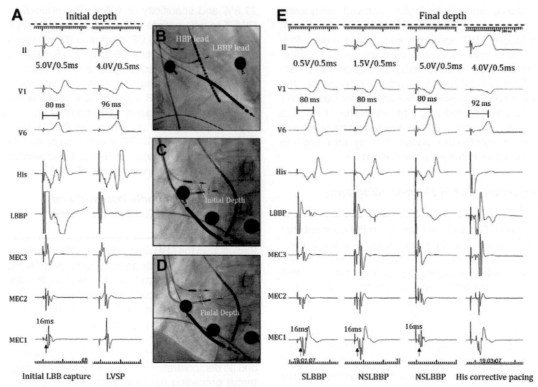

Fig. 6. (*A*) Demonstration of left conduction system potential using a multielectrode catheter during LBBP in a patient with baseline LBBB. Note at initial depth high output resulted in capture of LBB with manifest LCS potential. LVSP resulted in sudden prolongation of RWPT in lead V6 along with loss of LCS potential. (*B–D*) Fluoroscopic image showing the position of HBP lead, depth of LBBP lead, and multielectrode catheter in RAO 30° and LAO 30°. (*E*) At final depth short and constant RWPT of 80 ms along with manifest LCS potential could be demonstrated during both selective and nonselective LBB capture. His corrective pacing resulted in complete correction of LBBB and appearance of LBB potential. (*From* Wu S, Chen X, Wang S, et al. Evaluation of the Criteria to Distinguish Left Bundle Branch Pacing From Left Ventricular Septal Pacing. JACC Clin Electrophysiol. 2021;7(9):1166-1177. https://doi.org/10.1016/j.jacep.2021.02.018; with permission.)

V6-V1 Interpeak Interval

RV and LV activation patterns differ during selective LBB capture, nonselective LBB capture, and LV septal capture; this could change the duration of intrinsicoid deflection in lead V1 (surrogate of RV activation delay) and V6 (surrogate of LV activation delay). The V6-V1 interpeak interval could differentiate between LBB capture and LVSP.[20] The RV activation is delayed during transition from nonselective to selective LBB capture, as there is a loss of interventricular septal capture, whereas the LV activation remains unchanged (**Fig. 8**A). On the contrary, the LV activation is delayed during transition from nonselective to LVSP due to loss of LBB activation, whereas RV activation via the interventricular septum remains unchanged (**Fig. 8**B). Hence in patients with LV septal capture the paced QRS could be narrow and without right bundle branch block or LBBB despite lack of conduction system capture, as

there are 2 oppositely directed wavefronts. The time to intrinsicoid deflection in both V1 and V6 is delayed, as there is a delayed activation of both LV and RV.

Marek and colleagues[20] showed that the V6-V1 interpeak interval would be shortest during LVSP (26±8 ms), intermediate during nonselective LBB capture (41 ± 14 ms), and longest during selective LBB capture (62 ± 21 ms). A cutoff of 33 ms has the sensitivity of 71.8% and specificity of 90% for differentiating nonselective capture from LVSP. A cutoff value of greater than 44 ms has 100% specificity for confirming selective LBB capture at the cost of low sensitivity (see **Fig. 8**). Similarly, as the capture changes from nonselective to selective, lead V1 would show increase in R-wave duration and prolongation of RWPT. A cutoff of greater than or equal to 15 ms could differentiate LBB capture from LVSP with a specificity of 95.6% and specificity of 59.4%.

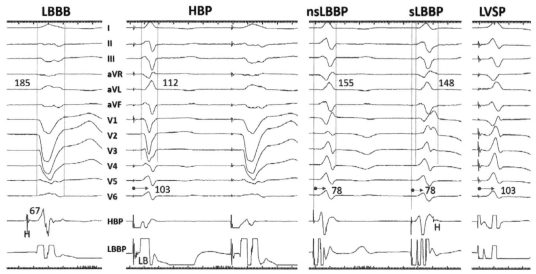

Fig. 7. R-wave peak time during His corrective pacing, selective LBBP, nonselective LBBP, and LVSP in a patient with baseline LBBB. ΔRWPT of 25 ms during LBBP confirmed LBB capture. (*From* Vijayaraman P, Jastrzebski M. Novel Criterion to Diagnose Left Bundle Branch Capture in Patients With Left Bundle Branch Block. JACC Clin Electrophysiol. 2021;7(6):808-810. https://doi.org/10.1016/j.jacep.2021.03.013; with permission.)

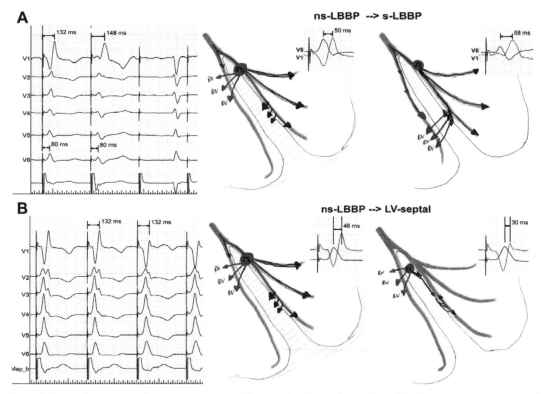

Fig. 8. (*A*) Nonselective to selective capture transition resulted in prolongation of lead-V1 RWPT, constant lead-V6 RWPT, and prolongation of V6-V1 interval. (*B*) Nonselective to septal transition showed no significant change in lead-V1 RWPT but prolonged the V6-RWPT due to loss of LBB capture. (*From* Jastrzębski M, Burri H, Kiełbasa G, et al. The V6-V1 interpeak interval: a novel criterion for the diagnosis of left bundle branch capture [published online ahead of print, 2021 Jul 12]. Europace. 2021;euab164. https://doi.org/10.1093/europace/euab164; with permission.)

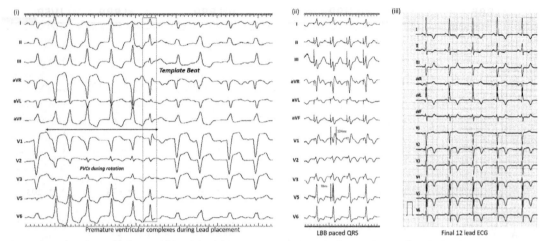

Fig. 9. Template beat during rapid lead deployment. Post-LBBP ECG after AV interval optimization to correct RBB delay showed QRS duration of 98 ms with T-wave memory.

Template or Fixation Beats

Rapid deployment of the lead in the proximal interventricular septum to capture the LBB would generate premature ventricular complexes (PVCs).[21] The morphology of the PVC would change from QS pattern to qR/rSR pattern in lead V1, as the lead traverses from the right side to left side of the septum (**Fig. 9**). A PVC with a morphology of right bundle branch delay pattern (qR/rSR in lead V1), labeled as template or fixation beat,[22,23] predicts the deployment of the lead in the LBB area. Fixation or template beats can predict the capture of LBB with the sensitivity of 96.4% and specificity of 97.3%.[23] PVC-guided lead deployment would help in reducing the fluoroscopy duration and myocardial injury and avoiding perforation into the LV cavity.[22]

Ultra-High Frequency Electrocardiography

Ultra-high frequency ECG (UHF-ECG) shows the time sequence of ventricular depolarization and describes electrical dyssynchrony.[9] UHF-ECG is

Fig. 10. Algorithm to confirm LBB capture.

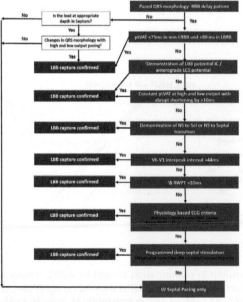

1. In rare instances, RBBB pattern in V1 may not be seen with NS LBB capture due to QS complexes from high left septal capture offsetting the RBBB pattern from LBB capture.
2. In native LBBB, LBB potentials may be seen with corrective HBP. LBB potentials with injury current is associated with LBB capture
3. Δ RWPT >10ms denotes the difference in RWPT during HBP and LBBP

used to calculate e-DYS (interventricular dyssynchrony) and Vd$_{mean}$ (mean local depolarization duration). Positive e-DYS indicates delayed LV activation, and a negative e-DYS indicates delayed RV activation. Curila and colleagues[9] showed that both LBB capture and LVSP reduced the transeptal conduction time associated with RV pacing. However, LBB capture was associated with earlier electrical activation of LV free wall compared with LVSP as reflected by shorter RWPT in lead V5. LVSP resulted in significant prolongation of local depolarization durations in lateral precordial leads due to slower myocardial cell-to-cell propagation without involvement of the conduction system. The interventricular dyssynchrony (e-DYS) was shorter during LVSP than during LBB capture. LBBP resulted in premature activation of LV, delayed activation under leads V1 to V3, and greater LV-RV dyssynchrony with a more negative e-DYS than during LVSP. Although LVSP produces lesser interventricular dyssynchrony, LV depolarization is delayed due to lack of conduction system capture.

SUMMARY

Although LBBP overcomes many of the limitations of the HBP, it is fraught with lack of definite LBB capture confirmation criteria. Paced QRS morphology alone is a poor predictor, as LVSP produces similar morphology with relatively narrow QRS duration. The authors propose a stepwise algorithm (**Fig. 10**); combining ECG- and electrogram-based criteria would help, as it is essential to confirm conduction system capture. Further, hemodynamics and clinical outcome-based studies are essential to confirm the superiority of LBB capture over LV septal-only pacing.

CLINICS CARE POINTS

- LBBP is a novel strategy which overcomes many of the limitations of His bundle pacing.
- Confirmation of LBB capture using ECG and intracardiac electrogram based criteria is warranted to obtain electrical and mechanical synchrony.
- The criteria described require validation in large scale studies.

ACKNOWLEDGMENT

None

DISCLOSURE

S.S. Ponnusamy—Consultant, Medtronic; P. Vijayaraman—Speaker, Consultant, Research, Fellowship support—Medtronic; Consultant—Abbott, Biotronik, Boston Scientific; Patent—HBP delivery tool.

REFERENCES

1. Kurshid S, Epstein AE, Verdino RJ, et al. Incidence and predictors of right ventricular pacing-induced cardiomyopathy. Heart Rhythm 2014;11(9):1619–25.
2. Poole JE, Singh JP, Birgersdotter-Green U. QRS duration or QRS morphology: what really matters in cardiac resynchronization therapy? J Am Coll Cardiol 2016;67:1104–17.
3. Kaye GC, Linker NJ, Marwick TH, et al. Effect of right ventricular pacing lead site on left ventricular function in patients with high-grade atrioventricular block: results of the Protect-Pace study. Eu Heart J 2015;36(14):856–62.
4. Deshmukh P, Casavant DA, Romanyshyn M, et al. Permanent, direct His-bundle pacing: a novel approach to cardiac pacing in patients with normalHis-Purkinje activation. Circulation 2000;101:869–77.
5. Vijayaraman P, Chung MK, Dandamudi G, et al. His bundle pacing. J Am Coll Cardiol 2018;72:927–47.
6. Huang W, Su L, Wu S, et al. A novel pacing strategy with low and stable output: pacing the left bundle branch immediately beyond the conduction block. Can J Cardiol 2017;33:1736.e1-3.
7. Vijayaraman P, Subzposh FA, Naperkowski A, et al. Prospective evaluation of feasibility, electrophysiologic and echocardiographic characteristics of left bundle branch area pacing. Heart Rhythm 2019;16:1774–82.
8. Ponnusamy SS, Arora V, Namboodiri N, et al. Left bundle branch pacing: a comprehensive review. J Cardiovasc Electrophysiol 2020;31(9):2462–73.
9. Curila K, Jurak P, Jastrzebski M, et al. The left bundle branch pacing compared to left ventricular septal myocardial pacing increases interventricular dyssynchrony but accelerates left ventricular lateral wall depolarization. Heart Rhythm 2021;18(8):1281–9.
10. Wu S, Chen X, Wang S, et al. Evaluation of the criteria to distinguish left bundle branch pacing from left ventricular septal pacing. J Am Coll Cardiol EP 2021;7(9):1166–77.
11. Su L, Xu T, Cai M, et al. Electrophysiological characteristics and clinical values of left bundle branch current of injury in left bundle branch pacing. J Cardiovasc Electrophysiol 2020;31(4):834–42.

12. Huang W, Wu S, Vijayaraman P, et al. Cardiac resynchronization therapy in patients with nonischemic cardiomyopathy using left bundle branch pacing. J Am Coll Cardiol EP 2020;6(7):849–58.

13. Qian Z, Wang Y, Hou X, et al. A pilot study to determine if left ventricular activation time is a useful parameter for left bundle branch capture: validated by ventricular mechanical synchrony with SPECT imaging. J Nucl Cardiol 2021;28(3):1153–61.

14. Vijayaraman P, Ponnusamy SS, Cano O, et al. Left bundle branch area pacing for cardiac resynchronization therapy: results from international LBBAP collaborative study group. JACC Clin Electrophysiol 2021;7(2):135–47.

15. Chen X, Wu S, Su L, et al. The characteristics of the electrocardiogram and the intracardiac electrogram in left bundle branch pacing. J Cardiovasc Electrophysiol 2019;30(7):1096–101.

16. Su L, Wang S, Wu S, et al. Long-term safety and feasibility of left bundle branch pacing in a large single-center study. Circ Arrhythm Electrophysiol 2021;14(2):e009261.

17. Jastrzebski M, Moskal P, Bednarek A, et al. Programmed deep septal stimulation - a novel maneuver for the diagnosis of left bundle branch capture during permanent pacing. J Cardiovasc Electrophysiol 2020;31:485–93.

18. Jastrzebski M, Keilbasa G, Curila K, et al. Physiology-based electrocardiographic criteria for left bundle branch capture. Heart Rhythm 2021;18(6):935–43.

19. Vijayaraman P, Jastrzebski M. Novel criterion to diagnose left bundle branch capture in patients with left bundle branch block. J Am Coll Cardiol EP 2021;7(6):808–10.

20. Jastrzebski M, Burri H, Kielbasa G, et al. The V6-V1 interpeak interval: a novel criterion for the diagnosis of left bundle branch capture. Europace 2022 Jan 4;24(1):40–7. https://doi.org/10.1093/europace/euab164.

21. Ponnusamy SS, Vijayaraman P. Left bundle branch pacing guided by premature ventricular complexes during implant. Heartrhythm Case Rep 2020;6(11):850–3.

22. Ponnusamy SS, Ganesan V, Syed T, et al. Template Beat: a novel marker for left bundle branch capture during physiological pacing. Circ Arrhythm Electrophysiol 2021;14(4):e009677.

23. Jastrzebski M, Keilbasa G, Moskal P, et al. Fixation beats: a novel marker for reaching the left bundle branch area during deep septal lead implantation. Heart Rhythm 2021;18(4):562–9.

What Intracardiac Tracings Have Taught Us About Left Bundle Branch Block

Jeremy S. Treger, MD, PhD, Gaurav A. Upadhyay, MD, FACC, FHRS*

KEYWORDS

- Conduction system pacing • His bundle pacing • Left bundle branch area pacing
- Left ventricular septal pacing

KEY POINTS

- Although multiple electrocardiogram (ECG) criteria for left bundle branch block (LBBB) are currently used in clinical practice, none were developed based on direct assessment of endocardial activation patterns.
- The surface ECG pattern of LBBB may subsume multiple electrophysiologic phenomena, including complete conduction block (CCB) of the left His and common left bundle, and also patients with intact Purkinje activation and distal fibrosis and conduction delay. Present criteria lack specificity for the identification of CCB.
- Electrophysiologic recordings of the left septum or endocardial activation maps allow for definitive assessment of conduction system physiology, and possible noninvasive alternatives are in ongoing development.
- Accurate identification of LBBB physiology secondary to CCB is important for appropriate patient selection for conduction system pacing.

INTRODUCTION

Left bundle branch block (LBBB) has been recognized as a clinical entity for over a century, following the pioneering work of Eppinger and Rothberger in a canine model.[1] Lewis is credited with the first recording of LBBB pattern (**Fig. 1**), although he had incorrectly attributed this to right bundle branch block at the time.[2] Building on work in canines, observation of similar patterns of bundle branch block were noted in human patients.[3] As early as 1939, it was noted in canine models that complete transection of the bundle branches was associated with a change in stroke volume distinct from nonspecific delayed excitation leading to wide QRS.[4] Since then, a considerable body of work has been assembled to elucidate the pathophysiologic causes of bundle branch block, as well as the prognostic implications of these conduction defects.[2]

HISTORICAL DEFINITIONS OF LEFT BUNDLE BRANCH BLOCK

Multiple definitions for LBBB based on a surface ECG have evolved over the years. The current American Heart Association/American College of Cardiology/Heart Rhythm Society (AHA/ACC/HRS) guidelines for ECG interpretation of interventricular conduction disturbances were published in 2009.[5] The LBBB criteria elaborated in that document were retained for the most recent guidelines for management of bradycardia and cardiac conduction delays, published in 2018.[6] These modern criteria had been adapted with minimal alterations from the 1985 World Health Organization (WHO) criteria for LBBB.[7] These criteria specify a QRS

The University of Chicago Medicine, Center for Arrhythmia Care, Heart and Vascular Center, Chicago, IL, USA
* Corresponding author. Section of Cardiology, Center for Arrhythmia Care, The University of Chicago Medicine, 5841 South Maryland Avenue| MC 9024, Chicago, IL 60637, USA.
E-mail address: upadhyay@uchicago.edu

Card Electrophysiol Clin 14 (2022) 203–211
https://doi.org/10.1016/j.ccep.2021.12.015
1877-9182/22/© 2021 Elsevier Inc. All rights reserved.

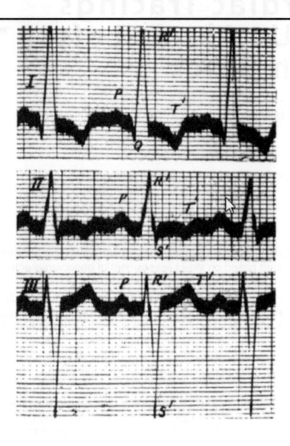

Fig. 1. Early surface ECG of LBBB. One of the earliest known ECG recordings of LBBB in humans. Although precordial leads were not yet in use, the widened QRS is evident. (*From* Lewis T. Philosophic Transactions of the Royal Society of London. Series B, Containing Papers of a Biological Character. Vol. 207 (1916), pp. 221310 (98 pages). Published By: Royal Society; with permission.)

duration of 120 ms as well as broad notched or slurred R waves in the left-sided leads I, aVL, V_5, and V_6; delayed time to R-wave peak; and several other criteria involving the ST segment and T-wave morphology (**Table 1**). The WHO criteria derive in turn from earlier criteria,[8] and the lineage of these criteria can be traced back in largely preserved form to work published in the 1940s and earlier

by Wilson and others.[9–11] The observations used to inform these criteria were primarily derived from in vitro canine models and limited intraprocedural recordings during early cardiac surgery.

The current European Society of Cardiology (ESC) criteria for LBBB were published in 2013 and are adapted from the AHA/ACC/HRS guidelines.[12] In particular, the ESC criteria use the

Table 1
Comparison of commonly used electrocardiogram criteria

	ACC/AHA/HRS Criteria (2009)[5]	ESC Criteria (2013)[12]	Strauss Criteria (2011)[15]
QRS duration	≥120 ms	≥120 ms	≥130 ms in women; ≥140 ms in men
Notched or slurred R wave	I, aVL, V_5, V_6	I, aVL, V_5, V_6	I, aVL, V_1, V_2, V_5, V_6
QS or rS pattern	—	V_1	V_1, V_2
Absent Q wave	I, V_5, V_6	V_5, V_6	—
Time to R-wave peak >60 ms	V_5, V_6	—	—
Discordant T wave	Usually present	—	—

A comparison of components of the most recent ACC/AHA/HRS criteria, the most recent ESC criteria, and the Strauss criteria for left bundle branch block.

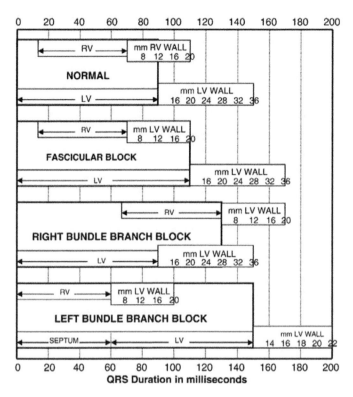

Fig 2. Modeled QRS durations in normal and pathologic hearts. The relative timings for electrical depolarization across different components of cardiac tissue in with normal conduction (top) as well as varying types of conduction block.[19] This work is calculated based on average conduction velocities in cardiac tissue, and it highlights that LBBB should cause QRS widening well greater than 120 ms. It also emphasizes that LVH can cause QRS prolongation that could potentially masquerade as LBBB. These calculations helped inform the Strauss criteria for LBBB.[15] (*From* Strauss DG, Selvester RH. The QRS complex–a biomarker that "images" the heart: QRS scores to quantify myocardial scar in the presence of normal and abnormal ventricular conduction. J Electrocardiol. 2009;42(1):85–96. https://doi.org/10.1016/j.jelectrocard.2008.07.011; with permission.)

same standards for QRS duration and left-sided R-wave morphology as the earlier AHA/ACC/HRS criteria (see **Table 1**). However, the ESC guidelines were strongly influenced by a 2011 reanalysis of the MADIT-CRT trial.[13] This analysis suggested that patients with reduced ejection fraction less than 30% and prolonged QRS greater than 130 ms derived greater benefit from cardiac resynchronization therapy (CRT) with defibrillator if they had an LBBB pattern compared with patients with non-LBBB QRS patterns (eg, right bundle branch block or nonspecific interventricular conduction delay). Importantly, this study incorporated the criterion of the presence of a QS or rS pattern in lead V_1, and it abandoned the criteria regarding time to R-wave peak and ST-segment and T-wave morphologies. These changes were then integrated into the 2013 ESC guideline definition of LBBB. Later in the same year, the large, randomized EchoCRT trial amplified the importance of QRS duration even further, as it identified a signal for harm if biventricular pacing was pursued in patients with QRS duration less than 130 ms.[14]

A third set of criteria for LBBB was proposed by Strauss and colleagues in 2011.[15] These new criteria were motivated in large part by mounting evidence that CRT gives the greatest benefit to patients with LBBB due to conduction block (rather

than other causes of apparent LBBB pattern such as hypertrophy), highlighting the importance of the accurate identification of these patients. In formulating their criteria, Strauss and colleagues noted that multiple prior studies suggested that approximately one-third of patients who meet conventional ECG criteria for LBBB did not, in fact, have complete LBBB.[16–18] In particular, one study showed that among patients with QRS duration greater than 120 ms, those with endocardial mapping that suggested LBBB due to conduction block demonstrated significantly longer QRS durations than patients whose mapping suggested no LBBB. Indeed, the fundamental difficulty they identified was distinguishing LBBB from patients with left ventricular hypertrophy (LVH) and nonspecific intraventricular conduction delay (IVCD). Using an approach based on average activation times (assuming conduction velocity of 30–40 cm/s) and anticipated transseptal activation times, they developed a mathematical model to estimate average QRS width (**Fig. 2**).[19] Based on this, they proposed modifications to the LBBB criteria to include a QRS duration of at least 130 ms in women or 140 ms in men, a QS or rS pattern in lead V_1 and V_2, and mid-QRS notching or slurring in at least 2 of the leads V_1, V_2, I, aVL, V_5, and V_6 (see **Table 1**).[15] Some studies have indicated that the Strauss criteria perform better than

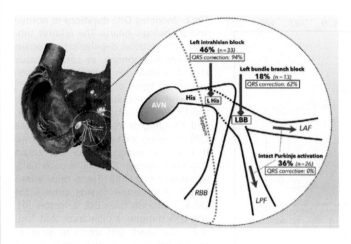

Fig. 3. Sites of conduction system block in patients with LBBB on surface ECG. The proximal His-Purkinje system in human hearts. Also shown are the relative frequency of patients with complete block found at the level of the His, complete block at the level of the left bundle branch, and absence of complete block (ie, intact Purkinje activation) in the studied patient population.[23] Along with these are shown the frequencies of successful QRS correction for each site of block when conduction system pacing is attempted. (*From* Upadhyay GA, Cherian T, Shatz DY, et al. Intracardiac Delineation of Septal Conduction in Left Bundle-Branch Block Patterns. Circulation. 2019;139(16):1876-1888. https://doi.org/10.1161/CIRCULATIONAHA.118.038648; with permission.)

other commonly accepted criteria with respect to distinguishing responders versus nonresponders to CRT,[20,21] whereas other works suggest that no specific definition performs significantly better.[22] Taken together, these observations suggest that there may be inherent limitations to the use of surface criteria in assessing level of conduction block.

INSUFFICIENCY OF SURFACE ELECTROCARDIOGRAM FOR ACCURATE IDENTIFICATION OF LEFT BUNDLE BRANCH BLOCK

The variety of extant surface ECG criteria for LBBB speaks to the difficulty of the accurate identification of a true LBBB, where there is interruption of conduction (ie, complete conduction block [CCB]) through the left bundle branch of the His-Purkinje system. In particular, it is frequently challenging to distinguish CCB from various forms of IVCD due to LVH or fibrosis, which also may lead to slowed or asynchronous conduction through the myocardial tissue, but in which conduction through the His-Purkinje system remains intact. This difficulty was first highlighted by a 2004 study by Auricchio and colleagues, wherein 24 patients who had LBBB morphology on ECG and met criteria for CRT implantation underwent an invasive electrophysiologic (EP) study to map their ventricular activation pattern.[18] It was found that approximately one-third of these patients had no significant delay between onset of activation of their right and left ventricles, implying persistent conduction of left bundle branch fibers.

A more recent study investigated a cohort of patients who had an indication for either device implantation or ventricular tachycardia (VT)

ablation.[23] These patients underwent intraprocedural mapping of left septal conduction to definitively assess whether or not they had intact conduction through their left-sided His-Purkinje system. Among these patients, left-sided septal recordings were obtained in 72 patients who met ACC/AHA/HRS criteria for LBBB.[5] It was found that only 64% of these patients demonstrated CCB of the left conduction system, whereas the remaining 36% had intact His-Purkinje activation of the left ventricle despite meeting standard surface ECG criteria for LBBB. When present, CCB was usually proximal in the left conduction system, at the level of the left-sided His (ie, where an atrial recording was still present), whereas block was in the common left bundle in the remainder (**Fig. 3**).

Taken together, these data suggest that although the sensitivity of the ACC/AHA/HRS criteria for LBBB is likely high, the specificity is poor. Indeed, up to one-third of the patients who meet ACC/AHA/HRS criteria for LBBB demonstrated intact activation of their ventricles via the His-Purkinje system. These findings are in agreement with the earlier work of Auricchio and others.[16–18] The study additionally investigated the performance of the stricter Strauss criteria in patients categorized as having LBBB by the ACC/AHA/HRS criteria. The sensitivity of the Strauss criteria remained high at 91% in this population; however, specificity was only 62% for correct identification of true LBBB as assessed by septal mapping. Among the components of the Strauss criteria, the presence of notching in the lateral leads demonstrated the highest negative predictive value (ie, CCB was unlikely to present in patients without notches) but with still only modest positive predictive value.

Intracardiac Patterns of Electrical Activation

Although LBBB and IVCD can frequently seem deceivingly similar on a surface ECG, they can be readily distinguished based on intracardiac recordings of ventricular activation patterns. **Fig. 4** shows surface ECG and intracardiac tracings for 3 different patients who all had wide QRS complexes and met traditional criteria for LBBB. In **Fig. 4**A, baseline morphology from the surface ECG shows a pattern consistent with LBBB, with a QRS width of 184 ms. A duodecapolar catheter positioned against the left ventricular septal wall captures His-Purkinje potentials on some leads but does not show clear conduction of the His-Purkinje signal down the length of the septum, consistent with LBBB secondary to CCB—here at the level of the left-sided His. Pacing from the proximal septum results in selective capture of the His-Purkinje fibers and leads to correction of the QRS duration to 121 ms with notable morphology change (**Fig. 4**D); this confirms the diagnosis of LBBB secondary to CCB.

In contrast is the patient shown in **Fig. 4**B. In this case, the baseline QRS duration is 134 ms, and the morphology is again consistent with an LBBB pattern. In this case, however, mapping of the left ventricular septum clearly shows intact His-Purkinje activation. This rules out LBBB secondary to CCB and establishes the diagnosis as IVCD. Consistent with this, selective pacing from the septal position is not able to provide any meaningful correction to QRS duration, which remains 132 ms with nearly identical QRS morphology to baseline (see **Fig. 4**E).

Finally, a third case is shown in **Fig. 4**C. Here, baseline QRS duration is extremely long at 251 ms and meets all criteria for LBBB. Septal mapping shows abrupt cessation of His-Purkinje activation, consistent with CCB. Selective pacing from the left ventricular septum was performed and in this case did show some narrowing of the QRS duration (see **Fig. 4**F). With pacing, QRS width was decreased to 153 ms with an accompanying morphology change and selective capture. On review of the tracing, one may question whether the paced QRS reflects correction of LBBB versus fortuitous narrowing through septal capture. Further decrement in pacing stimulus output (see **Fig. 4**F) for this patient revealed selective capture with no QRS correction and identical morphology as to the underlying QRS. When analyzed together, the findings suggest that multiple pathologies are present concurrently. The patient demonstrates CCB along with concomitant distal, myopathic delay and IVCD, which was "unmasked" once the LBBB was corrected. The persistently wide QRS due to IVCD remains present even after correction of the LBBB. As these 3 examples show, intracardiac mapping and pacing maneuvers can reliably distinguish between LBBB due to CCB and IVCD and may also be used to identify a combination of both phenomena. A patient with concomitant LBBB and IVCD may not derive substantial benefit from a conduction system pacing (CSP) strategy alone, although may uniquely benefit from a hybridized conduction system and biventricular pacing strategy such as combined His-bundle and LV lead pacing or combined left bundle branch area pacing and LV lead pacing.[24–26]

MODALITIES TO CONFIRM PRESENCE OR ABSENCE OF LEFT BUNDLE BRANCH BLOCK SECONDARY TO CONDUCTION BLOCK

There are several possibilities for more accurate assessment of the presence or absence of LBBB due to CCB. First, as discussed earlier, intracardiac EP recordings can definitively establish the presence or absence of LBBB.[27] However, although this remains the most rigorous modality for diagnosis, it is generally only used in patients who already have another indication for an invasive EP procedure, such as VT ablation or during EP study. It remains an open question whether operators will routinely perform left-sided septal mapping as an isolated diagnostic study in the absence of other relevant indications. Although invasive procedures always entail additional risk compared with noninvasive diagnostics, the risk profile of left ventricular septal mapping is likely comparable to routine diagnostic coronary angiography. An additional barrier may be the justification of economic costs and time associated with EP study to guide CRT implant. Presently, there are no published guidelines to suggest what patient populations would most benefit from invasive studies to further clarify their electrical activation pattern.

One attractive alternative to routine invasive mapping would be to develop more accurate criteria for the diagnosis of LBBB by surface ECG. Unfortunately, such criteria have remained elusive. As discussed earlier, even the stricter Strauss criteria suffer from lack of specificity. In a study performed at our center, 39% of patients with intact His-Purkinje activation on septal mapping nonetheless met Strauss criteria by surface ECG.[23] As indicated earlier, the most helpful single characteristic was mid-QRS notching in V_1, V_2, I, aVL, V_5, or V_6. The determination of a "notch," however, remains somewhat subjective with more interobserver variability than other ECG features.[28]

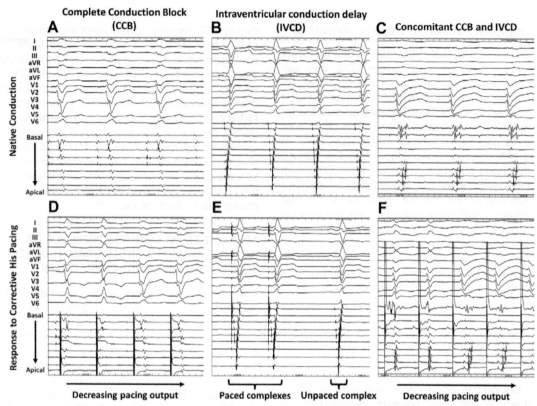

Fig. 4. Intracardiac tracings can distinguish between LBBB due to CCB and IVCD. (*A–C*) Natively conducted beats from 3 patients who all met standard ECG criteria for LBBB. Upper traces show surface ECG leads, and lower traces show intracardiac LV septal mapping. (*A*) The septal mapping for this patient shows conduction block at the level of the left-sided His fibers, consistent with LBBB due to CCB. (*B*) Septal mapping shows intact His-Purkinje activation down the length of the septum, demonstrating that this patient has IVCD rather than CCB. (*C*) Septal mapping for this patient also shows conduction block at the level of the left-sided His recordings, consistent with LBBB due to CCB. (*D–F*) Tracings for the same 3 patients while being paced from the LV septum. (*D*) Pacing just below the level of conduction block results in selective capture and correction of the QRS duration from 184 ms to 121 ms (left 2 beats). Decrement in pacing output results in selective capture with no QRS correction and a return to the original QRS morphology (right 2 beats). These findings suggest that the patient's LBBB pattern is due to CCB as the primary underlying pathophysiology. (*E*) Pacing from the right-sided His (not shown) results in selective capture of the left conduction system (left 2 beats), and identical QRS as to that of the natively conducted complex (rightmost beat); this is expected given the intact His-Purkinje activation and supports the diagnosis of wide QRS secondary to IVCD. (*F*) Here, pacing at the site of the left His recording demonstrated selective capture with significant QRS narrowing compared with baseline (left 2 beats, 153 ms vs 251 ms). Decremental pacing output shows selective capture with identical QRS morphology and duration to baseline (right 3 beats); this confirms the presence of LBBB due to CCB, which was corrected with left-sided pacing. However, the fact that the QRS cannot be fully corrected with septal pacing suggests the presence of concomitant distal disease or IVCD.

One potential solution to the lack of accuracy of traditional surface ECGs for identification of LBBB is the use of ultrahigh-frequency ECG (UHF-ECG; typically performed using the ventricular dyssynchrony imaging monitor).[29] In LBBB, the underlying desynchrony of ventricular activation leads primarily to alterations in the heart's electrical vector during depolarization. Accordingly, the QRS complex represents the main feature of interest for identification of LBBB, as evidenced by most of the guideline criteria relating to the QRS complex. Unfortunately,

the QRS complex is relatively brief, usually lasting less than 200 ms, and a standard ECG is typically acquired only with sufficient data rate to capture dynamics less than 100 Hz.[29] Thus, much of the nuance of ventricular activation is filtered out of a standard ECG. UHF-ECGs use a much higher acquisition frequency, up to 5 kHz, to allow for much more detailed understanding of electrical activity during ventricular depolarization (the period corresponding to the QRS complex, **Fig. 5**).[29,30] Early results show that this technique may hold

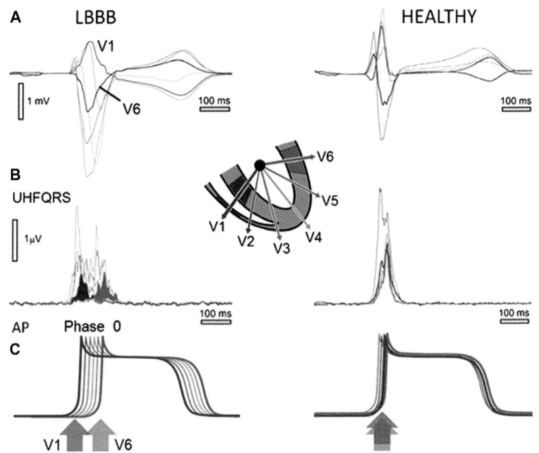

Fig. 5. UHF-ECG reveals hidden dynamics of the QRS. (*A*) Standard ECG precordial lead tracings from a patient with LBBB (*left*) and normal conduction (*right*). V_1 is shown in blue, V_2 to V_5 in gray, and V_6 in green. The low-frequency response of a standard ECG results in substantial overlap between the observed depolarizations of septal tissue (seen in V_1) and lateral wall tissue (in V_6), even though these do not occur simultaneously in LBBB. (*B*) UHF-ECG precordial lead tracings from the same patients as earlier. Here, the greater frequency response of the UHF-ECG clearly shows that depolarization of the septal tissue (V_1, blue) occurs before lateral tissue (V_6, green) in LBBB (left), whereas they are nearly simultaneous with normal conduction (right). (*C*) The relative timing of cardiac action potentials from different regions of tissue seen by the various precordial leads. (*From* Jurak P, Halamek J, Meluzin J, et al. Ventricular dyssynchrony assessment using ultra-high frequency ECG technique. J Interv Card Electrophysiol. 2017;49(3):245-254. https://doi.org/10.1007/s10840-017-0268-0; with permission.)

promise for more accurate selection of patients for resynchronization therapies. However, the discriminatory performance of high-frequency ECG has not yet been validated against intracardiac assessment of LBBB. Furthermore, the requirement for new ECG acquisition hardware may prove to be a barrier to widespread adoption of this technique in the immediate future.

IMPLICATIONS FOR CONDUCTION SYSTEM PACING

CSP has recently emerged as a potential alternative strategy to traditional biventricular (BiV) pacing as a means to deliver CRT.[31–33] Until recently,

however, it was unclear what patient populations would most benefit from this therapy relative to traditional BiV-CRT; this was exemplified by the design of the recent His-SYNC trial, which included both patients with LBBB by strict Strauss criteria, as well as patients who were judged to have IVCD.[34,35] This trial randomized 41 patients with an indication for CRT to either traditional biventricular pacing or His-bundle pacing. The trial suffered from significant crossover between groups, as nearly half of the patients assigned to receive His bundle pacing ultimately received biventricular pacing. The most common reason for this crossover was an inability to correct QRS widening in cases of IVCD. Notably, no patients with intact His-Purkinje activation on septal mapping (and thus proved IVCD rather than LBBB) were able to be corrected with His bundle pacing. Further subsequent work looked at a group of 72 patients who met ACC/AHA/HRS criteria for LBBB and found similar results (see **Fig. 3**).[23] Of the 46 patients confirmed to have true LBBB, 85% were successfully corrected to a QRS duration less than 130 ms using His bundle pacing. By contrast, of the 26 patients with intact His-Purkinje activation, none could be successfully corrected with His bundle pacing. These findings emphasize the importance of appropriate patient selection when considering a strategy of CSP. In patients who have intact His-Purkinje activation, CSP is unlikely to provide clinical benefit and the patient may be better served with a traditional BiV pacing strategy.

SUMMARY

Multiple criteria have been developed for identification of LBBB by surface ECG. These criteria have good sensitivity, but they generally suffer from poor specificity. With growing interest in applications for CSP, there is clinical need to accurately distinguish between patients with LBBB secondary to conduction block who are the most likely to benefit from CSP versus patients with wide QRS secondary to IVCD who are unlikely to benefit from a CSP strategy alone. Invasive EP studies with left-sided septal recording may be used to accurately assess conduction patterns, although this is associated with additional periprocedural risks and costs. Patients with combined LBBB and IVCD may uniquely benefit from hybrid approaches to CRT; using corrective CSP to circumvent focal conduction block synchronized with LV pacing helps correct more distal myopathic delay. The routine use of invasive EP study to guide pacing strategy, however, remains uncertain. Ongoing research into noninvasive approaches with new surface ECG criteria or the development of novel electrical assessment tools, such as UHF-ECG, is necessary to help refine patient selection and procedural planning for CSP and CRT.

CLINICS CARE POINTS

- Left bundle branch block (LBBB) pattern on ECG may not necessarily reflect underlying complete conduction block (CCB).
- Patients with CCB are more likely to respond to conduction system pacing.

DISCLOSURE

G.A. Upadhyay reports consulting and speaking fees from Abbott, BioTel, Biotronik, Medtronic, and Zoll Medical. J. Treger has no disclosures.

REFERENCES

1. Eppinger H, Rothberger CJ. Zur analyse des elektrokardiogramms. Wien Klin Wochenschr 1909; 22(1091):8.
2. Flowers NC. Left bundle branch block: a continuously evolving concept. J Am Coll Cardiol 1987; 9(3):684–97.
3. Carter EP. Clinical observations on defective conduction in the branches of the auriculoventricular bundle: a report of twenty-two cases, in which aberrant beats were obtained. Arch Intern Med 1914; XIII(5):803–40.
4. Braun-Menendez, Solari LA. Ventricular asynchronism in bundle branch block. Arch Intern Med 1939;63(5):830–47.
5. Surawicz B, Childers R, Deal BJ, et al. AHA/ACCF/HRS Recommendations for the Standardization and interpretation of the electrocardiogram: Part III: intraventricular conduction disturbances A Scientific Statement from the American heart association Electrocardiography and Arrhythmias Committee, Council on clinical Cardiology; the American College of Cardiology Foundation; and the heart Rhythm Society Endorsed by the international Society for Computerized Electrocardiology. J Am Coll Cardiol 2009;53(11):976–81.
6. ACC/AHA/HRS guideline on the Evaluation and management of patients with bradycardia and cardiac conduction delay: a report of the American College of Cardiology/American heart association Task Force on clinical practice guidelines and the heart Rhythm Society | Journal of the American College of Cardiology. 2018. Available at: https://www.jacc.org/doi/full/10.1016/j.jacc.2018.10.044. Accessed July 30, 2021.
7. Willems JL, Robles de MEO, Bernard R, et al. Criteria for intraventricular conduction disturbances and pre-excitation. J Am Coll Cardiol 1985;5(6): 1261–75.
8. Scott RC. Left bundle branch block—a clinical assessment Part I. Am Heart J 1965;70(4):535–66.
9. Wilson FN. Concerning the form of the QRS deflections of the electrocardiogram in bundle branch block. J Mt Sinai Hosp NY 1941;8:1110.
10. Wilson FN, Johnston FD, Rosenbaum FF, et al. The precordial electrocardiogram. Am Heart J 1944; 27(1):19–85.
11. ROSENMAN RH, PICK A, KATZ LN. Intraventricular block: review of the Literature. Arch Intern Med 1950;86(2):196–232.

12. Members AF, Brignole M, Auricchio A, et al. 2013 ESC Guidelines on cardiac pacing and cardiac re-synchronization therapyThe Task Force on cardiac pacing and resynchronization therapy of the European Society of Cardiology (ESC). Developed in collaboration with the European Heart Rhythm Association (EHRA). Eur Heart J 2013;34(29):2281–329.

13. Zareba W, Klein H, Cygankiewicz I, et al. Effectiveness of cardiac resynchronization therapy by QRS morphology in the Multicenter Automatic defibrillator implantation trial–cardiac resynchronization therapy (MADIT-CRT). Circulation 2011;123(10):1061–72.

14. Ruschitzka F, Abraham WT, Singh JP, et al. Cardiac-resynchronization therapy in heart failure with a narrow QRS complex. N Engl J Med 2013;369(15):1395–405.

15. Strauss DG, Selvester RH, Wagner GS. Defining left bundle branch block in the Era of cardiac resynchronization therapy. Am J Cardiol 2011;107(6):927–34.

16. Grant RP, Dodge HT. Mechanisms of QRS complex prolongation in man: left ventricular conduction disturbances. Am J Med 1956;20(6):834–52.

17. Vassallo JA, Cassidy DM, Marchlinski FE, et al. Endocardial activation of left bundle branch block. Circulation 1984;69(5):914–23.

18. Auricchio A, Fantoni C, Regoli F, et al. Characterization of left ventricular activation in patients with heart Failure and left bundle-branch block. Circulation 2004;109(9):1133–9.

19. Strauss DG, Selvester RH. The QRS complex—a biomarker that "images" the heart: QRS scores to quantify myocardial scar in the presence of normal and abnormal ventricular conduction. J Electrocardiol 2009;42(1):85–96.

20. Jastrzębski M, Kukla P, Kisiel R, et al. Comparison of four LBBB definitions for predicting mortality in patients receiving cardiac resynchronization therapy. Ann Noninvasive Electrocardiol 2018;23(5):e12563.

21. Caputo ML, van Stipdonk A, Illner A, et al. The definition of left bundle branch block influences the response to cardiac resynchronization therapy. Int J Cardiol 2018;269:165–9.

22. van Stipdonk AMW, Hoogland R, ter Horst HI, et al. Evaluating Electrocardiography-based identification of cardiac resynchronization therapy responders beyond current left bundle branch block definitions. JACC Clin Electrophysiol 2020;6(2):193–203.

23. Upadhyay GA, Cherian T, Shatz DY, et al. Intracardiac Delineation of septal conduction in left bundle-branch block patterns. Circulation 2019;139(16):1876–88.

24. Vijayaraman P, Herweg B, Ellenbogen KA, et al. His-optimized cardiac resynchronization therapy to Maximize electrical resynchronization. Circ Arrhythm Electrophysiol 2019;12(2):e006934.

25. Zweerink A, Zubarev S, Bakelants E, et al. His-optimized cardiac resynchronization therapy with ventricular Fusion pacing for electrical resynchronization in heart Failure. JACC Clin Electrophysiol 2021;7(7):881–92.

26. Jastrzębski M, Moskal P, Huybrechts W, et al. Left bundle branch–optimized cardiac resynchronization therapy (LOT-CRT): results from an international LBBAP collaborative study group. Heart Rhythm 2021. https://doi.org/10.1016/j.hrthm.2021.07.057.

27. Tung R, Upadhyay GA. Defining left bundle branch block patterns in cardiac resynchronisation therapy: a return to His bundle recordings. Arrhythmia Electrophysiol Rev 2020;9(1):28–33.

28. van Stipdonk AMW, Vanbelle S, ter Horst IAH, et al. Large variability in clinical judgement and definitions of left bundle branch block to identify candidates for cardiac resynchronisation therapy. Int J Cardiol 2019;286:61–5.

29. Jurak P, Halamek J, Meluzin J, et al. Ventricular dyssynchrony assessment using ultra-high frequency ECG technique. J Interv Card Electrophysiol 2017;49(3):245–54.

30. Jurak P, Curila K, Leinveber P, et al. Novel ultra-high-frequency electrocardiogram tool for the description of the ventricular depolarization pattern before and during cardiac resynchronization. J Cardiovasc Electrophysiol 2020;31(1):300–7.

31. Lustgarten DL, Calame S, Crespo EM, et al. Electrical resynchronization induced by direct His-bundle pacing. Heart Rhythm 2010;7(1):15–21.

32. Lustgarten DL, Crespo EM, Arkhipova-Jenkins I, et al. His-bundle pacing versus biventricular pacing in cardiac resynchronization therapy patients: a crossover design comparison. Heart Rhythm 2015;12(7):1548–57.

33. Ajijola OA, Upadhyay GA, Macias C, et al. Permanent His-bundle pacing for cardiac resynchronization therapy: Initial feasibility study in lieu of left ventricular lead. Heart Rhythm 2017;14(9):1353–61.

34. Upadhyay GA, Vijayaraman P, Nayak HM, et al. His corrective pacing or biventricular pacing for cardiac resynchronization in heart Failure. J Am Coll Cardiol 2019;74(1):157–9.

35. Upadhyay GA, Vijayaraman P, Nayak HM, et al. On-treatment comparison between corrective His bundle pacing and biventricular pacing for cardiac resynchronization: a secondary analysis of the His-SYNC Pilot Trial. Heart Rhythm 2019;16(12):1797–807.

What Body Surface Mapping Has Taught Us About Ventricular Conduction Disease Implications for Cardiac Resynchronization Therapy and His Bundle Pacing

Marc Strik, MD, PhD[a,b,*], Sylvain Ploux, MD, PhD[a,b],
Pierre Bordachar, MD, PhD[a,b]

KEYWORDS

- CRT • Electrocardiography • Mapping • Left bundle branch block • Right bundle branch block

KEY POINTS

- Two systems are currently used in clinical practice in cardiac resynchronization therapy (CRT) to noninvasively determine ventricular activation mapping: electrocardiographic (ECG) mapping and the ECG belt.
- In patients with left bundle branch block, the ventricular activation sequence is characterized by limited interindividual variability with relatively consistent patterns of activation.
- Patients with nonspecific intraventricular conduction disturbance on the surface ECG may demonstrate multiple sites of epicardial breakthrough, varying regions of delayed activation, and varying amounts of interventricular dyssynchrony.
- Although these systems have the potential to predict CRT responders, its clinical use remains limited.

INTRODUCTION

Cardiac resynchronization therapy (CRT) is an effective intervention in select patients with symptomatic heart failure, depressed left ventricular (LV) ejection fraction, and conduction disorders.[1,2] Current international guidelines for CRT selection rely on metrics of electrical dyssynchrony derived from the surface 12-lead electrocardiogram (ECG).[3,4] The degree and pattern of conduction disease seem determinant when assessing potential CRT candidates.[2,5] In patients with similar QRS duration, those with left bundle branch block (LBBB) respond significantly better than those with right bundle branch block (RBBB) or nonspecific intraventricular conduction disturbance (NICD). A limitation of the surface ECG is its inability to provide a precise pattern of regional electrical activity, the electrical substrate being depicted in only rudimentary fashion. In contrast, ECG body surface mapping provides detailed patient-specific information on ventricular

Funding This work received financial support from the French Government as part of the "Investments of the Future" program managed by the National Research Agency (ANR) [Grant number ANR-10-IAHU-04].
[a] Bordeaux University Hospital (CHU), Avenue de Magellan, Pessac F-33600, France; [b] IHU Liryc, Electrophysiology and Heart Modeling Institute, Av. du Haut Lévêque, 33600 Pessac, France
* Corresponding author. Service Pr Haïssaguerre, Hôpital cardiologique du Haut-Lévêque, Avenue de Magellan, Pessac 33600, France.
E-mail address: marc.strik@chu-bordeaux.fr
Twitter: @StrikMarc (M.S.)

Card Electrophysiol Clin 14 (2022) 213–221
https://doi.org/10.1016/j.ccep.2021.12.008
1877-9182/22/© 2021 Elsevier Inc. All rights reserved.

electrical activation and permits generation of activation maps and timings.[6] ECG mapping may be fundamental to precisely characterize the specificities of electrical substrate according to the ECG pattern and to elucidate the mechanisms involved in CRT response.

In the present review, the authors discuss the available noninvasive techniques that can be used to acquire ventricular activation time maps. They then describe what body surface mapping has taught us about LBBB, RBBB, intraventricular conduction delay (IVCD), and right ventricular (RV) pacing and discuss the ability of derived parameters of electrical dyssynchrony to predict long-term clinical response to CRT or His bundle pacing.

ELECTROCARDIOGRAPHIC BODY SURFACE MAPPING: TECHNICAL ASPECTS

Two systems are currently used in clinical practice in CRT to noninvasively determine ventricular activation mapping: ECG mapping and the ECG belt.

Electrocardiographic Mapping System (CardioInsight Technologies Inc, Cleveland, OH)

This system, pioneered by Dr Yoram Rudy's laboratory and acquired by Medtronic, provides noninvasive high-resolution electrical mapping of cardiac activation on the epicardial surface from body-surface ECG measurements.[7] Body surface potentials are collected from 252 electrodes supported in a single-use vest positioned around the entire surface of the thorax. A low-dose thoracic computed tomography (CT) scan is performed to define the heart-torso geometry in order to orientate each electrode to the epicardial mesh. The body surface potentials and radiologically acquired cardiac anatomy are then combined and processed to the inverse problem, allowing to reconstruct greater than 2500 epicardial unipolar electrograms from which isochrones can be constructed continuously on a beat-by-beat basis. **Fig. 1** shows the workflow of the ECG mapping system as used for the authors' CRT studies.

Ventricular activation times can be calculated from the onset of the QRS duration or the pacing spike to the maximal negative slope of each unipolar electrogram. **Fig. 2** shows examples of electrical activation maps from 2 patients with systolic heart failure without complete bundle branch block but with dyssynchronous contraction patterns on the echocardiogram. The activation maps show very limited asynchrony of the LV, and both patients did not clinically respond to CRT after 6 months. Multiple electrical asynchrony

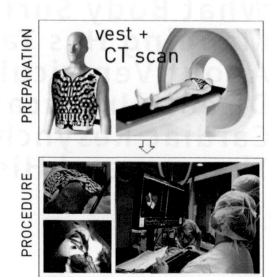

Fig. 1. Workflow of using electrocardiographic mapping during CRT implantation. In the preparation phase (*top panel*), the patient is equipped with the electrode vest and undergoes a CT scan. To enable a subclavian CRT implantation, the prepectoral area of the vest is removed (*bottom left panels*). Beat-to-beat mapping is possible during the procedure (*bottom right panels*), which enables mapping studies during CRT implantation.

indexes can be derived from acquired activation maps such as total activation time (duration from the earliest to the latest site of ventricular activation), ventricular electrical uncoupling (VEU; difference between the mean LV and RV activation times), and most recently the activation delay vector (3-dimensional representation of asynchrony magnitude and direction).[5,8–11] The system has been validated, both experimentally and in patients, under different physiologic and pathologic conditions, by comparison with direct epicardial mapping during open-heart surgery and with catheter intracardiac mapping. Reconstruction accuracy superior to 10 mm was consistently obtained in humans. A recent validation study showed poor overall agreement of ECG mapping and contact mapping.[12] However, the between-map correlation was good for wide QRS patterns such as seen during asynchronous ventricular activation in CRT candidates.[6]

Electrocardiographic Belt (Heartscape Technologies, Verathon, Seattle, Washington)

The ECG belt records unipolar electrograms using a 53-electrode body surface mapping system that wraps around the upper torso.[13] From the multi-electrode ECG data, the system provides beat-by-beat color-coded isochronal maps presented

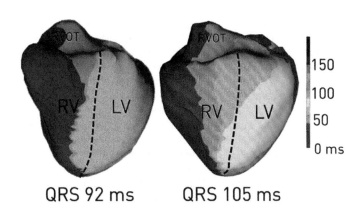

QRS 92 ms   QRS 105 ms

Fig. 2. Electrocardiographic maps of 2 patients with systolic heart failure without bundle branch block. Views are anteroposterior with the dashed line demarking the RV and LV.LV, left ventricle; RV, right ventricle; RVOT, RV outflow tract.

in 2 views (anterior and posterior) and quantifies 2 metrics of electrical heterogeneity: standard deviation of the activation times and LV activation time. **Fig. 3** shows ECG belt isochronal maps in normal subject, LBBB, RBBB, and NICD.

A CT scan is not required, which facilitates the workflow and reduces the radiation but decreases the resolution and the accuracy because the patient-specific cardiothoracic anatomy is not integrated in the analysis. The lack of detailed

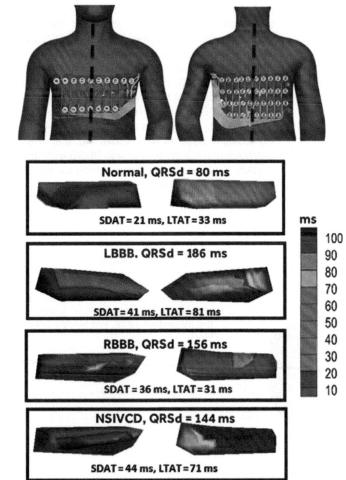

Fig. 3. ECG belt as applied on the torso. Dotted lines on the anterior and posterior indicate the sternal line and the spine, respectively, which were used to delineate the left and right sides of the thorax. Color-coded ECG belt isochronal maps in anterior and posterior views in normal subject, left bundle branch block (LBBB), right bundle branch block (RBBB), and nonspecific interventricular conduction disorder (NICD), along with corresponding values of standard deviation of activation times (SDAT) and average left thorax activation times (LTAT). (*From* Johnson WB, Vatterott PJ, Peterson MA, et al. Body surface mapping using an ECG belt to characterize electrical heterogeneity for different left ventricular pacing sites during cardiac resynchronization: Relationship with acute hemodynamic improvement. Heart Rhythm. 2017;14(3):385-391. https://doi.org/10.1016/j.hrthm.2016.11.017; with permission)

anatomic information limits its value in investigating the patient-specific electrical substrate in detail and limits the use of this tool to better understand the mechanisms involved in the response to resynchronization.

CHARACTERIZATION OF THE ELECTRICAL SUBSTRATE IN RESYNCHRONIZATION CANDIDATES

ECG mapping has been used to precisely analyze the activation sequence in patients with heart failure who are candidates for resynchronization with different ECG patterns.

Patients with LBBB on the surface ECG remain the principle candidates for CRT. In patients with LBBB, the ventricular activation sequence is characterized by limited interindividual variability with relatively consistent patterns of activation, making the map easily recognizable. As shown in **Fig. 4**, in 2 patients with LBBB, the main features of an activation map observed in a patient with left block include the following: (1) no LV breakthrough, (2) RV breakthrough with rapid and centrifugal spread of activation across the RV free wall, (3) the spread of the LV activation front is consistently impaired (both anteriorly and posteriorly) by areas of slow conduction, (4) the basal region of the LV is typically the latest area to be activated, and (5) a consistent delay of more than 50 milliseconds between the mean activation time of the 2 ventricles. Recently, the authors examined whether the QRS axis in patients with heart failure and LBBB is determined by electrophysiologic, structural, or anatomic characteristics. Using a combined cardiac MRI and ECG mapping approach, the results revealed a purely electrophysiological explanation for left axis deviation in patients with LBBB, with no discernible associations of structural characteristics (cardiac size, LV dimensions, or LV

mass) or cardiac anatomic axis with the QRS axis.[14] RV activation patterns were similar for patients with left or normal heart axis, with breakthrough activation from its free wall followed by circumferential spreading toward the LV. In contrast, LV activation differed in terms of patterns and latest activated area. LBBB with normal axis was associated with circumferential LV activation with the latest activation seen at the midlateral LV wall. In contrast, LBBB with leftward axis deviation demonstrated the latest activation at the basal lateral LV wall, resulting in an apex-to-base activation pattern. In fact, the apex-to-base activation delay correlated significantly with QRS axis ($R^2 = 0.67$), with a higher gradient associated with a more leftward axis. As a consequence, activation of the LV basal segments was more delayed in the leftward axis deviation group.

Patients with NICD on the surface ECG demonstrate more heterogeneous patterns of activation (**Fig. 5**), in contrast to patients with LBBB who display a "typical" activation pattern: (1) multiple sites of epicardial breakthrough may be seen (including the LV epicardium), (2) the site of latest activation is highly variable, (3) broad spectrum of interventricular delay, the LV relative to RV delay ranging from negative (RV delay) to positive (significant LV delay in some patients).

Patients with RBBB on the surface ECG demonstrate a typical right to left activation. Because patients with RBBB overall respond poorly to CRT, there are only limited data available on ECG imaging (ECGi) in patients with RBBB. **Fig. 6** shows 2 examples of ECGi in patients with RBBB with rapid breakthrough over a large area of the LV epicardium and with delayed and slow activation of the RV with a large area of latest activation.

Patients with RV apical pacing (RVAP) have delayed activation of the LV similar to patients with LBBB. In a study performed in 24 patients,

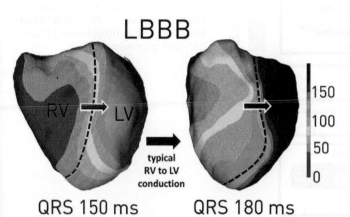

LBBB

QRS 150 ms   QRS 180 ms

typical RV to LV conduction

150
100
50
0

Fig. 4. Electrocardiographic maps of 2 patients with LBBB. Views are anteroposterior with the dashed line demarking the RV and LV. LBBB, left bundle branch block.

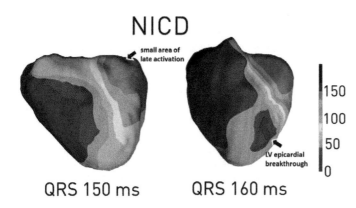

NICD

small area of
late activation

LV epicardial
breakthrough

150
100
50
0

QRS 150 ms   QRS 160 ms

Fig. 5. Electrocardiographic maps of 2 patients with NICD in anteroposterior views. NICD, nonspecific intraventricular conduction delay.

the authors compared qualitative and quantitative characteristics of ventricular electrical activation during LBBB and RVAP.[8] In order to eliminate anatomic substrate as a variable, within-patient comparisons were made. Despite obvious similarities in activation (interventricular and intra-LV dyssynchrony), significant differences in ventricular activation duration and patterns were observed: (1) the RV activation was significantly prolonged during RVAP vs LBBB, (2) the LV activation proceeded from apex to base with RVAP compared with circumferential activation during LBBB, (3) the LV activation was nearly twice as long during intrinsic LBBB activation as that during RVAP.

ELECTROCARDIOGRAPHIC IMAGING FOR PREDICTING CARDIAC RESYNCHRONIZATION THERAPY RESPONSE

The ability of different body surface mapping–derived parameters of electrical dyssynchrony to predict long-term clinical response to CRT was assessed in a first prospective study including 33 patients with heart failure and wide QRS duration.[10] The prolongation of the VEU was strongly associated with clinical CRT response and seemed to be a more powerful predictor than 12-lead ECG parameters. The area under the receiver-operating characteristic curve (AUC) indicated that VEU (AUC: 0.88) was significantly superior to QRS duration (AUC: 0.73) for predicting CRT response ($P < .05$). With a 50-ms cutoff value, VEU identified CRT responders with 90% sensitivity and 82% specificity, whether LBBB was present or not. Patients with a VEU greater than 50 ms had a 42-fold increase in the likelihood of being a responder ($P < .001$). Significant VEU was found in all patients with LBBB, which may account for the high rate of response to CRT in this subgroup. These results suggest that it is the magnitude of right-to-left activation delay that separates responders from nonresponders to CRT. This finding was later confirmed in a larger study where the ADV, a 3-dimensional approach to describing electrical asynchrony, performed equally to the VEU.[5] The diagnostic accuracy of the ECG belt to predict remodeling after 6 months of CRT was tested in 66 CRT candidates.[15] Patients with SDAT greater than or equal to 35 ms had greater improvement in ejection fraction (13 ± 8 vs 4 ± 9 units, $P < .01$) and LV end-systolic volume (-34 ± 28 vs $-13 \pm 29\%$, $P = .005$).

For the time being, the place of noninvasive mapping techniques in clinical practice to optimize the selection of candidates for resynchronization is extremely limited for various reasons. The

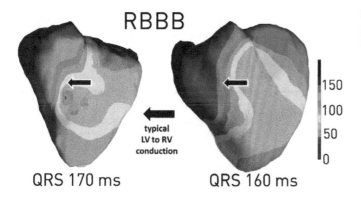

RBBB

typical
LV to RV
conduction

150
100
50
0

QRS 170 ms   QRS 160 ms

Fig. 6. Electrocardiographic maps of 2 patients with RBBB. RBBB, right bundle branch block.

complexity and cost of the system limit its use in routine patient selection. Moreover, validation of the interest of an asynchrony parameter measured with this technology cannot be carried out from the results of a single center and requires the realization of a randomized study on large numbers. Another group tested the predictive value of ECGi-derived parameters for volumetric response to CRT at 6 months. They found that the VVSync parameter (reverse of VEU) was significantly higher for the 10 patients with LBBB than for 14 patients without LBBB (−51 ± 19 vs18,4 ± 26 ms; P = .004). In this small cohort, none of the electrical dyssynchrony parameter was found to be associated with response, including the LBBB pattern on the 12-lead ECG (only 50% responders).[16] Nevertheless, the potential of the interventricular dyssynchrony (VEU) has been confirmed in a computational study that shows its interest for patient selection and patient-specific modeling.[17] The degree of response to CRT in patients with LBBB is very high, and the clinical value of VEU/VVsync in screening these patients may be modest and challenging to prove. ECG maps reveal highly homogeneous patterns of activation in patients with LBBB. Therefore, even if noninvasive cardiac mapping provides a more detailed depiction of the electrical substrate and helps in the understanding of the determinants of the CRT response, it would be difficult to demonstrate potential clinical additional benefit from noninvasive mapping in patients with LBBB. Contrarily, patients with a prolonged QRS duration on the surface ECG, but who do not display typical LBBB morphology, may respond to treatment with CRT. Additional selection criteria are clearly needed for identifying potential responders in this subgroup.[18] There may be a potential role for ECG mapping as a mean for screening non-LBBB or chronically RV-paced patients to identify individual patients with significant VEU, a fundamental component of the electrical substrate amenable to treatment with CRT. Randomized, multicentric, blinded studies are required to confirm this hypothesis.

LIMITATIONS OF BIVENTRICULAR PACING AND SEARCH FOR MORE PHYSIOLOGIC PACING

Based on detailed ventricular activation mapping, during both baseline conduction (patients with narrow QRS, LBBB, or IVCD) and CRT, the authors' results cast some light on mechanisms through which CRT alters cardiac performance. The ventricular activation time and pattern produced during CRT do not depend on the baseline ventricular conduction characteristics.[9] CRT provides similar activation features, whatever the underlying electrical substrate and induces a new stage of electrical dyssynchrony, which is roughly homogeneous regardless of the baseline QRS pattern. The mean amount of dyssynchrony is somewhere in between the baseline dyssynchrony values for patients with narrow QRS duration and those with LBBB. Thus the pacing-induced dyssynchrony can be worse than the baseline condition. CRT actually results in more dyssynchronous electrical ventricular activation when it is applied to patients with little or no electrical dyssynchrony. Because CRT results in similar ventricular activation regardless of the baseline conduction characteristics, improvement or worsening in function are mostly determined by the severity of the ventricular conduction impairment during baseline conduction, which also determines the extent to which dyssynchrony is corrected. Responders show significantly higher baseline electrical dyssynchrony parameters than do nonresponders but a similar degree of electrical dyssynchrony during CRT. Hemodynamic positive response and volumetric favorable remodeling can be expected as long as the degree of baseline electrical dyssynchrony with right-to-left delay exceeds the dyssynchrony induced by CRT. Conversely, in patients with insufficient intrinsic electrical dyssynchrony, iatrogenic electrical dyssynchrony is observed with prolongation of activation times associated with a deterioration in acute hemodynamic and volumetric responses.

The authors' results show that CRT does not eliminate electrical dyssynchrony but rather decreases it similarly, independent of the patient's underlying electrical substrate.[9] CRT does not fully reverse the conduction impairment induced by LBBB and does not return activation times and patterns to those seen in normal hearts with narrow QRS duration. Therefore, there is probably considerable potential in physiologic pacing modes for improving the effectiveness of resynchronization. His bundle pacing (HBP) could represent a very interesting alternative in this context. In patients with LBBB, noninvasive epicardial mapping (ECGi) was performed during conventional CRT and temporary HBP. It did not seem to be possible to shorten ventricular activation time in all patients with LBBB, the efficacy of HBP being restricted to patients with proximal conduction system disease. However, in 88% patients with LBBB, HBP successfully shortened the LV activation time.[19,20] Interestingly, in 33% in this study and in 52% in the His-Sync trial,[21] HBP resulted in complete ventricular resynchronization, with activation times and patterns indistinguishable from normal subjects. These results suggest that in certain patients, HPB may deliver the maximum potential ventricular resynchronization. Unfortunately, HBP is technically challenging, and it is associated with varying success rates (70%–90%), higher rates of lead displacement, higher pacing thresholds, lower R-wave amplitudes, atrial oversensing, and programming difficulties.[22,23] Fact remains that in up to half of patients with LBBB, the conduction block may lie beyond the His bundle and require distal pacing in the conduction system.[24] These arguments have motivated implanters to descend the pacing lead toward the left bundle branch area.[25,26] Left bundle branch pacing or pacing of the septum on the LV endocardium by advancing an active fixation lead through the septum is less demanding than HBP and has a similar directive: approaching physiologic depolarization of the LV.[27] The wide spread adaptation of left bundle branch area pacing and early studies on beneficial clinical outcomes may even position this pacing strategy over conventional RV pacing in future patients with bradycardia.[28] Mapping studies in left bundle branch area pacing remain anecdotal but left bundle branch area pacing consistently shows large decreases in LV dyssynchrony.[29–31] Using the ECG belt and compared with conventional CRT, LV septal pacing reduced electrical dyssynchrony similarly to HBP.[32] Potential explanations for this finding comes from previous animal experiments, which showed a sinus rhythm–like activation pattern when pacing into septal tissue below the point at which the his bundle penetrates the central fibrous body.[33,34] The slow transseptal conduction caused by LBBB and systolic heart failure is amendable by CRT but even more so by left bundle branch area pacing approaches.[35] During LV septal pacing, the transseptal conduction occurs in the rightward direction and simultaneous with the circumferential LV endocardial conduction, thus reducing total LV activation time significantly.[34,35] Although pacing the cardiac conduction system along Purkinje fibers and non-Purkinje LV endocardial fibers may provide an alternative to His bundle and conventional CRT, long-term clinical studies are needed to assess the utility of these pacing approaches to cardiac resynchronization therapy.

SUMMARY

Body surface mapping unravels the electrical substrate of patients with heart failure and ventricular conduction delay, amendable by CRT. Although it has the potential to predict CRT responders, its clinical use remains limited.

CLINICS CARE POINTS

- Twenty years into CRT, the surface ECG remains the principle tool for patient selection.
- ECGi improves patient selection, practical constraints limit it's clinical use.
- The major focus on improving CRT has moved from improving patient selection to conduction system pacing.

CONFLICT OF INTEREST

The authors declare no conflict of interest.

REFERENCES

1. Vernooy K, van Deursen CJM, Strik M, Prinzen FW. Strategies to improve cardiac resynchronization therapy. Nat Rev Cardiol 2014;11(8):481–93.
2. Strik M, Ploux S, Vernooy K, Prinzen FW. Cardiac resynchronization therapy: refocus on the electrical substrate. Circ J Off J Jpn Circ Soc 2011;75(6):1297–304.
3. Glikson M, Nielsen JC, Kronborg MB, et al. ESC Guidelines on cardiac pacing and cardiac resynchronization therapy: Developed by the Task Force on cardiac pacing and cardiac resynchronization therapy of the European Society of Cardiology (ESC) with the special contribution of the European Heart Rhythm Association (EHRA). Eur Heart J 2021;2021(ehab364). https://doi.org/10.1093/eurheartj/ehab364.
4. Kusumoto FM, Schoenfeld MH, Barrett C, et al. 2018 ACC/AHA/HRS guideline on the Evaluation and Management of patients with bradycardia and cardiac conduction delay: a Report of the American College of Cardiology/American heart association Task Force on clinical practice guidelines and the heart rhythm Society. Circulation 2019;140(8):e382–482.
5. Strik M, Ploux S, Huntjens PR, et al. Response to cardiac resynchronization therapy is determined by intrinsic electrical substrate rather than by its modification. Int J Cardiol 2018;270:143–8.
6. Bear LR, Huntjens PR, Walton RD, Bernus O, Coronel R, Dubois R. Cardiac electrical dyssynchrony is accurately detected by noninvasive electrocardiographic imaging. Heart Rhythm 2018;15(7):1058–69.
7. Rudy Y. Noninvasive electrocardiographic imaging of cardiac resynchronization therapy in patients with heart failure. J Electrocardiol 2006;39(4 Suppl):S28–30.
8. Eschalier R, Ploux S, Lumens J, et al. Detailed analysis of ventricular activation sequences during right ventricular apical pacing and left bundle branch block and the potential implications for cardiac

resynchronization therapy. Heart Rhythm 2015; 12(1):137–43.

9. Ploux S, Eschalier R, Whinnett ZI, et al. Electrical dyssynchrony induced by biventricular pacing: implications for patient selection and therapy improvement. Heart Rhythm 2015;12(4):782–91.

10. Ploux S, Lumens J, Whinnett Z, et al. Noninvasive electrocardiographic mapping to improve patient selection for cardiac resynchronization therapy: beyond QRS duration and left bundle branch block morphology. J Am Coll Cardiol 2013;61(24): 2435–43.

11. Lumens J, Ploux S, Strik M, et al. Comparative electromechanical and hemodynamic effects of left ventricular and biventricular pacing in dyssynchronous heart failure: electrical resynchronization versus left-right ventricular interaction. J Am Coll Cardiol 2013;62(25):2395–403.

12. Duchateau J, Sacher F, Pambrun T, et al. Performance and limitations of noninvasive cardiac activation mapping. Heart Rhythm 2019;16(3): 435–42.

13. Johnson WB, Vatterott PJ, Peterson MA, et al. Body surface mapping using an ECG belt to characterize electrical heterogeneity for different left ventricular pacing sites during cardiac resynchronization: Relationship with acute hemodynamic improvement. Heart Rhythm 2017;14(3):385–91.

14. Abu-Alrub S, Strik M, Huntjens P, et al. Left-axis deviation in patients with nonischemic heart failure and left bundle branch block is a purely electrical phenomenon. Heart Rhythm 2021;18(8):1352–60.

15. Gage RM, Curtin AE, Burns KV, Ghosh S, Gillberg JM, Bank AJ. Changes in electrical dyssynchrony by body surface mapping predict left ventricular remodeling in patients with cardiac resynchronization therapy. Heart Rhythm 2017;14(3):392–9.

16. Jackson T, Claridge S, Behar J, et al. Noninvasive electrocardiographic assessment of ventricular activation and remodeling response to cardiac resynchronization therapy. Heart Rhythm O2 2021;2(1): 12–8.

17. Huntjens PR, Ploux S, Strik M, et al. Electrical substrates driving response to cardiac resynchronization therapy: a combined clinical-computational evaluation. Circ Arrhythm Electrophysiol 2018; 11(4):e005647.

18. Eschalier R, Ploux S, Pereira B, et al. Assessment of cardiac resynchronisation therapy in patients with wide QRS and non-specific intraventricular conduction delay: rationale and design of the multicentre randomised NICD-CRT study. BMJ Open 2016; 6(11):e012383.

19. Arnold AD, Shun-Shin MJ, Keene D, et al. His resynchronization versus biventricular pacing in patients with heart failure and left bundle branch block. J Am Coll Cardiol 2018;72(24):3112–22.

20. Arnold AD, Shun-Shin MJ, Keene D, et al. Electrocardiographic predictors of successful resynchronization of left bundle branch block by His bundle pacing. J Cardiovasc Electrophysiol 2021;32(2): 428–38.

21. Upadhyay GA, Vijayaraman P, Nayak HM, et al. His corrective pacing or biventricular pacing for cardiac resynchronization in heart failure. J Am Coll Cardiol 2019;74(1):157–9.

22. Sharma PS, Dandamudi G, Herweg B, et al. Permanent His-bundle pacing as an alternative to biventricular pacing for cardiac resynchronization therapy: a multicenter experience. Heart Rhythm 2018;15(3):413–20.

23. Lustgarten DL, Crespo EM, Arkhipova-Jenkins I, et al. His-bundle pacing versus biventricular pacing in cardiac resynchronization therapy patients: a crossover design comparison. Heart Rhythm 2015; 12(7):1548–57.

24. Upadhyay GA, Cherian T, Shatz DY, et al. Intracardiac delineation of septal conduction in left bundle-branch block patterns. Circulation 2019; 139(16):1876–88.

25. Zhang W, Huang J, Qi Y, et al. Cardiac resynchronization therapy by left bundle branch area pacing in patients with heart failure and left bundle branch block. Heart Rhythm 2019;16(12):1783–90.

26. Huang W, Su L, Wu S, et al. A novel pacing strategy with low and stable output: pacing the left bundle branch immediately beyond the conduction block. Can J Cardiol 2017;33(12):1736.e1-3.

27. Ravi V, Hanifin JL, Larsen T, Huang HD, Trohman RG, Sharma PS. Pros and cons of left bundle branch pacing: a single-center experience. Circ Arrhythm Electrophysiol 2020;13(12):e008874.

28. Sharma PS, Patel NR, Ravi V, et al. Clinical outcomes of left bundle branch area pacing compared to right ventricular pacing: results from the geisinger-rush conduction system pacing registry. Heart Rhythm 2021. https://doi.org/10.1016/j.hrthm.2021.08.033. S1547-5271(21)02102-0.

29. Pujol -López M, Guasch E, Jim énez AR, San AR, Mont L, Tolosana JM. Left bundle branch pacing. JACC Case Rep 2020;2(14):2225–9.

30. Elliott MK, Mehta V, Sidhu BS, Niederer S, Rinaldi CA. Electrocardiographic imaging of His bundle, left bundle branch, epicardial, and endocardial left ventricular pacing to achieve cardiac resynchronization therapy. Hear Case Rep 2020;6(7):460–3.

31. Chan JYS, Huang WJ, Yan B. Non-invasive electrocardiographic imaging of His-bundle and peri-left bundle pacing in left bundle branch block. EP Eur 2019;21(6):837.

32. Salden FCWM, Luermans JGLM, Westra SW, et al. Short-term hemodynamic and electrophysiological effects of cardiac resynchronization by left ventricular septal pacing. J Am Coll Cardiol 2020;75(4):347–59.

33. Laske TG, Skadsberg ND, Hill AJ, Klein GJ, Iaizzo PA. Excitation of the intrinsic conduction system through his and interventricular septal pacing. Pacing Clin Electrophysiol 2006;29(4): 397–405.

34. Mills RW, Cornelussen RN, Mulligan LJ, et al. Left ventricular septal and left ventricular apical pacing chronically maintain cardiac contractile coordination, pump function and efficiency. Circ Arrhythm Electrophysiol 2009;2(5):571–9.

35. Strik M, van Deursen CJM, van Middendorp LB, et al. Transseptal conduction as an important determinant for cardiac resynchronization therapy, as revealed by extensive electrical mapping in the dyssynchronous canine heart. Circ Arrhythm Electrophysiol 2013;6(4):682–9.

Pacing Optimized by Left Ventricular dP/dt$_{max}$

Mark K. Elliott, MBBS[a,b,*], Vishal S. Mehta, MBBS[a,b], Christopher A. Rinaldi, MD, FHRS[a,b]

KEYWORDS

- Cardiac resynchronization therapy • Pressure wire • Acute hemodynamic response
- Device optimization • Endocardial left ventricular pacing • Conduction system pacing
- Multisite pacing • Multipoint pacing

KEY POINTS

- Left ventricular (LV) dP/dt$_{max}$ is measured invasively using a pressure-wire or pressure-volume catheter in the LV and provides a sensitive measure of the acute hemodynamic response to cardiac resynchronization therapy (CRT).
- Acute hemodynamic response is predictive of echocardiographic reverse remodeling 6 months after CRT implant.
- Pressure-wire guided LV lead implant improved response to CRT in the multicenter randomized RADI-CRT trial.
- A temporary pacing protocol using a pressure wire may be useful to help choose the optimal method of CRT delivery (including conduction system pacing and endocardial LV pacing) in nonresponders to conventional CRT, or in those who have risk factors for nonresponse.

INTRODUCTION

Cardiac resynchronization therapy (CRT) is an effective treatment for patients with heart failure and electrical dyssynchrony; however, despite 2 decades of clinical use, rates of nonresponse remain static at 30% to 50%.[1] The maximal rate of change in pressure within the left ventricle (LV dP/dt$_{max}$) is a useful acute measure of the hemodynamic response to CRT and is predictive of LV reverse remodeling at 6 months.[2,3] LV dP/dt$_{max}$ is measured invasively with a pressure wire or pressure-volume catheter inserted into the LV via either the radial or the femoral artery. LV dP/dt can also be measured noninvasively via echocardiography using the Doppler trace of mitral regurgitation, although this technique requires sufficient valvular regurgitation to perform, is operator dependent, and is impractical during device implantation. It is widely used as a research tool to investigate methods to improve CRT response, such as optimization of device programming, multisite pacing, targeting of LV lead placement, and alternative methods of CRT delivery. The clinical use of LV dP/dt$_{max}$ for CRT optimization is less well established; however, a beneficial effect of using a pressure wire to guide LV lead placement has recently been demonstrated in a multicenter randomized control trial.[3] In this review, the authors explore the methods of measuring LV dP/dt$_{max}$, discuss the relationship to long-term outcomes, and propose how it may be used clinically to improve CRT response.

MEASUREMENT OF LEFT VENTRICULAR HEMODYNAMICS

Invasive measurement LV dP/dt$_{max}$ can be performed with a pressure wire, for example, the wireless 0.014-in high-fidelity PressureWire X Guidewire (Abbott, St Paul, MN, USA), which is the same system used to measure fractional flow reserve in coronary angiography. The pressure wire is inserted into the LV using a retrograde aortic approach via the radial or femoral artery.

[a] School of Biomedical Engineering and Imaging Sciences, King's College London, London, UK; [b] Department of Cardiology, Guy's and St Thomas' NHS Foundation Trust, London, UK
* Corresponding author. School of Biomedical Engineering and Imaging Sciences, St Thomas' Hospital, London SE1 7EH, UK.
E-mail address: mark.elliott@kcl.ac.uk

Card Electrophysiol Clin 14 (2022) 223–232
https://doi.org/10.1016/j.ccep.2021.12.002
1877-9182/22/© 2021 Elsevier Inc. All rights reserved.

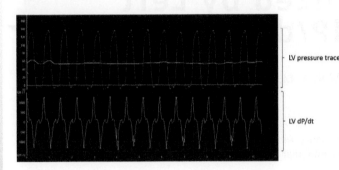

Fig. 1. LV pressure trace and dP/dt trace recorded via the CoroFlow software (Coroventis).

LV pressure trace

LV dP/dt

Insertion is generally contraindicated in patients with mechanical aortic valves or significant aortic stenosis. Heparinization is required, usually with a small-dose bolus of 2500 IU. An LV pressure trace is provided in real time via dedicated software (for example, CoroFlow; Coroventis, Uppsala, Sweden), from which the rate of change of pressure over time (dP/dt) is calculated, with its maximal (dP/dt_{max}) and minimal values (dP/dt_{min}), as shown in **Fig. 1**. LV dP/dt_{max} is generally averaged from multiple beats over a defined period of recording. It can also be measured using a pressure-volume conductance catheter, which provides a more comprehensive assessment of LV hemodynamics, including metrics such as cardiac output and stroke work; however, these catheters come at considerable cost, which likely restricts their use in clinical practice.

Invasive LV dP/dt_{max} measurement is susceptible to several sources of error, which need to be taken into consideration when determining acute hemodynamic response. Significant beat-to-beat variations in LV dP/dt_{max} can occur,[4] and an average of measurements over a predetermined period of time during a pacing protocol is recommended. In a study comparing different invasive hemodynamic protocols for atrioventricular (AV) optimization in CRT patients, there was poor reproducibility in absolute measurements of LV dP/dt_{max} and a significant improvement in reproducibility when relative changes between two different settings were used.[5] Expressing acute hemodynamic response as a percentage increase from baseline to a test setting is therefore recommended, rather than using absolute LV dP/dt_{max} values. LV dP/dt_{max} increases with heart rate,[6] and thus all measurements should be made at a fixed pacing rate, ideally 5 to 10 bpm above intrinsic, to avoid noncapture secondary to intrinsic rhythm. LV dP/dt_{max} is also sensitive to changes in preload and thus varies throughout the respiratory cycle and can drift significantly throughout a procedure, owing to changes in volume status and the use of vasoactive drugs. In

an acute hemodynamic protocol design study in 25 patients, the median effect of respiratory variation on LV dP/dt_{max} was found to be 6.4% (interquartile range [IQR] 4.1% to 9.9%), and the median drift from first to last baseline measurement was 5.0% (IQR 2.8% to 13.8%).[7] Respiratory variation can be addressed by averaging LV dP/dt_{max} over at least 2 respiratory cycles (typically ≥10 seconds). Drift is addressed by repeating baseline measurements throughout the protocol, and calculating relative change in LV dP/dt_{max} from baseline to test measurements at each time point. These considerations have been taken into consideration when designing the acute hemodynamic protocol used by the authors' group, which was also used for the multicenter RADI-CRT trial,[3] and is described in **Fig. 2**. Further improvement in reproducibility may be achieved by averaging multiple repetitions of the same test pacing configuration.[5,7,8]

Noninvasive measurement of LV dP/dt is feasible via echocardiography using the continuous-wave Doppler trace of a jet of mitral regurgitation. This is achieved using the "rate pressure rise" method.[9] In brief, the time interval of the velocity increase from 1 meter per second to 3 meters per second is measured on the Doppler trace (**Fig. 3**), and the corresponding pressure change (4 V^2 leading to 36–4 mm Hg), according to the Bernoulli equation, is divided by the time interval. It should be noted that there is a difference between LV dP/dt calculated by this method (which reflects the rate in change in pressure between two predefined points in the curve) and LV dP/dt_{max}, where the maximal rate of change in pressure can be defined. The latter of the two may therefore provide a more sensitive assessment of LV contractility. Although good correlation between invasive LV dP/dt_{max} and noninvasively measured LV dP/dt has been demonstrated,[10] there are significant limitations to this technique, which has restricted its widespread use in clinical practice. First, its measurement is only possible in patients with sufficient mitral regurgitation, and with adequate echocardiographic

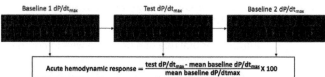

Fig. 2. Protocol for measurement of acute hemodynamic response. AF, atrial fibrillation; CHB, complete heart block; RV, right ventricular.

acoustic windows. Second, averaging of measurements from sequential beats throughout the respiratory cycle can be technically challenging. Third, error can be introduced if the imaging beam is not aligned exactly parallel with the mitral regurgitation jet, which can be difficult in eccentric or complex regurgitation. Finally, performing echocardiography during device implantation is challenging because of the sterile field, which can limit its use for providing real-time intraprocedural measurements.

RELATIONSHIP BETWEEN LEFT VENTRICULAR dP/DT$_{MAX}$ AND LONG-TERM OUTCOMES

Although LV dP/dt$_{max}$ is often used as a gold-standard acute assessment of CRT response, studies correlating acute hemodynamic response with long-term outcomes after CRT have shown conflicting results. An early echocardiography-based study of patients with dilated cardiomyopathy undergoing CRT found that improvement in noninvasive LV dP/dt measurements from baseline to CRT were predictive of symptomatic response to CRT.[11] In a nonrandomized study of 33 patients in which LV dP/dt$_{max}$ was used to guide LV lead placement during CRT implant, the authors' group demonstrated that acute hemodynamic response greater than 10% was predictive of echocardiographic reverse remodeling ($\geq$15% reduction in LV end-systolic volume [ESV]) at 6 months with a high degree of sensitivity (0.94) and specificity (0.86).[2] This association was seen for both

ischemic and nonischemic heart failure causes, and acute hemodynamic response greater than 10% was similarly predictive of symptomatic improvement after CRT. In a subsequent study of 41 patients who underwent more complex hemodynamic assessment with a pressure-volume loop measurement before CRT implant, acute change in LV dP/dt$_{max}$ was not significantly different between patients who displayed reverse remodeling at 6 months and those who did not.[12] In contrast, stroke work was found to be predictive of remodeling. Pressure-volume loop assessments performed by the authors' group in 9 patients undergoing CRT found significant acute improvements in both LV dP/dt$_{max}$ and stroke volume in echocardiographic responders, but not nonresponders. In the RADI-CRT study, whereby 281 patients undergoing CRT were randomized to standard implant versus pressure-wire guidance of LV lead placement, LV dP/dt$_{max}$ was predictive of reverse remodeling at 6 months, and 84% of patients with an acute hemodynamic response greater than 10% demonstrated a reduction in LV ESV $\geq$15% versus only 28% with an acute hemodynamic response less than 10% (P<.001).

In a feasibility study of CRT for patients with narrow QRS and echocardiographic evidence of dyssynchrony, 47 patients underwent invasive pressure-wire study to optimize AV delays. The maximal acute hemodynamic response achieved with CRT in this cohort was minor (2% $\pm$ 2%) and reflected the lack of improvement in either

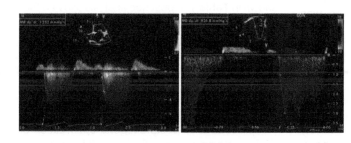

Fig. 3. Calculation of left ventricular dP/dt from the mitral regurgitation (MR) continuous-wave Doppler trace on transthoracic echocardiography. The marked points represent 1 meter per second (4 mm Hg) and 3 meters per second (36 mm Hg). dP/dt is calculated by dividing the fixed pressure change (36–4 mm Hg) by the measured time interval between these 2 points. (*From* Tissot C, Singh Y and Sekarski N (2018) Echocardiographic Evaluation of Ventricular Function—For the Neonatologist and Pediatric Intensivist. Front. Pediatr. 6:79. https://doi.org/10.3389/fped.2018.00079)

symptomatic or echocardiographic indices at 6 and 12 months.[13] When data were combined with previous acute hemodynamic studies of CRT in patients with broad QRS (excluding right bundle branch block),[14,15] a positive correlation between acute change in LV dP/dt_{max} and baseline QRS duration was noted. These findings were predictive of the subsequent randomized EchoCRT trial, in which CRT did not reduce the composite outcome of death or heart failure hospitalization in a similar cohort of patients with narrow QRS and echocardiographic dyssynchrony, with a higher reported death rate in the CRT group.[16] Although the acute hemodynamic and long-term mortality data were from different studies, this is an interesting observation and highlights the potential use of hypothesis-generating feasibility studies using LV dP/dt_{max} to guide large randomized trials.

The direct correlation between acute change in LV dP/dt_{max} and hard clinical end points, such as mortality and hospitalization, is less clear. In a study of 53 patients undergoing CRT, acute change in LV dP/dt derived noninvasively from echocardiography was predictive of the composite end point of all-cause mortality or hospitalizations at 12 months.[17] In contrast, in a subsequent a study of 68 CRT patients undergoing invasive pressure-wire assessment, although baseline LV dP/dt_{max} was found to be an independent predictor of the same composite end point, acute change in LV dP/dt_{max} from baseline to CRT was not.[18] Similarly, in a larger retrospective study of 285 patients in whom invasive LV dP/dt_{max} was measured during a temporary pacing procedure before CRT implantation, LV dP/dt_{max} at baseline and during CRT was predictive of a composite end point of all-cause mortality, heart transplantation, or LV assist device at 12 months; however, acute change in LV dP/dt_{max} was not.[19]

Discrepancies in the outcomes of these studies may be related to different acute hemodynamic protocols used, with potential sources of error and bias as previously discussed. The fact that the use of a pressure wire alone to guide LV lead placement, regardless of whether an acute hemodynamic response greater than 10% was achieved, resulted in higher rates of reverse remodeling in the randomized RADI-CRT study suggests that acute changes in LV dP/dt_{max} are indeed a useful indicator of longer-term outcomes after CRT.[3] The studies assessing mortality and hospitalization may have been underpowered to detect a significant association with acute hemodynamic response, particularly with a relatively short follow-up period of 1 year,[18,19] and longer-term post hoc analyses of the randomized RADI-CRT study may prove useful.

GUIDANCE OF LEFT VENTRICULAR LEAD PLACEMENT

Intraprocedural use of a pressure wire to compare acute hemodynamic performance of different LV lead positions within the coronary sinus tributaries has been investigated in several mechanistic studies.[2,20–24] Although lateral and posterolateral lead positions were generally associated with higher acute hemodynamic response compared with anterior locations,[2,20,22] there was marked variation in the optimal lead position between patients.[2,21,23,24] Optimal LV lead location is dependent on a variety of factors, including myocardial scar, coronary sinus anatomy, the site of latest mechanical activation, and avoidance of phrenic nerve stimulation. The use of a pressure wire to test various lead positions and choose the optimal coronary sinus branch at the time of implantation may therefore prove superior to empirical lead placement. In an initial feasibility study of 33 patients, the authors' group demonstrated a significant improvement in LV dP/dt_{max} during CRT between the worst and best LV lead positions (792 ± 160 mm Hg per second vs 924 ± 203 mm Hg per second; $P<.001$), with no single lead position being optimal in every patient.[2] As previously discussed, an acute hemodynamic response greater than 10% was predictive of reverse remodeling at 6 months. The clinical utility of pressure-wire guided LV lead placement was subsequently assessed in the multicenter randomized controlled RADI-CRT trial.[3] 281 patients across 12 centers were randomized 1:1 to either a pressure-wire guided CRT implant or standard care. In the pressure-wire guided arm, LV dP/dt_{max} was assessed during biventricular pacing in multiple coronary sinus tributaries, and the optimal position was selected according to the highest acute hemodynamic response, provided pacing thresholds were acceptable and there was no phrenic nerve stimulation. The pressure-wire guided approach resulted in a significantly higher rate of reverse remodeling (≥15% reduction in LV ESV) compared with conventional CRT (73% vs 60%; $P = .02$), as shown in **Table 1**. A post hoc analysis showed that the benefit of a pressure-wire guided approach was higher in patients with ischemic cause of heart failure.

OPTIMIZATION OF DEVICE PROGRAMMING

Another potential clinical use of LV dP/dt_{max} is the intraprocedural or postprocedural optimization of CRT programming, specifically AV delay, ventriculoventricular (VV) delay, and LV pacing vector optimization. Several small mechanistic studies of

Table 1
Efficacy outcomes from the RADI-CRT trial

Outcome	Conventional Arm (N = 139)	Pressure-Wire Guided Arm (N = 139)	P Value
Echo-responder, n (%)	83 (60)	101 (73)	.02
Clinical responder (based on CCS)	93 (67)	106 (76)	.06
ΔLVESV (%)	−21 ± 29	−29 ± 32	.03
ΔLVEF	4 ± 9	7 ± 8	.003
ΔQOL score	−18 ± 23	−19 ± 22	.71
Δ6-min walk (m)	43 ± 98	68 ± 77	.02
ΔNT-proBNP (pg/mL)	−909 ± 1102	−1129 ± 1099	.09

Abbreviations: CCS, clinical composite score; LVEF, left ventricular ejection fraction; LVESV, left ventricular end-systolic volume; NT-proBNP, N-terminal pro B-type natriuretic peptide; QOL, quality of life.
From Sohal M, Hamid S, Perego G, et al. A multicenter prospective randomized controlled trial of cardiac resynchronization therapy guided by invasive dP/dt. *Heart Rhythm O2.* 2021;2(1):19-27; with permission

pressure-wire guided optimization have demonstrated significant improvements in acute hemodynamic response from the worst to best AV intervals, and considerable interpatient variability in the optimal settings.[25–27] VV optimization has also been shown to improve acute hemodynamic response, and although interpatient variability is observed, a degree of LV preexcitation is associated with a higher acute hemodynamic response in most patients.[6,28,29] Although pressure-wire guided optimization of AV and VV delays is therefore feasible, echocardiographic techniques remain more commonplace. There is good correlation between the two techniques, with a study of 30 patients who underwent both invasive and echocardiographic AV optimization demonstrating that the optimal AV delay determined by invasive LV dP/dt$_{max}$ and by Doppler echocardiography (via the velocity time integral of the mitral valve inflow trace) was the same for 29/30 patients (R = 0.96).[30] In addition, since the widespread adoption of quadripolar LV leads, multiple pacing vectors are available for LV pacing, and pressure-wire guidance is one potential method to determine the optimal pacing vector. In a study of 16 patients who underwent pressure-wire assessment of different pacing vectors after CRT implant with a quadripolar LV lead, a 10% incremental benefit in acute hemodynamic response was observed between the worst and best pacing vector.

It should be noted that the clinical value of AV and VV optimization after CRT implant remains unclear. In a small nonrandomized study of 41 patients, LV ejection fraction and New York Heart Association funcation class were significantly greater at 6 months in patients who underwent echocardiography-guided AV optimization (using dP/dt from the MR Dopper trace), compared to those programmed to an empirical AV delay of 120 milliseconds.[31] However, in a large randomized trial of more than 1000 patients, echocardiographic optimization of AV delays after CRT implant failed to show a significant clinical benefit over empirical programming of 120 milliseconds.[32] More recently, studies using device-based algorithms to automatically optimize AV delays have shown more promise[33,34] and suggest that dynamic alteration of settings may provide more benefit than programming of a fixed delay that has been determined to be "optimal" at a given time point.

MULTISITE AND MULTIPOINT PACING

The use of more than one lead in the coronary sinus (multisite pacing) or pacing from multiple points within the same coronary sinus tributary using a quadripolar lead (multipoint pacing) has been theorized to improve CRT response by increasing the volume of stimulated LV myocardium and thus achieving more rapid ventricular activation and effective resynchronization.[35] Improvements in acute hemodynamic response over conventional CRT have been demonstrated in small observational studies with both multisite pacing and multipoint pacing.[36–39] However, this has not translated into a consistent benefit in randomized studies, with significant variation in outcomes between trials. A recent meta-analysis showed that there was no overall benefit for multipoint pacing over conventional CRT when only randomized studies were included.[40] Although two small randomized trials showed benefits for multisite pacing over conventional CRT,[41,42] two larger multicenter trials have since had negative results.[43,44] Mechanistic studies from the authors' group have demonstrated that the acute hemodynamic benefits of both multipoint and multisite pacing appear to be restricted to patients who are not acute responders to conventional CRT,[45] or in those with a significant burden of myocardial scar.[46] These findings are supported by animal model studies of left bundle branch block (LBBB), in which improvements in LV dP/dt$_{max}$ with multisite and multipoint pacing were only demonstrated in cases where the response to single-site LV pacing was suboptimal.[47,48] This may explain why these strategies fail to show consistent clinical benefit in all-comers in randomized studies, although trials that included only CRT nonresponders[43] or those with intermediate QRS prolongation (120–150 milliseconds) also failed to show benefit.[44] There may be subsets of patients in whom multisite or multipoint pacing is superior to conventional CRT, and measuring invasive LV dP/dt$_{max}$ intraprocedurally to identify such patients may prove useful.

ALTERNATIVE METHODS OF DELIVERING CARDIAC RESYNCHRONIZATION THERAPY
Endocardial Left Ventricular Pacing

Endocardial LV pacing is an alternative to conventional CRT for nonresponders, or in those in whom pacing the LV via a lead in the coronary sinus is not feasible. Although lead-based endocardial LV pacing may be limited by thromboembolic complications, leadless LV pacing via the WiSE-CRT system (EBR Systems, Sunnyvale, CA, USA) mitigates these risks, as the endocardial electrode becomes endothelialized, and has been demonstrated as a feasible and effective method of CRT delivery.[49] Mechanistic studies in humans have consistently shown superior acute hemodynamic response during endocardial LV pacing compared with conventional epicardial CRT.[50–53] Some of this benefit likely comes from the ability to pace anywhere within the LV during endocardial pacing, unrestricted by coronary sinus anatomy, thus allowing the avoidance of scar and targeting of the latest activation site. However, in a study by the authors' group, 8 patients with ischemic cardiomyopathy underwent temporary pacing at several different epicardial and endocardial sites within the LV, and superior acute hemodynamic response was demonstrated when pacing at the same location endocardially versus epicardially.[54] This suggests that the hemodynamic benefits of endocardial LV pacing go beyond optimal pacing

location, and computational modeling studies have suggested that this benefit is explained by access to fast conducting endocardial tissue and/or the distal Purkinje network.[55]

Given the wide variety of LV endocardial sites available for electrode placement, pressure-wire guidance may be of particular use to select the optimal site. Indeed, studies have shown that the optimal site for endocardial LV pacing varies greatly between patients,[51–55] suggesting a targeted, rather than empirical, approach may be warranted. The authors' group has previously reported high echocardiographic response rates of 90% after WiSE-CRT implantation when a guided approach was used for electrode placement.[56] In this multicenter study, a total of 26 patients across 3 centers underwent a guided implant, with a variety of techniques used to identify a target site in the LV, including echocardiography with speckle-tracking radial strain analysis, electrical latency (Q-LV), electroanatomic mapping, and cardiac MRI. A pressure wire was used in each case to measure the acute hemodynamic response during pacing at the target site and could be used alone to identify the optimal location for endocardial pacing within the LV. The authors' group has previously reported the utility of using a pressure wire to determine optimal location for the endocardial electrode during WiSE-CRT implantation.[57]

Conduction System Pacing

His bundle pacing (HBP) and left bundle branch area pacing (LBBAP) have recently emerged as novel methods of delivering CRT. These techniques may provide more physiologic ventricular activation compared with conventional biventricular pacing. HBP has been shown to achieve superior LV activation times and acute hemodynamic response in a temporary pacing study of 23 patients with LBBB, although systolic blood pressure was used as the hemodynamic end point, rather than LV dP/dt$_{max}$.[58] In a similar study comparing temporary LV septal pacing with conventional CRT, although improvements in electrical resynchronization metrics (measured using an electrocardiographic belt) were noted, there was no improvement in acute hemodynamic response (measured by LV dP/dt$_{max}$).[59] In this study, the LV septum was paced empirically, without mapping and targeting of the left bundle branch, which likely resulted in a variety of selective and nonselective LBBAP and pure septal pacing, which may have affected the results. Further study of both the acute hemodynamic and the long-term benefits of conduction system pacing techniques is required.

Table 2
Potential uses of left ventricular dP/dt$_{max}$ to optimize response to cardiac resynchronization therapy

Preprocedure	Intraprocedure	Postprocedure

• Temporary pacing study to determine optimal method of CRT delivery:
  ○ Conventional CRT
  ○ Endocardial LV pacing
  ○ HBP
  ○ LBBAP
  ○ Multisite pacing
	• Guidance of LV lead placement in coronary sinus tributaries
	• Guidance of endocardial electrode placement in WiSE-CRT implant
		• Optimization of device programming:
		  ○ AV interval
		  ○ VV interval
		  ○ LV pacing vector
		  ○ Multipoint pacing
		• Temporary pacing study to determine alternative method of CRT delivery in nonresponders

Selection of the Optimal Method of Delivering Cardiac Resynchronization

Large-scale randomized trials comparing the efficacy of endocardial LV pacing and conduction system pacing techniques with conventional CRT are lacking. However, it is likely that the optimal technique to deliver CRT will vary depending on the underlying substrate. In a study of 85 patients who underwent mapping of the LV septum, the ability of HBP to correct LBBB varied significantly according to the level of conduction block. Although HBP achieved LBBB correction in 94% of patients with left intra-Hisian block, success rates were only 62% when block was located within the left bundle branch, and 0% when intact Purkinje activation was observed.[60] Another factor to be considered is the burden and location of myocardial scar, as significant infarction in the lateral wall may reduce the efficacy of endocardial pacing with a conventional lateral electrode position, whereas septal scar may attenuate response to conduction system pacing. A temporary pacing procedure may potentially be useful in nonresponders after conventional CRT, with the use of a pressure wire to assess acute hemodynamic response during different methods of CRT delivery. The authors' group has recently demonstrated the feasibility of such a technique, comparing temporary conventional CRT, endocardial LV pacing, HBP, and LBBAP in the same patient cohort, using both acute hemodynamic response and electrocardiographic imaging.[61,62] Similarly, in CRT-naïve patients who have borderline indications or significant risk factors for nonresponse, a temporary pacing procedure before implant may be useful to identify the technique most likely to provide effective resynchronization. The authors have also demonstrated the feasibility of performing leadless LBBAP using the WiSE-CRT system and used a pressure wire to compare the acute hemodynamic response between pacing in the septum and at the lateral wall.[57] This suggests that both conduction system pacing and endocardial LV pacing may be achievable via the WiSE-CRT system, and pressure-wire guidance during implant may prove useful in selecting the optimal choice for each patient.

SUMMARY

LV dP/dt$_{max}$ is typically measured invasively via a pressure-wire or pressure-volume catheter placed in the LV and provides a highly sensitive acute assessment of changes in cardiac contractility. Although an acute hemodynamic response of greater than 10% has been shown to be predictive of reverse remodeling at 6 months, further study of its correlation with longer-term and hard clinical end points is required. It is unlikely that the use of a pressure wire will be required in all patients undergoing CRT. Pressure-wire assessment of LV dP/dt$_{max}$ is an invasive procedure and comes with risks that must be weighed against any potential benefit to the patient. Additional costs must also be taken into consideration. In the RADI-CRT study, the pressure-wire guided arm had significantly higher procedural time (142 ± 39 vs 104 ± 39 minutes; $P<.001$) and fluoroscopy time (28 ± 15 vs 20 ± 16 minutes; $P<.001$) compared with the conventional implant arm, although there was no significant difference in complication rates between the two groups. LV dP/dt$_{max}$ is likely to be of most clinical use in patients who do not respond to conventional CRT, or in those who have borderline indications or risk factors for nonresponse. In such cases, LV dP/dt$_{max}$ may be useful to help guide LV lead placement, to optimize device programming (including multipoint pacing), and to select the best alternative method of delivering CRT, such as endocardial LV pacing or conduction system pacing (**Table 2**). Ideally, acute hemodynamic response could be assessed noninvasively, to minimize risk to patients. Although LV dP/dt can be measured via echocardiography, this requires sufficient mitral regurgitation and has significant limitations as previously discussed. Further work is required to develop noninvasive acute hemodynamic protocols that are reproducible and can successfully predict long-term outcomes after CRT.

CONFLICT OF INTEREST

The department is supported by the Wellcome/EPSRC Center for Medical Engineering (WT203148/Z/16/Z). Outside of the submitted work, M.K. Elliott and V.S. Mehta have received fellowship funding from Abbott. C.A. Rinaldi receives research funding and/or consultation fees from Abbott, Medtronic, Boston Scientific, Spectranetics, and MicroPort outside of the submitted work.

REFERENCES

1. Sieniewicz BJ, Gould J, Porter B, et al. Understanding non-response to cardiac resynchronisation therapy: common problems and potential solutions. Heart Fail Rev 2019;24(1):41–54.

2. Duckett SG, Ginks M, Shetty AK, et al. Invasive acute hemodynamic response to guide left ventricular lead implantation predicts chronic remodeling in patients undergoing cardiac resynchronization therapy. J Am Coll Cardiol 2011;58(11):1128–36.

3. Sohal M, Hamid S, Perego G, et al. A multicenter prospective randomized controlled trial of cardiac resynchronization therapy guided by invasive dP/dt. Heart Rhythm O2 2021;2(1):19–27.

4. Niederer S, Walker C, Crozier A, et al. The impact of beat-to-beat variability in optimising the acute hemodynamic response in cardiac resynchronisation therapy. Clin Trials Regul Sci Cardiol 2015;12:18–22.

5. Whinnett ZI, Francis DP, Denis A, et al. Comparison of different invasive hemodynamic methods for AV delay optimization in patients with cardiac resynchronization therapy: implications for clinical trial design and clinical practice. Int J Cardiol 2013;168(3):2228–37.

6. van Gelder BM, Meijer A, Bracke FA. Stimulation rate and the optimal interventricular interval during cardiac resynchronization therapy in patients with chronic atrial fibrillation. Pacing Clin Electrophysiol 2008;31(5):569–74.

7. Thibault B, Dubuc M, Karst E, et al. Design of an acute dP/dt hemodynamic measurement protocol to isolate cardiac effect of pacing. J Card Fail 2014;20(5):365–72.

8. Pabari PA, Willson K, Stegemann B, et al. When is an optimization not an optimization? Evaluation of clinical implications of information content (signal-to-noise ratio) in optimization of cardiac resynchronization therapy, and how to measure and maximize it. Heart Fail Rev 2011;16(3):277–90.

9. Tissot C, Singh Y, Sekarski N. Echocardiographic evaluation of ventricular function-for the neonatologist and pediatric intensivist. Front Pediatr 2018;6(April):1–12.

10. Bargiggia GS, Bertucci C, Recusani F, et al. A new method for estimating left ventricular dP/dt by continuous wave Doppler-echocardiography. Validation studies at cardiac catheterization. Circulation 1989;80(5):1287–92.

11. Oguz E, Dagdeviren B, Bilsel T, et al. Echocardiographic prediction of long-term response to biventricular pacemaker in severe heart failure. Eur J Heart Fail 2002;4(1):83–90.

12. de Roest GJ, Allaart CP, Kleijn SA, et al. Prediction of long-term outcome of cardiac resynchronization therapy by acute pressure-volume loop measurements. Eur J Heart Fail 2013;15(3):299–307.

13. Donahue T, Niazi I, Leon A, et al. Acute and chronic response to CRT in narrow QRS patients. Journal of Cardiovascular Translational Research 2012;5(2):232–41. https://doi.org/10.1007/s12265-011-9338-3. In this issue.

14. Niazi I, Kiemen JOANN, Yong P, et al. Hemodynamic superiority of dual-site left ventricular stimulation over conventional biventricular stimulation in heart failure patients. The Journal of Innovations in Cardiac Rhythm Management 2011;2(August):412–8.

15. Gold MR, Niazi I, Giudici M, et al. A prospective comparison of AV delay programming methods for hemodynamic optimization during cardiac resynchronization therapy. J Cardiovasc Electrophysiol 2007;18(5):490–6.

16. Ruschitzka F, Abraham WT, Singh JP, et al. Cardiac-resynchronization therapy in heart failure with narrow QRS complexes. N Engl J Med 2013;369(15):1395–405.

17. Tournoux FB, Alabiad C, Fan D, et al. Echocardiographic measures of acute haemodynamic response after cardiac resynchronization therapy predict long-term clinical outcome. Eur Heart J 2007;28(9):1143–8.

18. Suzuki H, Shimano M, Yoshida Y, et al. Maximum derivative of left ventricular pressure predicts cardiac mortality after cardiac resynchronization therapy. Clin Cardiol 2010;33(12). https://doi.org/10.1002/clc.20683.

19. Bogaard MD, Houthuizen P, Bracke FA, et al. Baseline left ventricular dP/dt max rather than the acute improvement in dP/dt max predicts clinical outcome in patients with cardiac resynchronization therapy. Eur J Heart Fail 2011;13(10):1126–32.

20. Butter C, Auricchio A, Stellbrink C, et al. Effect of resynchronization therapy stimulation site on the

systolic function of heart failure patients. Circulation 2001;104(25):3026–9.

21. Gold MR, Auricchio A, Hummel JD, et al. Comparison of stimulation sites within left ventricular veins on the acute hemodynamic effects of cardiac resynchronization therapy. Heart Rhythm 2005;2(4): 376–81.

22. de Roest GJ, Allaart CP, de Haan S, et al. Effects of QRS duration and pacing location on pressure-volume loop evaluation of cardiac resynchronization therapy in end-stage heart failure. Am J Cardiol 2011;108(11):1581–8.

23. Stockinger J, Staier K, Schiebeling-RÖmer J, et al. Acute hemodynamic effects of right and left ventricular lead positions during the implantation of cardiac resynchronization therapy defibrillators. Pacing Clin Electrophysiol 2011;34(11):1537–43.

24. Zanon F, Baracca E, Pastore G, et al. Multipoint pacing by a left ventricular quadripolar lead improves the acute hemodynamic response to CRT compared with conventional biventricular pacing at any site. Heart Rhythm 2015;12(5):975–81.

25. Kass DA, Chen CH, Curry C, et al. Improved left ventricular mechanics from acute VDD pacing in patients with dilated cardiomyopathy and ventricular conduction delay. Circulation 1999;99(12):1567–73.

26. Auricchio A, Stellbrink C, Block M, et al. Effect of pacing chamber and atrioventricular delay on acute systolic function of paced patients with congestive heart failure. Circulation 1999;99(23):2993–3001.

27. van Gelder BM, Bracke FA, van der Voort PH, et al. Optimal sensed atrio-ventricular interval determined by paced QRS morphology. Pacing Clin Electrophysiol 2007;30(4):476–81.

28. Kurzidim K, Reinke H, Sperzel J, et al. Invasive optimization of cardiac resynchronization therapy: role of sequential biventricular and left ventricular pacing. Pacing Clin Electrophysiol 2005;28(8):754–61.

29. van Gelder BM, Meijer A, Bracke FA. The optimized V-V interval determined by interventricular conduction times versus invasive measurement by LVdP/dtMAX. J Cardiovasc Electrophysiol 2008;19(9): 939–44.

30. Jansen AHM, Bracke FA, van Dantzig JM, et al. Correlation of echo-Doppler optimization of atrioventricular delay in cardiac resynchronization therapy with invasive hemodynamics in patients with heart failure secondary to ischemic or idiopathic dilated cardiomyopathy. Am J Cardiol 2006;97(4):552–7.

31. Morales MA, Startari U, Panchetti L, et al. Atrioventricular delay optimization by Doppler-derived left ventricular dP/dt improves 6-month outcome of resynchronized patients. Pacing Clin Electrophysiol 2006;29(6):564–8.

32. Ellenbogen KA, Gold MR, Meyer TE, et al. Primary results from the SmartDelay determined AV optimization: a comparison to other AV delay methods used in cardiac resynchronization therapy (SMART-AV) trial: a randomized trial comparing empirical, echocardiography- guided, and algorithmic atrioventricular delay programming in cardiac resynchronization therapy. Circulation 2010;122(25):2660–8.

33. Starling RC, Krum H, Bril S, et al. Impact of a novel adaptive optimization algorithm on 30-day readmissions. Evidence from the adaptive CRT trial. JACC Heart Fail 2015;3(7):565–72.

34. Varma N, Hu Y, Connolly AT, et al. Gain in real-world cardiac resynchronization therapy efficacy with SyncAV dynamic optimization: heart failure hospitalizations and costs. Heart Rhythm 2021. https://doi.org/10.1016/j.hrthm.2021.05.006.

35. Rinaldi CA, Burri H, Thibault B, et al. A review of multisite pacing to achieve cardiac resynchronization therapy. Europace 2014;17(1):7–17.

36. Thibault B, Dubuc M, Khairy P, et al. Acute haemodynamic comparison of multisite and biventricular pacing with a quadripolar left ventricular lead. Europace 2013;15(7):984–91.

37. Pappone C, Ćalović Ž, Vicedomini G, et al. Multipoint left ventricular pacing improves acute hemodynamic response assessed with pressure-volume loops in cardiac resynchronization therapy patients. Heart Rhythm 2014;11(3):394–401.

38. Umar F, Taylor RJ, Stegemann B, et al. Haemodynamic effects of cardiac resynchronization therapy using single-vein, three-pole, multipoint left ventricular pacing in patients with ischaemic cardiomyopathy and a left ventricular free wall scar: the MAESTRO study. Europace 2016;18(8): 1227–34.

39. Zanon F, Marcantoni L, Baracca E, et al. Optimization of left ventricular pacing site plus multipoint pacing improves remodeling and clinical response to cardiac resynchronization therapy at 1 year. Heart Rhythm 2016;13(8):1644–51.

40. Mehta VS, Elliott MK, Sidhu BS, et al. Multipoint pacing for cardiac resynchronisation therapy in patients with heart failure: a systematic review and meta-analysis. J Cardiovasc Electrophysiol 2021;32(9): 2577–89.

41. Rogers DPS, Lambiase PD, Lowe MD, et al. A randomized double-blind crossover trial of triventricular versus biventricular pacing in heart failure. Eur J Heart Fail 2012;14(5):495–505.

42. Leclercq C, Gadler F, Kranig W, et al. A randomized comparison of triple-site versus dual-site ventricular stimulation in patients with congestive heart failure. J Am Coll Cardiol 2008;51(15):1455–62.

43. Bordachar P, Gras D, Clementy N, et al. Clinical impact of an additional left ventricular lead in cardiac resynchronization therapy nonresponders: the V3 trial. Heart Rhythm 2018;15(6):870–6.

44. Gould J, Claridge S, Jackson T, et al. Standard care versus TRIVEntricular pacing in Heart Failure

(STRIVE HF): a prospective multicenter randomized control trial of triventricular pacing versus conventional biventricular pacing in patients with heart failure and intermediate QRS LBBB. Europace 2021. Accepted (In press).

45. Sohal M, Shetty A, Niederer S, et al. Mechanistic insights into the benefits of multisite pacing in cardiac resynchronization therapy: the importance of electrical substrate and rate of left ventricular activation. Heart Rhythm 2015;12(12):2449–57.

46. Jackson T, Lenarczyk R, Sterlinski M, et al. Left ventricular scar and the acute hemodynamic effects of multivein and multipolar pacing in cardiac resynchronization. IJC Heart and Vasculature 2018;19:14–9.

47. Ploux S, Strik M, van Hunnik A, et al. Acute electrical and hemodynamic effects of multisite left ventricular pacing for cardiac resynchronization therapy in the dyssynchronous canine heart. Heart Rhythm 2014; 11(1):119–25.

48. Heckman LIB, Kuiper M, Anselme F, et al. Evaluating multisite pacing strategies in cardiac resynchronization therapy in the preclinical setting. Heart Rhythm O2 2020;1(2):111–9.

49. Sieniewicz BJ, Betts TR, James S, et al. Real-world experience of leadless left ventricular endocardial cardiac resynchronization therapy: a multicenter international registry of the WiSE-CRT pacing system. Heart Rhythm 2020;17(8):1291–7.

50. Spragg DD, Dong J, Fetics BJ, et al. Optimal left ventricular endocardial pacing sites for cardiac resynchronization therapy in patients with ischemic cardiomyopathy. J Am Coll Cardiol 2010;56(10): 774–81.

51. Derval N, Steendijk P, Gula LJ, et al. Optimizing hemodynamics in heart failure patients by systematic screening of left ventricular pacing sites. the lateral left ventricular wall and the coronary sinus are rarely the best sites. J Am Coll Cardiol 2010;55(6):566–75.

52. Padeletti L, Pieragnoli P, Ricciardi G, et al. Acute hemodynamic effect of left ventricular endocardial pacing in cardiac resynchronization therapy: assessment by pressure-volume loops. Circ Arrhythmia Electrophysiol 2012;5(3):460–7.

53. Shetty AK, Sohal M, Chen Z, et al. A comparison of left ventricular endocardial, multisite, and multipolar epicardial cardiac resynchronization: an acute haemodynamic and electroanatomical study. Europace 2014;16(6):873–9.

54. Behar JM, Jackson T, Hyde E, et al. Optimized left ventricular endocardial stimulation is superior to optimized epicardial stimulation in ischemic patients with poor response to cardiac resynchronization therapy: a combined magnetic resonance imaging, electroanatomic contact mapping, and hemodynamic study to target endocardial lead placement. JACC Clin Electrophysiol 2016;2(7):799–809.

55. Hyde ER, Behar JM, Claridge S, et al. Beneficial effect on cardiac resynchronization from left ventricular endocardial pacing is mediated by early access to high conduction velocity tissue: electrophysiological simulation study. Circ Arrhythmia Electrophysiol 2015;8(5):1164–72.

56. Sieniewicz BJ, Behar JM, Gould J, et al. Guidance for optimal site selection of a leadless left ventricular endocardial electrode improves acute hemodynamic response and chronic remodeling. JACC Clin Electrophysiol 2018;4(7):860–8.

57. Elliott M, Jacon P, Sidhu BS, et al. Technical feasibility of leadless left bundle branch area pacing for cardiac resynchronisation: a case series. Eur Heart J Case Rep 2021;5(11):ytab379. Accepted (In press).

58. Arnold AD, Shun-Shin MJ, Keene D, et al. His resynchronization versus biventricular pacing in patients with heart failure and left bundle branch block. J Am Coll Cardiol 2018;72(24):3112–22.

59. Salden FCWM, Luermans JGLM, Westra SW, et al. Short-term hemodynamic and electrophysiological effects of cardiac resynchronization by left ventricular septal pacing. J Am Coll Cardiol 2020;75(4): 347–59.

60. Upadhyay GA, Cherian T, Shatz DY, et al. Intracardiac delineation of septal conduction in left bundle-branch block patterns. Circulation 2019; 139(16):1876–88.

61. Elliott MK, Mehta V, Sidhu BS, et al. Electrocardiographic imaging of His bundle, left bundle branch, epicardial, and endocardial left ventricular pacing to achieve cardiac resynchronization therapy. HeartRhythm Case Rep 2020;6(7):460–3.

62. Elliott M, Strocchi M, Sidhu B, et al. Acute hemodynamic response of epicardial and endocardial cardiac resynchronization therapy, His bundle pacing and left bundle branch pacing. EP Europace 2021; 23(Suppl_3):2021.

Role of Electrical Delay in Cardiac Resynchronization Therapy Response

Zain S. Gowani, MD[1], Brett Tomashitis, MD[1], Chau N. Vo, MD,
Michael E. Field, MD, Michael R. Gold, MD, PhD*

KEYWORDS

- Cardiac resynchronization therapy • Left ventricular pacing • Electrical delay

KEY POINTS

- We review measures of electrical delay: QLV, RV-LV, and QRV.
- Pacing at sites of prolonged electrical delay, assessed by QLV and RV-LV, are associated with improved CRT response.
- Pacing from LV electrodes with longer electrical delay as well as programming to achieve fusion of LV paced complexes with intrinsic conduction can improve CRT outcomes.

Cardiac resynchronization therapy (CRT) is a well-established therapy for patients with symptomatic heart failure (HF), left ventricular (LV) systolic dysfunction, and intraventricular delay with prolonged QRS duration (QRSd). Pivotal, randomized trials have established that CRT reduces HF hospitalizations and mortality, improves quality of life, and promotes reverse LV remodeling.[1–7] Patient characteristics associated with improved CRT response include female gender, longer unpaced QRSd, and nonischemic HF cause.[8,9] Several device-related factors that are also associated with CRT response rate include LV lead position and programmed atrioventricular (AV) timing.

Traditionally, LV lead position was guided by anatomic criteria largely based on acute hemodynamic studies, showing that pacing from the lateral wall of the LV was associated with improved hemodynamic response.[10] However, retrospective analyses from major CRT clinical trials revealed little effect of LV lead position on outcomes, other than noting worse outcomes with apical positions.[11–13] Given the poor correlation of CRT outcomes with anatomically guided LV lead placement, focus shifted toward more physiologic predictors such as targeting the areas of delayed mechanical and electrical activation.

Earliest studies attempted to assess the benefit of mechanical activation patterns and location of scar. Several investigators showed that pacing near scar was associated with worse outcomes,[14] whereas pacing in areas of late LV contraction had better CRT response.[15] Subsequently, 2 randomized trials, using speckle tracking echocardiography, showed improved CRT outcomes pacing at sites of late LV mechanical activation.[16,17] These important studies demonstrated the value of directing pacing based on measures of late contraction. However, they did not gain wide clinical adoption, likely because of the challenges of reliably performing speckle tracking, the resources needed to do these measurements, and the challenges of translating echo images to fluoroscopic views of the coronary sinus venous system. Subsequently, focus turned to electrical measures of dyssynchrony. Specifically, measures of intraventricular and interventricular conduction delay were evaluated as an alternative assessment of mechanical activation patterns. This chapter focuses on such measures, which are now

Department of Medicine, Medical University of South Carolina, 25 Courtenay Drive, MS-492, Charleston, SC 29425, USA

[1] Signifies co-first authorship

* Corresponding author. Division of Cardiology, MUSC, 25 Courtenay Drive, MS-492, Charleston, SC 29425.
E-mail address: goldmr@musc.edu

Card Electrophysiol Clin 14 (2022) 233–241
https://doi.org/10.1016/j.ccep.2021.12.013

commonly used in CRT implantation and incorporated in many commercial devices.

MEASURES OF ELECTRICAL DELAY AND AN ELECTRICAL DELAY–ORIENTED STRATEGY

A CRT strategy focused on electrical delay is based on the principle of electromechanical coupling: pacing in the area with the greatest delayed activation improves electrical and mechanical synchrony.[18] The ability to identify electrical delay by noninvasive and invasive markers could help with both patient selection for CRT and optimal LV lead location. Simple markers based on the surface electrocardiogram (ECG) such as the QRSd were initially chosen. Although this remains the part of the standard criteria in clinical practice guidelines for CRT patient selection,[19] studies showed that QRSd does not always correlate with mechanical dyssynchrony. For example, even patients with normal QRSd may have mechanical dyssynchrony,[20] yet in these patients, CRT is associated with harm.[21] Similarly, many patients with a wide QRSd in an right bundle branch block (RBBB) pattern do not have mechanical dyssynchrony, but others do, so therefore a better measure of electrical dyssynchrony was needed.[22] As was later discovered, the delay in left ventricular activation interval (QLV) or interventricular activation interval (RV-LV) are associated with CRT response, even after adjusting for QRSd or morphology.[23,24] As a result, alternative measures of electrical delay were studied using the combination of surface and intracardiac electrocardiographic measures of electrical activation.

Compared with the initiation of the QRS on the surface ECG, electrical delay may occur with activation of the LV, right ventricle (RV), or both ventricles. QRSd is a surface electrocardiographic marker of electrical delay. The QLV interval is defined as the time from the onset of QRS on surface ECG until the first major peak of LV activation on the LV lead electrogram (EGM) or the time it takes for the ventricular electrical wavefront to reach the LV pacing site.[23,25] This interval can be measured as either an absolute duration or as the QLV ratio, which is the QLV as a percentage of the QRS duration.[18] The QRV interval is defined as the time between the onset of QRS on surface ECG until RV activation on RV lead EGM or the time it takes for the ventricular electrical wavefront to reach the RV pacing site.[25] The RV-LV interval is defined as the time between LV and RV activation on the LV and RV leads in the same QRS complex or the delay in ventricular activation between the RV and LV pacing sites[25];this is also the difference between QLV and QRV and may be measured during spontaneous native rhythm or during pacing.[26] Representative measurements of the QLV, QRV, and RV-LV intervals on EGM are shown in **Fig. 1**.

Despite the physiologic principles underlying electrical delay in CRT pacing, the electromechanical relationship in ventricular dyssynchrony is still not fully understood. Mechanical dyssynchrony due to delayed electrical activation of the left ventricle is the target of CRT. However, electromechanical uncoupling can occur in cardiomyopathies, such as regional differences in contractile or diastolic properties of the ventricular myocardium.[27] As noted previously, CRT pacing in

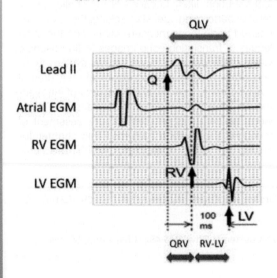

QLV, RV-LV and QRV Interval Measurement

Fig. 1. Example of RV-LV, QLV, and QRV measurements, measured from the onset of the QRS complex on ECG to the first positive or negative peak in the left ventricular EGM. The RV-LV is always shorter than the QLV, as the RV electrogram comes after the onset of the QRS complex. The QRV is also the difference between the QLV and RV-LV. (*From* Field, M. E., et al. "Comparison of measures of ventricular delay on cardiac resynchronization therapy response." Heart Rhythm 2020; 17(4): 615-620; with permission. (Figure 1 in original).)

mechanical dyssynchrony without delayed activation may cause harm.[21] As such, although electrical activation time correlates well with peak mechanical ventricular contraction, more heterogeneity exists when accounting for mechanical dyssynchrony.[28] Accounting for regional variations in electromechanical decoupling in CRT pacing, on an individual and widespread level, is still being studied. In addition, more complex measures of electrical activation are being tested in clinical studies using body surface mapping rather than simply a single measure at the site of the LV pacing electrode.[29]

COMPARISON OF ELECTRICAL DELAY MEASURES

Direct comparisons of electrical delay are limited in the literature. Both QLV and QLV ratio (QLV/QRSd) show similar impacts on outcomes and have not been evaluated in comparison. Comparison between QLV and RV-LV was studied as a part of the SMART-AV trial.[25] In this study of 419 patients with a mean QRSd of 150 ms (75% left bundle branch block [LBBB]), with LV lead location placed without electrical delay guidance, QLV and RV-LV intervals were highly correlated with each other and CRT response independently (defined as reduction in left ventricular end-systolic volume [LVESV] $\geq$ 15%), but only RL-LV was associated with CRT response on multivariate analysis.[25] QRV was highly correlated with presence of RBBB and CRT nonresponse.[25] There was a signal for added benefit of increased QLV in patients with decreased RV-LV.[25] Finally, this study showed that specific measures of electrical delay were correlated with conduction delay patterns present on the surface ECG. In patients with LBBB, QLV and RV-LV were similarly predictive of CRT response; in patients with intraventricular conduction delay (IVCD), RV-LV and QRV were predictive of CRT response; in patients with RBBB, only QRV was predictive of response.[25]

The results of the SMART-AV trial suggest that the location and duration of electrical delay is pivotal for improving response to CRT. RV-LV duration is most highly correlated with response to CRT in this study, likely due to the parameter itself and the predominant LBBB population in the cohort. RV-LV duration is unaffected by the QRV interval. However, QLV is the sum of RV-LV + QRV. Because RV-LV depends on both LV and RV lead positions, both leads can be adjusted to increase the RV-LV interval during device implantation. Whether repositioning the RV lead to increase interventricular delay will improve response has not been studied. Furthermore,

because RV-LV is measured entirely from intracardiac electrograms, device algorithms for measurement and optimization continue to be evaluated. Finally, in patients with increased QRSd, morphology of conduction delay pattern (LBBB, IVCD, RBBB) may be important in helping to determine which markers of electrical delay to measure and optimize.

In addition, the ability to optimize the benefit of prolonged electrical delay may be enhanced by selecting the electrode configuration on a quadripolar lead with the longest electrical delay, assuming that there are adequate pacing characteristics with that vector. It has been shown that the odds ratio for a CRT reverse remodeling response (>15% reduction in left ventricular end systolic volume index) increased about 11.3% for every 10 msec increase in RV-LV duration.[30] In CRT patients, both QLV and RV-LV durations were longer in the proximal versus distal pair of electrodes in patients with LBBB and highly correlated,[31] such that the additional prolongation afforded by using the proximal electrode pair over the distal electrode pair would be expected to improve the response rate for CRT reverse remodeling by about 10%. In patients without LBBB conduction delay, RV-LV but not QLV, was increased in the proximal pair of electrodes, and RV-LV and QLV poorly correlated, suggesting greater variance in this population.[31]

IMPACT ON ACUTE AND LONG-TERM OUTCOMES

A considerable percentage of patients receiving CRT fail to respond hemodynamically or clinically by traditional cutoff values of response.[32] More recent studies have challenged the value of dichotomizing CRT response metrics and instead have focused on maximizing response.[5,33] Nevertheless, a suboptimal response is multifactorial in cause, attributed to preprocedural selection criteria, intraprocedural implantation techniques, postprocedural programming variations, and quality of follow-up care. Improving CRT response continues to be an essential goal. There are several studies that have evaluated the association of electrical delay on CRT response.

HEMODYNAMICS RESPONSE

CRT seems most beneficial in patients with abnormal baseline ventricular electrical activation and reduced LV contractility (evidenced by dP/dt_{max}), and correspondingly, the magnitude of change in dP/dt_{max} begets the acute impact of CRT on global systolic function.[34] In this regard, measures of electrical delay (QLV, RV-LV) are associated with improved acute hemodynamic response, independent of pacing mode.[30] QLV correlates directly with acute hemodynamic changes. Simple measures such as baseline QRSd or postpacing QRS shortening do not translate into either acute or long-term hemodynamic benefit.[35] Several metrics of increased LV contractility (%LV dP/dt$_{max}$, %SW) have been evaluated in relation to electrical delay optimization.[11,23,36,37] A QLV interval of greater than or equal to 95 ms is associated with greater CRT response rates[38] and furthermore is highly predictive of increases in contractility, of between 10%[36] and greater than or equal to 25%.[18] Larger responses are observed in the nonischemic cardiomyopathies. Further multivariate analyses have shown that with biventricular pacing, QLV is an independent predictor of hemodynamic response, with a 1.7% increase in %LV dP/dt$_{max}$ for every 10 ms prolongation of QLV, independent of pacing modality.[30] In the era of quadripolar LV leads, this relationship has become more complex. Although maximizing electrical delay (QLV, RV-LV) is associated with advantageous hemodynamic responses and may be used for optimal anatomic quadripolar LV lead placement, it does not predict the specific quadripolar lead electrode with the largest hemodynamic response (as defined by %SW) on an individual patient level.[37]

MIDTERM AND LONG-TERM OUTCOMES

Comprehensive data for the association of QLV and long-term CRT outcomes have also been studied. A strong relationship is noted across a variety of measures including reverse remodeling endpoints (eg, LVESV, left ventricular end-diastolic volume, left ventricular ejection fraction [LVEF]), CRT response, and clinical events including quality-of-life (QOL) metrics.

Increased QLV (≥40% native QRSd) predicts long-term event-free survival among patients with ischemic and nonischemic cardiomyopathy receiving CRT and even patients with anatomically suboptimal lead positioning.[18] QLV is strongly associated with advantageous reverse remodeling, specifically LVESV (>15% reduction in LVESV), and QOL metrics, as shown in **Fig. 2**. A QLV value of greater than or equal to 95 ms seems optimal based on receiver operating characteristic analysis for LVESV and QOL. Longer QLV have a 3.2-fold increase in odds of a reverse remodeling response after correcting for QRSd, bundle branch block type, and clinical characteristics by multivariate logistic regression analysis.[23] Many other studies have validated this relationship.[18,26,39] LV

electric delay correlates with the composite clinical endpoint of time to first HF hospitalization and the composite outcome of all-cause mortality, HF hospitalization, LV assist device implantation, and cardiac transplantation at 3 years.[40]

Improving response in the population of patients without an LBBB remains a challenge. Most large clinical trial have only a minority of patients without LBBB, so identifying strategies to improve efficacy in this population is limited. Limited data exist for improving outcomes from large randomized clinical trials on CRT effectiveness in patients without LBBB. The potential for using an implantation strategy to select an LV lead location based on intraprocedural QLV measurement in patients without LBBB was studied in the ENHANCE-CRT study.[41] This study was a prospective, randomized trial of 248 patients that evaluated an electrical delay (QLV)-oriented approach versus conventional anatomic approach to LV lead implantation, for the primary endpoint of a clinical composite score (NYHA functional class, patient global assessment, HF events, and cardiovascular death). All patients had a QRS greater than or equal to 120 ms with a non-LBBB morphology, received a quadripolar LV lead, and were followed for an average of 12 months postimplantation. The ENHANCE-CRT study revealed marked improvement in clinical composite score, QOL, and LVEF predominantly in patients with NYHA III HF with severely reduced LVEF and non-LBBB prolonged QRSd. However, differences in outcomes between an electrical delay–oriented strategy versus conventional anatomic approach were nonsignificant: primary clinical compositive score (67% vs 73%, respectively) and secondary QOL score (18.6 vs 19.4, respectively) or LVEF (6.0% vs 6.9%, respectively). The high response rate in this cohort was surprising and supports the practice of implanting selective patients without LBBB. The lack of benefit in the QLV arm may reflect the relatively short QLV intervals in this cohort (mean 87.7 ms). Roubiceck and colleagues[42] revealed the direct relationship between QLV and QLV ratio and clinical CRT response; QLV durations in the ENHANCE CRT study would have fallen in the lowest Roubicek's QLV tertiles. In addition, despite the different approaches (electrical delay vs anatomic) to which patients were randomized in this study, there was substantial overlap in the final anatomic locations in both study arms, predominantly in the lateral (51% QLV, 59% control) region. Finally, the patient population studied may have played a role. The large proportion of patients with QRSd less than 150 ms likely contributed to the shorter QLV durations, as well as the large proportion of patients

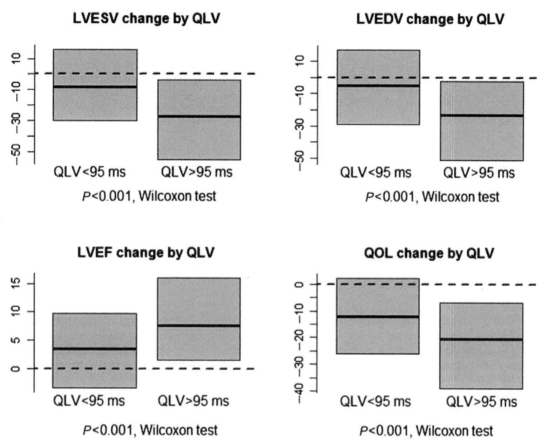

Fig. 2. Comparison of the changes in left ventricular end systolic volume, end-diastolic volume, ejection fraction, and quality of life from implant baseline to 6 months for the 2 QLV groups separated by median value ± inter-quartile range. (*From* Gold, M. R., et al. "The relationship between ventricular electrical delay and left ventricular remodelling with cardiac resynchronization therapy." Eur Heart J 2011; **32**(20): 2516-2524; with permission. (Figure 2 in original).)

with RBBB. Finally, QLV (as opposed to RV-LV, QRV) may be an incomplete metric of electrical delay in these patients.[25]

Longer-term outcomes using LV-RV as a marker of electrical delay have also been studied. In a post hoc analysis of the Pacing Evaluation-Atrial SUpport Study (PEGASUS) trial, RV-LV duration (eg, a longer intraventricular delay) is also a strong predictor of CRT clinical response, QOL, clinical composite score, and the composite of HF hospitalization and mortality. An RV-LV greater than the median duration (≥67 ms) is associated with improved HF-free survival, visualized in the Kaplan-Meier curve in **Fig. 3**, as well as death or HF hospitalizations, via spline analysis as shown in **Fig. 4**.[24] On further evaluation, when separated by quartiles based on interventricular delay, the magnitudes of LV volumes (LVESV 30% to 75%), LVEF, and the QOL measure (50% to 65% improved response rates) increased significantly with prolongation of RV-LV delay. Patients in the

highest quartile of RV-LV had a 6-fold increase in their odds of a reverse remodeling response, with female sex, ischemic cause, and baseline LV end-systolic volume being the other independent predictors of response.[30]

Interestingly, this association was not limited to traditional parameters of CRT success (LBBB; QRS ≥150 ms) but also translated to patients without LBBB or QRS less than 150 ms. In total, irrespective of QRSd or conduction disorder type, RV-LV duration remains an independent predictor of response and supports the strategy of evaluating and maximizing RV-LV intervals to improve clinical outcomes.[24]

PROGRAMMING CONSIDERATIONS

Most current AV optimization algorithms are designed to achieve fusion of LV paced complexes with intrinsic conduction. For several of the algorithms, the RV-LV duration is used in part

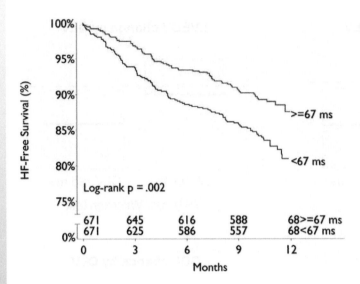

Fig. 3. Heart failure-free survival stratified by long and short RV-LV groups over 12 months. (*From* Gold, M. R., et al. "The role of interventricular conduction delay to predict clinical response with cardiac resynchronization therapy." Heart Rhythm 2017; **14**(12): 1748-1755; with permission. (Figure 3 in original).)

to decide on ventricular pacing chamber. A long RV-LV time is a surrogate for LBBB, so LV-only pacing is used, whereas a negative RV-LV time indicates RBBB and a short RV-LV time may represent an IVCD. In these scenarios, biventricular pacing is used. The Smart CRT trial is a prospective, randomized study comparing the Smart Delay algorithm with normal AV delays in patients with a prolonged AV delay. All patients are required to have an interventricular delay on at least one LV

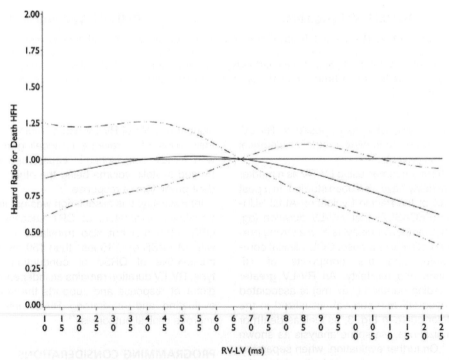

Fig. 4. Spline analysis of the relationship between the RV-LV interval and the hazard ratio for death or HFH. The response was normalized for the median RV-LV interval of 67 ms, and the model was adjusted for age, sex, NYHA class, QRS morphology, duration, LEVF, LV lead location, and HF cause. (*From* Gold, M. R., et al. "The role of interventricular conduction delay to predict clinical response with cardiac resynchronization therapy." Heart Rhythm 2017; **14**(12): 1748-1755; with permission. (Figure 4 in original).)

electrode greater than 70 ms, as longer RV-LV delays are associated with better response to an optimization algorithm to achieve fusion of paced and intrinsic activation.[43–45]

SUMMARY

Improving CRT response remains a priority for this therapy. Strategies include better patient selection, optimizing implant strategies, programming, and follow-up. Fundamentally, the target of resynchronization is stimulating the area of electrical delay, and indeed clinical trial data support that LV pacing at sites of prolonged electrical delay, assessed by the QLV and RV-LV, are associated with improved CRT response. Particular challenges remain, including identifying how to optimize the approach to patients without LBBB or those with other markers of poor response such as history of prior myocardial infarction. Additional opportunities for improvement include using noninvasive mapping technology to guide lead placement, vector selection, and device programming, as well as novel approaches for endocardial pacing of the left ventricle.

CLINICS CARE POINTS

- A long QLV or RV-LV interval are associated with robust acute hemodynamic and long-term outcomes of CRT response. Cutoffs of 95 msec and 67 msec showed strong responses.

- Improving CRT response in non-LBBB patterns remains a challenge; however, in both LBBB and non-LBBB patients, RV-LV was an independent predictor of improved outcomes.

- Use of proximal versus distal pairs of electrodes on quadripolar leads often affords longer measurements of electrical delay and therefore improved response to CRT.

REFERENCES

1. Abraham WT, Fisher WG, Smith AL, et al. Cardiac resynchronization in chronic heart failure. N Engl J Med 2002;346(24):1845–53.
2. Bristow MR, Saxon LA, Boehmer J, et al. Cardiac-resynchronization therapy with or without an implantable defibrillator in advanced chronic heart failure. N Engl J Med 2004;350(21):2140–50.
3. Cazeau S, Leclercq C, Lavergne T, et al. Effects of multisite biventricular pacing in patients with heart failure and intraventricular conduction delay. N Engl J Med 2001;344(12):873–80.
4. Cleland JG, Daubert JC, Erdmann E, et al. The effect of cardiac resynchronization on morbidity and mortality in heart failure. N Engl J Med 2005;352(15):1539–49.
5. Gold MR, Rickard J, Daubert JC, et al. Redefining the classifications of response to cardiac resynchronization therapy: results from the REVERSE study. JACC Clin Electrophysiol 2021;7(7):871–80.
6. Moss AJ, Hall WJ, Cannom DS, et al. Cardiac-resynchronization therapy for the prevention of heart-failure events. N Engl J Med 2009;361(14):1329–38.
7. Ypenburg C, van Bommel RJ, Borleffs CJ, et al. Long-term prognosis after cardiac resynchronization therapy is related to the extent of left ventricular reverse remodeling at midterm follow-up. J Am Coll Cardiol 2009;53(6):483–90.
8. Linde C, Abraham WT, Gold MR, et al. Predictors of short-term clinical response to cardiac resynchronization therapy. Eur J Heart Fail 2017;19(8):1056–63.
9. Rickard J, Michtalik H, Sharma R, et al. Predictors of response to cardiac resynchronization therapy: a systematic review. Int J Cardiol 2016;225:345–52.
10. Butter C, Auricchio A, Stellbrink C, et al. Effect of resynchronization therapy stimulation site on the systolic function of heart failure patients. Circulation 2001;104(25):3026–9.
11. Singh JP, Klein HU, Huang DT, et al. Left ventricular lead position and clinical outcome in the multicenter automatic defibrillator implantation trial-cardiac resynchronization therapy (MADIT-CRT) trial. Circulation 2011;123(11):1159–66.
12. Thebault C, Donal E, Meunier C, et al. Sites of left and right ventricular lead implantation and response to cardiac resynchronization therapy observations from the REVERSE trial. Eur Heart J 2012;33(21):2662–71.
13. Saxon LA, Olshansky B, Volosin K, et al. Influence of left ventricular lead location on outcomes in the COMPANION study. J Cardiovasc Electrophysiol 2009;20(7):764–8.
14. Bleeker GB, Kaandorp TA, Lamb HJ, et al. Effect of posterolateral scar tissue on clinical and echocardiographic improvement after cardiac resynchronization therapy. Circulation 2006;113(7):969–76.
15. Ypenburg C, van Bommel RJ, Delgado V, et al. Optimal left ventricular lead position predicts reverse remodeling and survival after cardiac resynchronization therapy. J Am Coll Cardiol 2008;52(17):1402–9.
16. Khan FZ, Virdee MS, Palmer CR, et al. Targeted left ventricular lead placement to guide cardiac resynchronization therapy: the TARGET study: a randomized, controlled trial. J Am Coll Cardiol 2012;59(17):1509–18.
17. Saba S, Marek J, Schwartzman D, et al. Echocardiography-guided left ventricular lead placement for cardiac resynchronization therapy: results of the

Speckle Tracking Assisted Resynchronization Therapy for Electrode Region trial. Circ Heart Fail 2013; 6(3):427–34.

18. Singh JP, Fan D, Heist EK, et al. Left ventricular lead electrical delay predicts response to cardiac resynchronization therapy. Heart Rhythm 2006;3(11): 1285–92.

19. Writing Group M, Tracy CM, Epstein AE, et al. 2012 ACCF/AHA/HRS focused update of the 2008 guidelines for device-based therapy of cardiac rhythm abnormalities: a report of the American College of Cardiology Foundation/American Heart Association Task Force on Practice Guidelines. J Thorac Cardiovasc Surg 2012;144(6):e127–45.

20. Yu CM, Sanderson JE, Marwick TH, et al. Tissue Doppler imaging a new prognosticator for cardiovascular diseases. J Am Coll Cardiol 2007;49(19): 1903–14.

21. Ruschitzka F, Abraham WT, Singh JP, et al. Cardiac-resynchronization therapy in heart failure with a narrow QRS complex. N Engl J Med 2013;369(15): 1395–405.

22. Hara H, Oyenuga OA, Tanaka H, et al. The relationship of QRS morphology and mechanical dyssynchrony to long-term outcome following cardiac resynchronization therapy. Eur Heart J 2012;33(21):2680–91.

23. Gold MR, Birgersdotter-Green U, Singh JP, et al. The relationship between ventricular electrical delay and left ventricular remodelling with cardiac resynchronization therapy. Eur Heart J 2011;32(20):2516–24.

24. Gold MR, Yu Y, Wold N, et al. The role of interventricular conduction delay to predict clinical response with cardiac resynchronization therapy. Heart Rhythm 2017;14(12):1748–55.

25. Field ME, Yu N, Wold N, et al. Comparison of measures of ventricular delay on cardiac resynchronization therapy response. Heart Rhythm 2020;17(4): 615–20.

26. Sassone B, Gabrieli L, Saccà S, et al. Value of right ventricular-left ventricular interlead electrical delay to predict reverse remodelling in cardiac resynchronization therapy: the INTER-V pilot study. Europace 2010;12(1):78–83.

27. Kass DA. An epidemic of dyssynchrony: but what does it mean? J Am Coll Cardiol 2008;51(1):12–7.

28. Mafi-Rad M, Van't Sant J, Blaauw Y, et al. Regional left ventricular electrical activation and peak contraction are closely related in candidates for cardiac resynchronization therapy. JACC Clin Electrophysiol 2017;3(8):854–62.

29. Rickard J, Jackson K, Biffi M, et al. The ECG Belt for CRT response trial: design and clinical protocol. Pacing Clin Electrophysiol 2020;43(10):1063–71.

30. Gold MR, Singh JP, Ellenbogen KA, et al. Interventricular electrical delay is predictive of response to cardiac resynchronization therapy. JACC Clin Electrophysiol 2016;2(4):438–47.

31. Koerber SM, Field ME, Cobb DB, et al. Electrical delays in quadripolar leads with cardiac resynchronization therapy. J Cardiovasc Electrophysiol 2021; 32(9):2498–503.

32. Yu CM, Bleeker GB, Fung JW, et al. Left ventricular reverse remodeling but not clinical improvement predicts long-term survival after cardiac resynchronization therapy. Circulation 2005;112(11):1580–6.

33. Mullens W, Auricchio A, Martens P, et al. Optimized implementation of cardiac resynchronization therapy: a call for action for referral and optimization of care: a joint position statement from the Heart Failure Association (HFA), European Heart Rhythm Association (EHRA), and European Association of Cardiovascular Imaging (EACVI) of the European Society of Cardiology. Eur J Heart Fail 2020;22(12):2349–69.

34. Kolias TJ, Aaronson KD, Armstrong WF. Doppler-derived dP/dt and -dP/dt predict survival in congestive heart failure. J Am Coll Cardiol 2000;36(5): 1594–9.

35. Molhoek SG, VAN Erven L, Bootsma M, et al. QRS duration and shortening to predict clinical response to cardiac resynchronization therapy in patients with end-stage heart failure. Pacing Clin Electrophysiol 2004;27(3):308–13.

36. Zanon F, Baracca E, Pastore G, et al. Determination of the longest intrapatient left ventricular electrical delay may predict acute hemodynamic improvement in patients after cardiac resynchronization therapy. Circ Arrhythm Electrophysiol 2014;7(3): 377–83.

37. van Everdingen WM, Zweerink A, Cramer MJ, et al. Can we use the intrinsic left ventricular delay (QLV) to optimize the pacing configuration for cardiac resynchronization therapy with a quadripolar left ventricular lead? Circ Arrhythm Electrophysiol 2018; 11(3):e005912.

38. Ellenbogen KA, Gold MR, Meyer TE, et al. Primary results from the SmartDelay determined AV optimization: a comparison to other AV delay methods used in cardiac resynchronization therapy (SMART-AV) trial: a randomized trial comparing empirical, echocardiography-guided, and algorithmic atrioventricular delay programming in cardiac resynchronization therapy. Circulation 2010;122(25):2660–8.

39. Yagishita D, Shoda M, Yagishita Y, et al. Time interval from left ventricular stimulation to QRS onset is a novel predictor of nonresponse to cardiac resynchronization therapy. Heart Rhythm 2019;16(3): 395–402.

40. Kandala J, Upadhyay GA, Altman RK, et al. QRS morphology, left ventricular lead location, and clinical outcome in patients receiving cardiac resynchronization therapy. Eur Heart J 2013;34(29): 2252–62.

41. Singh JP, Berger RD, Doshi RN, et al. Targeted left ventricular lead implantation strategy for non-left

bundle branch block patients: the ENHANCE CRT study. JACC Clin Electrophysiol 2020;6(9):1171–81.

42. Roubicek T, Wichterle D, Kucera P, et al. Left ventricular lead electrical delay is a predictor of mortality in patients with cardiac resynchronization therapy. Circ Arrhythm Electrophysiol 2015;8(5):1113–21.

43. Gold MR, Auricchio A, Leclercq C, et al. The rationale and design of the SMART CRT trial. Pacing Clin Electrophysiol 2018;41(9):1212–6.

44. Gold MR, Yu Y, Singh JP, et al. Effect of interventricular electrical delay on atrioventricular optimization for cardiac resynchronization therapy. Circ Arrhythm Electrophysiol 2018;11(8):e006055.

45. Gold MR, Yu Y, Singh JP, et al. The effect of left ventricular electrical delay on AV optimization for cardiac resynchronization therapy. Heart Rhythm 2013;10(7):988–93.

Programming Algorithms for Cardiac Resynchronization Therapy

Niraj Varma, MA, MD, PhD, FRCP

KEYWORDS

- Cardiac resynchronization therapy • Electrical dyssynchrony • Left bundle branch block
- Programming • Algorithms

KEY POINTS

- Cardiac resynchronization therapy (CRT) is an effective therapy for patients with heart failure (HF) with electrical dyssynchrony, but almost 30% of patients do not gain benefit.
- Increased probability and degree of response to CRT may require improved delivery of pacing therapy, but device-based algorithms have not been effective. This may be because these algorithms have been incomplete.
- A strategy of electrically optimizing pacing prescription on an individualized basis and accommodating ambulatory physiologic variations in AV interval may increase CRT efficacy (SyncAV CRT).

INTRODUCTION/HISTORY/DEFINITIONS/BACKGROUND

Cardiac resynchronization therapy (CRT) is an electrical therapy designed with the objective of correcting delayed LV activation among patients with heart failure (HF) with dyssynchrony thereby improving hemodynamic function.[1] This has been shown to suppress HF decompensation and improve patient survival which are important clinical outcomes. However, CRT benefit is not uniform and patient responses vary.[2,3] This in part may be due to incomplete electrical resynchronization. Methods to improve and maintain the quality of delivered CRT are needed. There is recent awareness that therapy has to be patient individualized. This requires attention to both electrical substrate (ie the disease being treated) and prescription of appropriate pacing therapies. Novel technologies may offer solutions.

The target condition is the electrical substrate created by the left bundle branch block (LBBB; **Fig. 1**).[4] Important features to note are intact right bundle branch (RBB), transseptal conduction delay, but normal (ie rapid) left ventricular (LV)-free wall activation. Ventricular resynchronization is traditionally restored with atrio-biventricular pacing that is, atrial, right ventricular (RV), and LV leads (**Fig. 2**). These components merit individual discussion.

Right Ventricular Pacing in Cardiac Resynchronization Therapy

RV pacing alone was deleterious among patients with HF.[5] This has led to a debate about the role of RV pacing in CRT. A result was the production of a device-based pacing algorithm that sought to minimize RV pacing during CRT (AdaptivCRT, **Table 1**).[6] When tested in a trial, it seemed to be noninferior to traditional biventricular pacing seeming to indicate the RV pacing was unnecessary. Although this may apply to small cohort studies with restricted selection criteria (see later in discussion), some individuals may benefit from the inclusion of RV pacing (ie biventricular pacing). This is because RV stimulation exerts variable effects in patients with HF with LBBB, some of which may facilitate biventricular resynchronization.[7,8] Although committing left ventricular activation

Funding: This study received no funding
Heart and Vascular Institute, Cleveland Clinic, Cleveland, OH 44195, USA
E-mail address: Varman@ccf.org

Card Electrophysiol Clin 14 (2022) 243–252
https://doi.org/10.1016/j.ccep.2021.12.018
1877-9182/22/© 2021 Elsevier Inc. All rights reserved.

A ECG

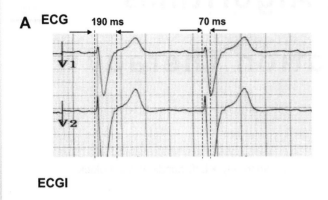

ECGI

B

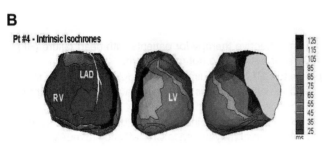

Pt #4 - Intrinsic Isochrones

Fig. 1. Electrical characteristics of LBBB. Representative ECG and ECGI maps during intrinsic conduction in a heart failure patient with ischemic cardiomyopathy (LVEF 35%) and preserved atrioventricular conduction with LBBB. (*A*) ECG. The QRS duration is 190 ms. In V1 and V2, the rS wave duration of 70 ms indicates rapid intrinsic forces that is, the rapid development of myocardial activation wavefront via intact right bundle branch conduction. (*B*) Ventricular activation map using electrocardiographic imaging (ECGI: algorithmic transformation of body surface electrograms using a multi-electrode vest to visually depict biventricular epicardial isochronal activation) maps of epicardial surfaces of both ventricles are displayed in 3 views: anterior (AP) which depicts the free wall of the RV, left lateral (LAO 90), and posterior (PA) projections. There is overlap between adjacent views. The left anterior descending (LAD) coronary artery is marked for orientation (scale: isochrones marked from QRS onset). RV epicardial free wall breakthrough (*) occurs laterally within 25 ms of QRS onset. Following this, RV activation is even and rapid (indicated by widely spaced isochrones) and occurs in a radial fashion. Free wall depolarization is largely completed within 45 ms of QRS onset. Following RV activation, the left ventricle is depolarized from apex to base. Thick black markings indicate line/region of conduction slowing in the septum. (*From* Varma N, Jia P, Ramanathan C, Rudy Y. RV electrical activation in heart failure during right, left, and biventricular pacing. JACC Cardiovasc Imaging. 2010;3(6):567-575. https://doi.org/10.1016/j.jcmg.2009.12.017; with permission)

totally to RV stimulation likely underlies the detrimental effects seen among patients with LBBB and LV dysfunction, some initial components of RV stimulation-specifically septal activation-may be useful to CRT (**Fig. 3**A) (see later in discussion).

Left Ventricular Pacing in Cardiac Resynchronization Therapy

LV pacing is the core component of CRT. Its purpose is to preexcite the LV, timed to RV activation to restore biventricular synchrony. Although conceptualized to restore confluent LV depolarization (see **Fig. 3**B) this rarely occurs[9]-instead LV paced effects are highly variable (see **Figs. 3** and **4**). LV epicardial stimulation does not replicate rapid intrinsic conduction even in normal ventricles.[10] In diseased hearts, wavefront propagation may be further retarded by scar and LV enlargement.[11,12] Paced responses to LV stimulation varies from patient to patient and can vary dramatically in an individual patient with a minor change in position of LV stimulation[13–16] (**Fig. 4**). This unpredictability may limit the ability to effectively pace, let alone restore biventricular resynchronization,

and needs to be accounted for during device programming.

The importance of paced effect was shown by reduction in CRT efficacy when LV pacing resulted in slow LV activation (eg, from scar) manifesting with wide paced QRS (>200 ms) or by the prolongation of transventricular activation time (measured by LV paced to RV sensed interval).[17,18] These challenges may be mitigated by multipolar LV leads.[19] Not only do these improve the success of achieving acceptable pacing thresholds and avoiding PNS[19] but also permit electrical optimization by the selection of most effective pacing vector (see **Fig. 4**).[20] Further, pacing from 2 electrodes simultaneously (multipoint pacing (see later in discussion)) may "jump" conduction barriers or increased the span of ventricular stimulation.[21] This may be useful in LV enlargement[22] (**Fig. 5**).

Atrioventricular Interval in Cardiac Resynchronization Therapy

The role of the atrial lead is traditionally to maintain atrioventricular (AV) synchrony and atrial support

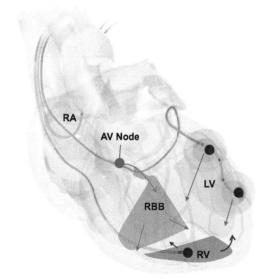

Fig. 2. Interplay of propagated wavefronts during CRT. Schematic showing the 3 pacing components of CRT. The atrial lead permits timing with ventricular pacing and thereby contribution of RBB mediated depolarization. RV pacing may mitigate the transseptal conduction barrier created by LBBB. The LV lead is used to preexcite delayed LV activation and its paced effects may be promoted by using multipolar leads (a quadripolar lead is depicted here). The term "triple fusion" refers to the incorporation of all 3 elements together during CRT delivery.

pacing similarly to its role during DDD pacing for pacemakers. However, control of the AV interval fulfills another important role in CRT when the RBB is intact by determining the degree of RBB mediated ventricular depolarization (see **Fig. 1**).[23] This is illustrated by the demonstration of the "fusion band." During biventricular (or left ventricular) pacing, the AV interval is set to minimal (typically 20–30 ms) then progressively elongated until intrinsic conduction supervenes.[24] Typically the QRS duration narrows then prolongs indicating various levels of fusion of biventricular (or LV) paced wavefronts with RBB-mediated activation. The AV interval providing the narrowest QRS may be considered the optimized AV interval. This highlights another challenge. The intrinsic AV conduction normally is subject to ambulatory variations in response to natural changes in physiologic and autonomic conditions.[25] These variations may upset optimized settings that have been so carefully selected and programmed at rest. Accommodating these and preserving optimized settings requires a device-based solution. Automated dynamic control dramatically improves the "quality" of delivered CRT.[26,27]

DISCUSSION

Coordinating these multiple and variegate effects to produce an optimized CRT prescription is complex, particularly as it has to be tailored to each individual (see **Fig. 3**). Hence, devices commonly are left at nominal settings, irrespective of intrinsic AV and/or interventricular (VV) intervals.[28] However, there is an advantage in achieving postimplant electrical optimization. Studies deliberately targeting electrical resynchronization (eg, QRS narrowing) as a goal showed changes in acute hemodynamics or chronic ventricular reverse remodeling superior to echocardiographic optimization or nominal device settings.[23,24,29–31] Nevertheless, this still requires significant operator input. An automatic device-based algorithm to manage this entire range of variations in substrate and paced effects is appealing. However, most incorporate some but not all the required features and apply a "one size fits all" solution. Unsurprisingly, these algorithms have yielded neutral results (see **Table 1**). They are briefly reviewed later in discussion.

Device-Based Algorithms

SMART delay integrates intrinsic AV intervals, QRS duration, and LV lead location.[32] Correlation between maximal achievable hemodynamic response (% change in LV dP/dt$_{max}$) and the AV delay predicted by the algorithm was excellent in acute studies. However, the algorithm did not result in chronically improved outcomes when tested in a randomized trial.[33] The reason may be that despite promoting electrical resynchronization, SMART Delay exerts no control over changing AV intervals which can lead to variable LV capture.[26]

The AdaptivCRT algorithm seeks to promote the fusion of LV activation during LV pacing with RBB activation of the RV. It aims to achieve this by pacing at a predetermined fraction (approx. 70%) of the intrinsic AV interval, and maintaining this by recalibrating the AV interval every 56 beats after reevaluating intrinsic conduction.[6] This dynamic control was successful in maintaining effective LV capture.[26] However, the algorithm was noninferior to standard biventricular pacing in a randomized trial.[6] Similarly, the event-driven AdaptResponse trial has not finished despite several years of follow-up (due to the lack of events) suggesting equipoise.[34] The reasons for this may be multiple. The algorithm is restricted to patients with LBBB and PR interval less than 200 ms (ie, a CRT group already with better prognosis). It may have no advantage when QRS duration is >150 ms.[35] This is because the main source

Table 1
Automatic device-based CRT algorithms

	QuickOpt (SJM)	SmartDelay (BSC)	AdaptivCRT (MDT)	SyncAV (Abbott)
Basis	IEGM	IEGM	IEGM	IEGM
Programmability (AV/VV)	√	X	X	√
Dynamic (Ambulatory)	X	X	√ (per minute)	√ (every 256 beats)
Trial	FREEDOM	SMART-AV	AdaptivCRT	SyncAV
Safety	√	√	√	Pending
Efficacy	NON-INFERIOR vs Empiric	EQUIVALENT vs ECHO-guided or Empiric	NON-INFERIOR vs Echo BiV	Pending

of LV delay in LBBB is intraseptal conduction delay-based and maintained (and not resolved) by RBB activation (see **Fig. 1**). On the other hand, this barrier may be mitigated by the initial effects of RV pacing-that is, biventricular pacing is more effective (see **Figs. 3**A and **6**).[36] Results of fusion optimization have shown that LV only fusion pacing is best in only a minority and that the AV interval that best delivers this varies among individuals with LBBB.[24] Thus, the main limitations of this algorithm are that it does not permit individual programming of the AV interval, nor the inclusion of RV pacing with LV pacing (or interventricular timing) and thus fails to deliver individualized electrical optimization.

SyncAV

As past data indicate that a universal programmed strategy (eg, nominal, LV fusion, etc[6]) may have limited value, the SyncAV algorithm was designed to enable *both* electrical optimization and dynamic AV interval control. Delivery of electrical optimization can be patiently individualized by permitting BiV or LV pacing as required, in patients with PR intervals up to 300 ms[37]. At the same time, these optimized settings may be preserved with the

automatic dynamic AV control feature. Briefly, SyncAV functions as follows. Every 256 beats, the algorithm automatically extends the paced and sensed AV delay for 3 beats, during which it measures the intrinsic AV interval. With the default SyncAV offset, 50 ms is subtracted from the measured intrinsic AV interval, and the result is applied as the paced AV interval for the following 255 beats (ie, SyncAV paced AVD = Intrinsic AV interval – 50 ms). The cycle repeats every 256 beats thus permitting the dynamic adjustment of the paced AV interval. The offset value may be reprogrammed across a wide range of offsets (10–120 ms). Additionally, ventricular pacing configuration may be changed from simultaneous biventricular ("BiV", default) to introduce interventricular timing delay or commit to LV only. Thus, any selected set (AV and VV) optimized settings in any individual may be preserved during ambulatory variations in AV interval resulting from changes in heart rate or autonomic tone.

Clinical Studies with SyncAV

The importance of dynamic (but programmable) AV interval optimization was illustrated in an acute electrical optimization study. Intrinsic PR intervals

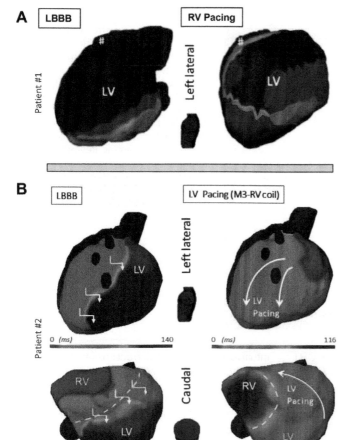

Fig. 3. Effects of RV and LV pacing on ventricular activation in LBBB. (*A*) RV pacing elicits early apical LV breakthrough by overcoming the transeptal conduction barrier. This effect is rarely observed. (*B*) LV pacing reversed all effects of LBBB, including transeptal delay indicating its functional basis. (*Adapted from* Varma N. Left ventricular electrical activation during right ventricular pacing in heart failure patients with LBBB: visualization by electrocardiographic imaging and implications for cardiac resynchronization therapy. J Electrocardiol. 2015;48(1):53-61. https://doi.org/10.1016/j.jelectrocard.2014.09.002; with permission; and Varma N., When left ventricular-only pacing reverses effects of left bundle branch block, EP Europace, 2021;, euab103, https://doi.org/10.1093/europace/euab103; with permission)

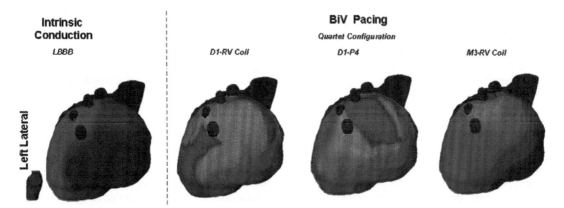

Fig. 4. Dependence of LV activation on stimulation site. ECGI mapping (Posterior view showing LV free wall. red: earliest and blue latest activation). Black dots represent the electrode positions of a quadripolar lead (interelectrode spacing (mm) D1-M2 20; M2-M3 10: and M3-P4 17 mm). (A) Left image shows intrinsic conduction in LBBB with early RV and delayed LV activation. The large blue area indicates a large area of terminal activation. Activation (or "qLV") is similar at each electrode site. (B) LV depolarization (area of earliest activation and pattern of subsequent LV depolarization) differs significantly among paced vectors. D1-P4 pacing activates the LV midsegment early. Stimulation from the anterobasal position (M3-RV coil) produces a small area of early activation locally at electrode site but also the generation of an area of slower conductor inferolateral to generate intra-LV dyssynchrony. Notably, these large variations were elicited despite little or no change in qLV along the quadripolar electrodes. Thus, slight positional changes in LV pacing site can generate large variations in ventricular depolarization, which are unrelated to baseline activation. Selection of vector eliciting most rapid and confluent LV activation may improve CRT efficacy. (*From* Varma N. Multipolar LV leads to optimize CRT-qLV or LV paced effect? *J Cardiovasc Electrophysiol.* 2020;31(1):238-239. https://doi.org/10.1111/jce.14306; with permission)

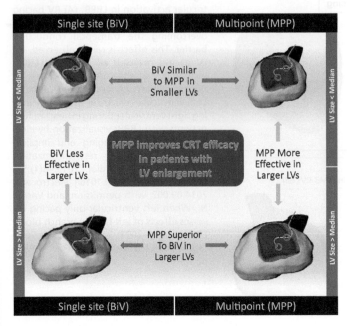

Fig. 5. Contrasting effects of multipoint versus single-site LV pacing in patients with differing LV size. C- LV epicardial pacing elicits slowly propagating wavefronts which reduce the ability to rapidly activate an LV that is grossly enlarged in heart failure. Multipoint pacing may overcome these limitations. (*From* Varma N, Baker J 2nd, Tomassoni G, et al. Left Ventricular Enlargement, Cardiac Resynchronization Therapy Efficacy, and Impact of MultiPoint Pacing. Circ Arrhythm Electrophysiol. 2020;13(11):e008680. https://doi.org/10.1161/CIRCEP.120.008680; with permission)

varied widely (range 117–300 ms) among CRT candidates with LBBB and optimized LV lead placement. Out-of-the-box static settings (which do not account for intrinsic PR) narrowed the QRS duration overall, though only by modest margins, and widened in some candidates—generated further electrical dyssynchrony (see **Fig. 6**).[37] Default SyncAV which adapts to intrinsic PR interval by pacing at approximately 80% of its measured value ("50 ms offset" Mode II) produces longer AV paced intervals which more consistently abbreviated QRS duration, and to a greater degree compared with static settings. When individually optimized, SyncAV narrowed QRSd in *every* patient and resulted in a maximal decrement in the whole cohort. Notably, optimized settings varied-the SyncAV offsets most frequently associated with the narrowest QRSd (ie, offsets used for Mode III) were between 30 and 50 ms, illustrating the value of AV interval control. LV only fusion pacing was best in only a minority (<15%) confirming prior observations.[23,24] In contrast, by permitting LV and RV timing as well as AV delay control, adjustments can promote "triple fusion."[24,36,38] These results indicate that postimplant electrical optimization could be significantly improved in otherwise electrically well-selected patients (LBBB and LV lead position) with patient-tailored programming facilitated with the SyncAV dynamic algorithm.

Clinical Outcome

These observations have clinical value. Electrical optimization with the goal of QRS narrowing is intuitive as CRT aims to correct an electrical disorder and systematic reviews support its predictive value.[39] A shorter LV paced QRS duration (index of rapid LV paced effect) was shown to be a strong predictor of clinical response following logistic regression analysis (AUC = 0.74).[17] In one recent RCT, patient-individualized electrical resynchronization improved outcomes measured by structural remodeling compared with nominal settings.[24] Interestingly, electrical optimization was largely dependent on the AV interval and usually required BiV (ie, RV and LV) rather than LV only pacing to deliver "triple fusion" (BiV pacing at longer AV intervals permits contribution of native RBB conduction[36,38]). One large, real-world investigation of patients with CRT reported that application of SyncAV generated a significant reduction in the rate of postimplant HFH, additive to the effect of CRT alone[40] and accompanying reduction in expenditure of health care resources (**Fig. 7**). Furthermore, SyncAV was associated with a reduction in the number of patients with multiple HF events and with 30-day HF rehospitalizations. SyncAV is currently being evaluated in a large international prospective multicenter randomized clinical trial (ClinicalTrials.gov Identifier: NCT04100148).

FUTURE

Opportunities for enhanced electrical resynchronization are being explored. Intracardiac paced intervals for example, RV paced to LV sense, and its reciprocal, may direct best programming strategies[14,18]. The use of multipoint pacing may improve LV activation, especially important when

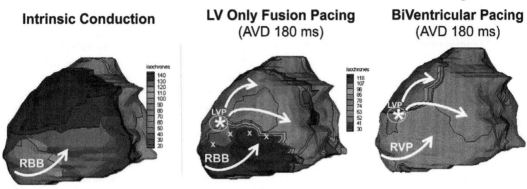

Intrinsic Conduction

LV Only Fusion Pacing
(AVD 180 ms)

BiVentricular Pacing
(AVD 180 ms)

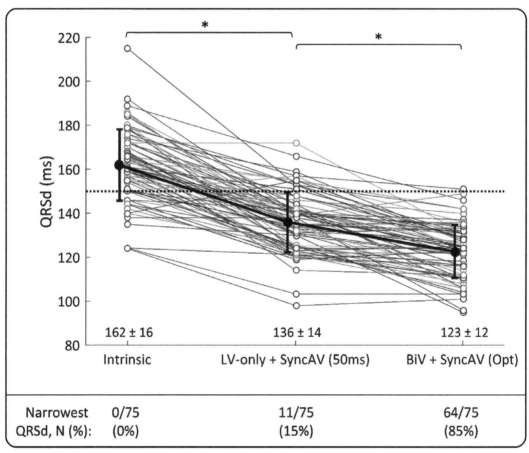

Narrowest QRSd, N (%):	0/75 (0%)	11/75 (15%)	64/75 (85%)

Fig. 6. Contrasting effects of LV-only versus biventricular pacing on ventricular activation. *Top* ECGI imaging of a male with ischemic cardiomyopathy (LVEF 10%), typical LBBB (QRS 184 ms), and PR 200 ms treated with CRT and laterally placed LV lead was (qLV 160 ms). LV pacing fails to generate confluent rapid LV activation (Middle). As a result, LV fusion pacing (at 180 ms AVD) was insufficient in restoring electrical synchrony, which was accomplished by adding RV pacing (BiV at the same AVD). Transseptal delay-the source of LV delay in LBBB—may have a functional basis that can be mitigated by RV pacing.[13,50] Resolution of conduction delay permits recruitment of a greater proportion of the LV and diminished total activation time, effects which improve hemodynamic function.[21] *Bottom* Among 75 patients with LBBB and LV lead location at terminally activated LV regions, Left ventricular (LV)–only fusion pacing reduced QRS duration (QRSd) by 15.6% relative to intrinsic, but individualized biventricular pacing (BiV) fusion pacing produced a greater effect (23.9% reduction, *P* < .001 vs LV fusion pacing). **P* < .001. Thus, biventricular stimulation at longer AV intervals introduces the initial effects of RV pacing as well as capturing intrinsic RBB conduction to deliver "triple fusion".[38] (*From* Varma N. Therapy for cardiac resynchronization: When left ventricular-only "fusion" pacing is not enough. HeartRhythm Case Rep. 2020;6(12):963-964. Published 2020 Aug 31. https://doi.org/10.1016/j.hrcr.2020.08.020; with permission; and Varma N, O'Donnell D, Bassiouny M, et al. Programming Cardiac Resynchronization Therapy for Electrical Synchrony: Reaching Beyond Left Bundle Branch Block and Left Ventricular Activation Delay. J Am Heart Assoc. 2018;7(3):e007489. Published 2018 Feb 6. https://doi.org/10.1161/JAHA.117.007489; with permission)

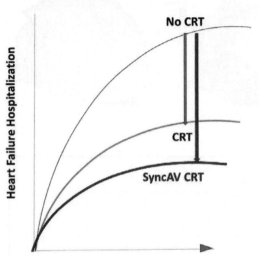

Hospitalizations for heart failure

No CRT

CRT

SyncAV CRT

Heart Failure Hospitalization

Fig. 7. Incremental benefit of SyncAV on CRT outcomes. Cumulative heart failure hospitalizations are compared for 2 years post-implant. (*A*) Whole cohort. CRT reduced the HFH rate dramatically. (*B*) SyncAV OFF CRT maintains a reduction in HFH rate. SyncAV ON CRT demonstrated the strongest suppression of HFH following treatment (HR = 0.70 [0.55, 0.89], *P* = .003). (*Adapted from* Varma N, Hu Y, Connolly AT, et al. Gain in real-world cardiac resynchronization therapy efficacy with SyncAV dynamic optimization: Heart failure hospitalizations and costs. Heart Rhythm. 2021;18(9):1577-1585. https://doi.org/10.1016/j.hrthm.2021.05.006; with permission)

the LV is enlarged or scarred (see **Fig. 5**).[41] This may be visualized with ECGI mapping to show patterns of wavefront propagation and their modulation by conduction barriers.[11,13,42] Functional conduction barriers to LV-paced wavefronts may develop without underlying scar and limit electrical resynchronization unless there is careful programming.[11,13,36] The SyncAV algorithm, though designed for traditional CRT using LV leads delivered via CS tributaries which remains the only approved therapy for patients with HF and a wide QRS duration, may be adapted to other delivery platforms under current investigation for example, endocardial LV[43,44]; or His/LBB area pacing.[45]

SUMMARY

Current expert consensus documents offer little guidance for postimplant management of CRT recipients beyond maximizing %BiV pacing because past CRT optimization trials have yielded neutral results.[46,47] The AUC associated with following a qLV > 95 ms was modest for predicting CRT reverse remodeling, and attempts at siting leads

at the point of latest LV activation did not improve results in the prospective ENHANCE CRT trial.[48,49] Ultimately qLV reports substrate for CRT but not the effects of therapy (see **Fig. 4**). Recent thinking advances the notion that CRT paced effect should be optimized to enable "triple fusion" to result in the best acute hemodynamic effects and chronic structural remodeling[24,36,38] while accommodating individual variations and changing conditions (AV interval, heart remodeling, etc.). This is logical as CRT represents an electrical solution for an electrical disorder. The currently enrolling SyncAV CRT trial investigates the incremental value of optimizing electrical treatment by the delivery of properly timed and dynamically maintained CRT pacing on patient outcomes.

CLINICS CARE POINTS

- CRT is an electrical therapy for an electrical disorder. It is logical that electrically optimized CRT delivery will enhance CRT efficacy and this is supported by studies.
- CRT optimization has to be individualized and automated
- Implementing device-based optimization algorithms may improve the ability of CRT to improve outcomes for example, reduced heart failure

DISCLOSURE

Speaking and consulting fees from Abbott, Biotronik, Boston Scientific, and Medtronic. ECGI studies sponsored by CardioInsight.

REFERENCES

1. Wells G, Parkash R, Healey JS, et al. Cardiac resynchronization therapy: a meta-analysis of randomized controlled trials. CMAJ 2011;183:421–9.
2. Daubert C, Behar N, Martins RP, et al. Avoiding nonresponders to cardiac resynchronization therapy: a practical guide. Eur Heart J 2017;38:1463–72.
3. Varma N, Boehmer J, Bhargava K, et al. Evaluation, management, and outcomes of patients Poorly responsive to cardiac resynchronization device therapy. J Am Coll Cardiol 2019;74:2588–603.
4. Varma N, Jia P, Ramanathan C, et al. RV electrical activation in heart failure during right, left, and biventricular pacing. JACC Cardiovasc Imaging 2010;3:567–75.
5. Wilkoff BL, Cook JR, Epstein AE, et al. Dual-chamber pacing or ventricular backup pacing in patients with an implantable defibrillator: the Dual Chamber

and VVI Implantable Defibrillator (DAVID) Trial. Jama 2002;288:3115–23.

6. Martin DO, Lemke B, Birnie D, et al. Investigation of a novel algorithm for synchronized left-ventricular pacing and ambulatory optimization of cardiac resynchronization therapy: results of the adaptive CRT trial. Heart Rhythm 2012;9:1807–14.

7. Varma N. Left ventricular conduction delays in response to right ventricular apical pacing. Influence of LV dysfunction and bundle branch block. J Cardiovasc Electrophsyiology 2008;19:114–22.

8. Varma N. Left ventricular electrical activation during right ventricular pacing in heart failure patients with LBBB: visualization by electrocardiographic imaging and implications for cardiac resynchronization therapy. J Electrocardiol 2015;48:53–61.

9. Varma N. When left ventricular-only pacing reverses effects of left bundle branch block. Europace 2022 Jan 4;24(1):164. https://doi.org/10.1093/europace/euab103.

10. Wiggers CJ. THE muscular reactions of the mammalian ventricles to artificial surface stimuli. Am J Physiol 1925;73:346–78.

11. Jia P, Ramanathan C, Ghanem RN, et al. Electrocardiographic imaging of cardiac resynchronization therapy in heart failure: observation of variable electrophysiologic responses. Heart Rhythm 2006;3:296–310.

12. Leyva F, Foley PW, Chalil S, et al. Cardiac resynchronization therapy guided by late gadolinium-enhancement cardiovascular magnetic resonance. J Cardiovasc Magn Reson 2011;13:29.

13. Varma N, Ploux S, Ritter P, et al. Noninvasive mapping of electrical dyssynchrony in heart failure and cardiac resynchronization therapy. Card Electrophysiol Clin 2015;7:125–34.

14. Wisnoskey B, Varma N. Left ventricular paced activation in CRT patients with LBBB and relationship to its electrical substrate. Heart Rhythm O2 2020;1:85–95.

15. van Everdingen WM, Zweerink A, Salden OAE, et al. Pressure-volume Loop analysis of multipoint pacing with a quadripolar left ventricular lead in cardiac resynchronization therapy. JACC Clin Electrophysiol 2018;4:881–9.

16. Varma N. Multipolar LV leads to optimize CRT-qLV or LV paced effect? J Cardiovasc Electrophysiol 2020;31:238–9.

17. Kobe J, Dechering DG, Rath B, et al. Prospective evaluation of electrocardiographic parameters in cardiac resynchronization therapy: detecting nonresponders by left ventricular pacing. Heart Rhythm 2012;9:499–504.

18. Ueda N, Noda T, Nakajima I, et al. Clinical impact of left ventricular paced conduction disturbance in cardiac resynchronization therapy. Heart Rhythm 2020;17:1870–7.

19. van Everdingen WM, Cramer MJ, Doevendans PA, et al. Quadripolar leads in cardiac resynchronization therapy. JACC Clin Electrophysiol 2015;1:225–37.

20. Varma N. Variegated left ventricular electrical activation in response to a novel quadripolar electrode: visualization by non-invasive electrocardiographic imaging. J Electrocardiol 2014;47:66–74.

21. Menardi E, Ballari GP, Goletto C, et al. Characterization of ventricular activation pattern and acute hemodynamics during multipoint left ventricular pacing. Heart Rhythm 2015;12:1762–9.

22. Varma N, Baker J 2nd, Tomassoni G, et al. Left ventricular enlargement, cardiac resynchronization therapy efficacy, and impact of MultiPoint pacing. Circ Arrhythm Electrophysiol 2020;13:e008680.

23. Arbelo E, Tolosana JM, Trucco E, et al. Fusion-optimized intervals (FOI): a new method to achieve the narrowest QRS for optimization of the AV and VV intervals in patients undergoing cardiac resynchronization therapy. J Cardiovasc Electrophysiol 2014;25:283–92.

24. Trucco E, Tolosana J, Arbelo E, et al. Improvement of reverse remodeling using ECG Fusion-Optimized Intervals in cardiac resynchronization therapy: a randomized study. JACC: Clin Electrophysiol 2018;4:181–9.

25. Cheng A, Landman SR, Stadler RW. Reasons for loss of cardiac resynchronization therapy pacing: insights from 32 844 patients. Circ Arrhythm Electrophysiol 2012;5:884–8.

26. Varma N, Stadler RW, Ghosh S, et al. Influence of automatic frequent pace-timing adjustments on effective left ventricular pacing during cardiac resynchronization therapy. Europace 2017;19:831–7.

27. Brugada J, Delnoy PP, Brachmann J, et al. Contractility sensor-guided optimization of cardiac resynchronization therapy: results from the RESPOND-CRT trial. Eur Heart J 2017;38:730–8.

28. Lunati M, Magenta G, Cattafi G, et al. Clinical Relevance of systematic CRT device optimization. J Atr Fibrillation 2014;7:1077.

29. Tamborero D, Vidal B, Tolosana JM, et al. Electrocardiographic versus echocardiographic optimization of the interventricular pacing delay in patients undergoing cardiac resynchronization therapy. J Cardiovasc Electrophysiol 2011;22:1129–34.

30. Vatasescu R, Berruezo A, Mont L, et al. Midterm 'super-response' to cardiac resynchronization therapy by biventricular pacing with fusion: insights from electro-anatomical mapping. Europace 2009;11:1675–82.

31. Lecoq G, Leclercq C, Leray E, et al. Clinical and electrocardiographic predictors of a positive response to cardiac resynchronization therapy in

advanced heart failure. Eur Heart J 2005;26: 1094–100.

32. Gold MR, Niazi I, Giudici M, et al. A prospective comparison of AV delay programming methods for hemodynamic optimization during cardiac resynchronization therapy. J Cardiovasc Electrophysiol 2007;18:490–6.

33. Ellenbogen KA, Gold MR, Meyer TE, et al. Primary results from the SmartDelay determined AV optimization: a comparison to other AV delay methods used in cardiac resynchronization therapy (SMART-AV) trial: a randomized trial comparing empirical, echocardiography-guided, and algorithmic atrioventricular delay programming in cardiac resynchronization therapy. Circulation 2011;122:2660–8.

34. Filippatos G, Birnie D, Gold MR, et al. Rationale and design of the AdaptResponse trial: a prospective randomized study of cardiac resynchronization therapy with preferential adaptive left ventricular-only pacing. Eur J Heart Fail 2017;19:950–7.

35. Yamasaki H, Lustgarten D, Cerkvenik J, et al. Adaptive CRT in patients with normal AV conduction and left bundle branch block: Does QRS duration matter? Int J Cardiol 2017 Aug 1;240:297–301. https://doi.org/10.1016/j.ijcard.2017.04.036.

36. Varma N. Therapy for cardiac resynchronization: when left ventricular–only "fusion" pacing is not enough. Heart Rhythm Case Rep 2020;6(12):963–4.

37. Varma N, O'Donnell D, Bassiouny M, et al. Programming cardiac resynchronization therapy for electrical synchrony: Reaching beyond left bundle branch block and left ventricular activation delay. J Am Heart Assoc 2018;7:e007489.

38. Ter Horst IAH, Bogaard MD, Tuinenburg AE, et al. The concept of triple wavefront fusion during biventricular pacing: using the EGM to produce the best acute hemodynamic improvement in CRT. Pacing Clin Electrophysiol 2017;40:873–82.

39. Bazoukis G, Naka KK, Alsheikh-Ali A, et al. Association of QRS narrowing with response to cardiac resynchronization therapy-a systematic review and meta-analysis of observational studies. Heart Fail Rev 2020;25:745–56.

40. Varma N, Hu Y, Connolly AT, et al. Gain in real-world cardiac resynchronization therapy efficacy with SyncAV dynamic optimization: heart failure hospitalizations and costs. Heart Rhythm 2021;18:1577–85.

41. O'Donnell D, Wisnoskey B, Badie N, et al. Electrical synchronization achieved by multipoint pacing combined with dynamic atrioventricular delay. J Interv Card Electrophysiol 2020;61(3):453–60.

42. Ginks MR, Shetty AK, Lambiase PD, et al. Benefits of endocardial and multisite pacing are dependent on the type of left ventricular electric activation pattern and presence of ischemic heart disease: insights from electroanatomic mapping. Circ Arrhythm Electrophysiol 2012;5:889–97.

43. Reddy VY, Miller MA, Neuzil P, et al. Cardiac resynchronization therapy with Wireless left ventricular endocardial pacing: the SELECT-LV study. J Am Coll Cardiol 2017;69:2119–29.

44. Morgan JM, Biffi M, Geller L, et al. ALternate Site Cardiac ResYNChronization (ALSYNC): a prospective and multicentre study of left ventricular endocardial pacing for cardiac resynchronization therapy. Eur Heart J 2016;37:2118–27.

45. Huang W, Wu S, Vijayaraman P, et al. Cardiac resynchronization therapy in patients with Nonischemic cardiomyopathy using left bundle branch pacing. JACC Clin Electrophysiol 2020;6:849–58.

46. Brignole M, Auricchio A, Baron-Esquivias G, et al. 2013 ESC Guidelines on cardiac pacing and cardiac resynchronization therapy: the Task Force on cardiac pacing and resynchronization therapy of the European Society of Cardiology (ESC). Developed in collaboration with the European Heart Rhythm Association (EHRA). Europace 2013;15: 1070–118.

47. Daubert JC, Saxon L, Adamson PB, et al. 2012 EHRA/HRS expert consensus statement on cardiac resynchronization therapy in heart failure: implant and follow-up recommendations and management. Europace 2012;14:1236–86.

48. Gold MR, Birgersdotter-Green U, Singh JP, et al. The relationship between ventricular electrical delay and left ventricular remodelling with cardiac resynchronization therapy. Eur Heart J 2011;32:2516–24.

49. Singh JP, Berger RD, Doshi RN, et al. Targeted left ventricular lead Implantation strategy for non-left bundle branch block patients: the ENHANCE CRT study. JACC Clin Electrophysiol 2020;6:1171–81.

50. Derval N, Duchateau J, Mahida S, et al. Distinctive left ventricular activations associated with ECG pattern in heart failure patients. Circ Arrhythm Electrophysiol 2017;10.

Multisite Left Ventricular Pacing in Cardiac Resynchronization Therapy

Sandeep K. Jain, MD[a], Samir Saba, MD[b],*

KEYWORDS

- Cardiac resynchronization therapy • Multisite pacing • Multipoint pacing • Heart failure • Response

KEY POINTS

- Many patients do not respond to conventional cardiac resynchronization therapy (CRT).
- Multisite pacing (MSP) has shown promise in improving response rates to CRT.
- Data from prospective trials have shown divergent results regarding the role of MSP in the management of patients with heart failure.

INTRODUCTION

Cardiac resynchronization therapy (CRT) is an established treatment option for patients with heart failure with reduced ejection fraction and ventricular conduction abnormalities despite optimal guideline-directed medical therapy.[1–4] Large randomized clinical trials[2–4] have demonstrated the beneficial impact of CRT on the end point of death or heart failure hospitalizations or events and on enhancing left ventricular (LV) reverse remodeling on echocardiographic imaging.[5]

Despite its salutary effects, it is estimated that up to 40% of patients do not respond to CRT and most reports estimate the rate of nonresponse to be around one-third of patients.[6–9] Echocardiographic response has been shown to be independently associated with improved survival.[10] Retrospective analyses have implicated patients' characteristics in predicting the rates of nonresponse to CRT.[1,11–14] These have included the morphology and width of the QRS complex with patients who have non–left bundle branch block QRS patterns and a QRS duration less than 150 milliseconds having lower response rates and therefore lower CRT indication levels, according to published guidelines.[1] In addition, other features have also been associated with lower rates of response to CRT, including the type of cardiomyopathy, with patients with heart failure with ischemic causes and high scar burden having worse CRT response rates compared with those with nonischemic causes.[15–17] Demographic criteria have also been implicated as predictors of response to CRT.[18–20] Lastly, intraoperative strategies applied at the time of the CRT device implantation (discussed later) have also been shown to improve the rates of response to CRT.[21,22] Still, the number of patients who do not extract clear benefit from CRT remains substantial.[6–9] LV multisite pacing (MSP) has been proposed and tested as an additional tool that could improve response to CRT and positively impact patient outcomes (**Table 1**).

LEFT VENTRICULAR PACING AT THE SITE OF LATEST MECHANICAL OR ELECTRICAL ACTIVATION

To increase the proportion of patients who extract clinical benefit from CRT, implantation strategies have been tested to examine if targeting the site of latest mechanical[21–23] or electrical[24] activation is superior to conventional LV lead placement in

a Cardiac Electrophysiology, Heart and Vascular Institute, University of Pittsburgh Medical Center, 200 Lothrop Street, South Tower E352.6, Pittsburgh, PA 15213, USA; b Cardiology, Heart and Vascular Institute, University of Pittsburgh Medical Center, 200 Lothrop Street, South Tower E355.6, Pittsburgh, PA 15213, USA
* Corresponding author.
E-mail address: sabas@upmc.edu

Card Electrophysiol Clin 14 (2022) 253–261
https://doi.org/10.1016/j.ccep.2021.12.003
1877-9182/22/© 2021 Elsevier Inc. All rights reserved.

Table 1
Multisite pacing studies enrolling a minimum of 50 patients

	Study Type	Groups	Findings
Zanon et al,[43] 2016	Single center, retrospective (n = 110)	Three groups: STD: standard bipolar LV OPT: optimized electrical + hemodynamics MPP: MPP + optimized hemodynamics	End-systolic volume reduction in STD 56%, OPT 72%, MPP 90% NYHA response in STD 59%, OPT 67%, MPP 90%
Niazi et al,[39] 2017 The MPP Trial	Multicenter, prospective randomized, double blind (n = 381)	Nonresponders at 3 mo randomized to MPP or continued BiV	Safety end point met at 93% ITT with equal response rates with MPP but those with anatomically separate electrode pacing with higher response (MPP 87% vs BiV 65%) and higher conversion from nonresponder to responder at 9 mo (100% vs 49%)
Forleo et al,[44] 2017 IRON-MPP	Multicenter, prospective nonrandomized, observational (n = 232)	6-mo echocardiographic follow-up in MPP (n = 94) vs standard BiV (n = 138)	At 6 mo, ejection fraction higher in MPP group (39.1% vs 34.7%) Clinical composite score improved in MPP patients more than BiV (56% vs 38%)
Leclerq et al,[41] 2019 MORE-CRT MPP Phase 1	Multicenter, prospective randomized (n = 544)	Nonresponders (<15% decrease in LVESV at 6-mo post-CRT) randomized to MPP (n = 236) vs BiV (n = 231)	At 6 mo postrandomization of nonresponders, no significant increase in echo response with MPP compared with BiV MPP-AS (30 mm or more pacing electrode separation) did have higher nonresponder conversion rate (46% vs 26%)
Christos-Konstantinos et al,[45] 2021 HUMVEE Trial	Multicenter, prospective single arm, nonrandomized (n = 80)	Sequential optimized CRT (1 mo) and MPP (7 mo) postimplant	MSP superior to optimized conventional CRT in 6-min-walk test results, quality of life scores, and echocardiographic parameters including LV stroke volume and ejection fraction, in addition to left atrial size, right ventricular strain, and pulmonary artery systolic pressure.
Saba et al,[46] 2021 SMART-MSP	Multicenter, prospective single arm, nonrandomized (n = 102)	Nonresponders at 6 mo (by clinical composite score) had MPP turned on and followed for additional 6 mo with outcomes of safety and effectiveness	MSP-related complication-free rate of 99.0% Battery impact of 3–4 mo Improved CCS score from 6–12 mo at 51.3% Proximal electrode use was predictor of response

Abbreviations: BiV, biventricular ; CCS, clinical composite score; ITT, intention to treat; LVESV, left ventricular end systolic volume; MPP, multipoint pacing; NYHA, New York Heart Association; OPT, optimized; STD, standard.

reducing mortality or heart failure hospitalization. Our group conducted the STARTER trial[22] at the University of Pittsburgh Medical Center. STARTER enrolled 187 CRT-eligible patients and randomized them to a strategy of echocardiography-guided LV lead placement at or close to the site of latest mechanical activation as determined by speckle tracking echocardiographic techniques versus conventional LV lead placement without image guidance. Our results demonstrated that the echocardiography-guided strategy leads to significant improvement in the composite end point of death or heart failure hospitalization and in other echocardiographic end points. These results confirmed the independent results of the TARGET trial[21] conducted in the United Kingdom, which had been published a few months earlier. Together, these two randomized controlled trials[21,22] demonstrate that pacing the LV at or adjacent to the site of latest mechanical activation leads to improved clinical response among CRT recipients. Although not randomized, data also support that pacing the LV close to the site of the latest electrical activation (site of longest Q-LV) is associated with improved response to CRT.[24] These data taken together support the mechanistic concept that in patients with heart failure who are eligible for CRT, there is an optimal LV site that should be targeted for pacing to increase the rate of response to CRT and maximize that response.

CONCEPTUAL MECHANISM OF INCREMENTAL BENEFIT FROM LEFT VENTRICULAR MULTISITE PACING

MSP of the LV has been proposed as a means of improving patients' response to CRT.[25–28] As opposed to conventional CRT where pacing is delivered from the right ventricular lead and one LV site, in LV MSP pacing is additionally delivered through a second LV site, usually on the same quadripolar LV lead (**Fig. 1**). Conceptually, LV MSP could provide better resynchronization to the LV during its systolic contraction by decreasing the LV activation time. With an electrical wavefront originating in the right ventricle and from two separate LV sites, the systolic contraction the LV is likely to complete is a shorter ejection time leading to a more synchronous ventricular contraction. In addition, pacing the LV at two separate sites increases the probabilistic chance of one of the two pacing electrodes being at or close to the LV optimal pacing site, through "electrical repositioning,"[29] which may mechanistically account for the potential incremental benefits of MSP.

LEFT VENTRICULAR MULTISITE PACING: PRECLINICAL STUDIES

In a porcine model of acute left bundle branch block induction and pacing, Heckman and colleagues[30] demonstrated that, compared with

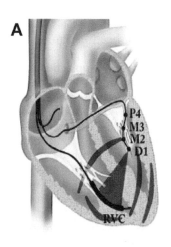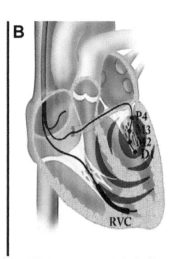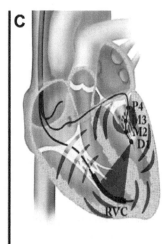

Fig. 1. Theoretic premise for the improved synchrony achieved through multipoint pacing as compared with conventional CRT. Initial extent of LV activation, based on initial pulse direction and subsequent propagation following the use of D1-RVC extended dipole (*A*), D1-P4 local dipole (*B*), and a combination of D1-RVC and M2-P4 (*C*). D1, distal pole; M2, second most distal pole; M3, middle electrode number 3; P4, proximal pole; RVC, right ventricle coil. (*From* Antoniou CK, Dilaveris P, Chrysohoou C, et al. Multipoint left ventricular pacing effects on hemodynamic parameters and functional status: HUMVEE single-arm clinical trial (NCT03189368) [published online ahead of print, 2021 Mar 4]. Hellenic J Cardiol. 2021;S1109-9666(21)00049-X. https://doi.org/10.1016/j.hjc.2021.02.012; with permission)

conventional single-site CRT, LV MSP significantly shortened the LV activation time and increased mechanical contractility as measured by LV dP/dt$_{Max}$, primarily when the reduction in LV activation time with conventional CRT was small (in the lowest quartile). In that study,[30] the authors reported no difference in the incremental value of MSP pacing whether the two active LV electrodes were located in the same or in two separate veins of the coronary sinus. Importantly, the highest increase in LV dP/dt$_{Max}$ was observed when the separation between the two LV pacing electrodes was larger than 5 cm.

LEFT VENTRICULAR MULTISITE PACING: CLINICAL STUDIES

Several studies (see **Table 1**) have examined the impact of LV MSP compared with conventional biventricular pacing in CRT recipients using a variety of clinical end points. Siciliano and colleagues[31] demonstrated in 11 consecutive patients that MSP improves LV mechanics and fluid dynamics by reducing end-diastolic and end-systolic LV volumes and improving LV ejection fraction and cardiac output, as assessed by echocardiography. In a single-center study of 27 patients with heart failure, Osca and colleagues[32] demonstrated an improved acute response rate (85.2% vs 62.9%; $P < .001$) with LV MSP compared with conventional CRT, defined as a greater than or equal to 10% improvement in cardiac output index. In a study of 14 patients with chronic atrial fibrillation and cardiomyopathy, Zanon and colleagues[33] examined the impact of higher number of LV pacing sites on acute hemodynamic and electrical signals, showing significant increase in LV dP/dt$_{Max}$ and decrease in QRS width with higher number of LV pacing sites. Similar results were documented in other studies[34,35] that have also highlighted the importance of tailoring biventricular MSP to the individual patient needs based on hemodynamic assessment.[34] In addition, Akerstrom and colleagues[36] evaluated the impact of MSP activation on estimated device battery longevity and found that, except when the programmed output was low ($\leq$1.5 V), the impact on battery longevity was significant, on the order of 1.5 to 1.9 years for the life of the device.

In a large single-center prospective study from Greece (NTC03189368), the heart failure trial of MSP effects on ventriculoarterial coupling (HUM-VEE)[37] enrolled 80 patients and examined the impact of MSP on patients' 6-minute-hallway-walk test, quality of life, and on echocardiographic parameters and serum markers of heart failure (eg, N-terminal pro–brain natriuretic peptide). In this trial,[37] MSP was shown to be superior to optimized conventional CRT in 6-minute-walk test results, quality of life scores, and echocardiographic parameters including LV stroke volume and ejection fraction, in addition to more favorable measures of left atrial size, right ventricular strain, and pulmonary artery systolic pressure.

It is worth mentioning that although most studies have demonstrated an incremental acute hemodynamic benefit from LV MSP over conventional CRT, few did not. In 24 CRT recipients with quadripolar LV leads, Sterlinski and colleagues[38] reported no increase in LV dP/dt$_{Max}$ compared with conventional CRT using any LV electrode configuration, and demonstrated a poor correlation between measures of LV contractility and QRS width or electrical delay at the site of LV pacing.

LEFT VENTRICULAR MULTISITE PACING: LARGE MULTICENTER PROSPECTIVE TRIALS

The MultiPoint Pacing (MPP) trial[39] (https://clinicaltrials.gov/ct2/show/NCT01786993?term=01786993&rank=1) is a multicenter randomized controlled study of CRT recipients who, 3 months after device implantation, were randomized 1:1 to MSP or conventional biventricular pacing and were followed for 6 months. The primary safety end point of this study was freedom from system-related complications and the primary effectiveness end point was noninferiority of MSP to conventional CRT with respect to the clinical composite score (CCS). The MPP trial[39] randomized 381 patients with heart failure to MSP (n = 201) or conventional CRT (n = 180) (**Fig. 2**). Through 9 months of follow-up, the rate of freedom from system-related complications was 93.2%, which easily cleared the predetermined performance goal of 75%. As far as the effectiveness end point, although MSP was noninferior to conventional biventricular pacing, it trended toward a higher rate of nonresponse by intention-to-treat analysis at 6 months (29.9% vs 25%). On subgroup analyses, patients randomized to MSP from anatomically distant electrodes had a significantly higher response rate (87% vs 65%; $P = .003$) and conversion rate from nonresponder to responder (100% vs 49%; $P = .014$) at 9 months, compared with patients with other MSP configurations involving smaller active electrode separation.

The Strategic Management to Improve CRT using Multisite Pacing (SMART-MSP, NCT02006069) trial, which was presented as a late-breaking clinical trial at the scientific sessions of the Heart Rhythm Society (Boston, July 2021), is a

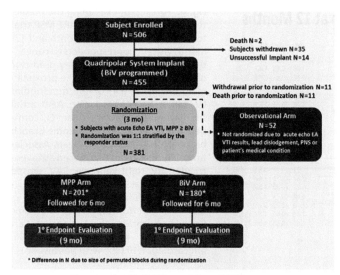

Fig. 2. MPP trial design and enrollment. BiV, biventricular; EA VTI, velocity-time integral of the transmitral flow; PNS, Phrenic nerve stimulation. (*From* Niazi I, Baker J 2nd, Corbisiero R, et al. Safety and Efficacy of Multipoint Pacing in Cardiac Resynchronization Therapy: The MultiPoint Pacing Trial. JACC Clin Electrophysiol. 2017;3(13):1510-1518. https://doi.org/10.1016/j.jacep.2017.06.022; with permission).

Responder Definition at 3 and 9 Mo
*Relative to 3-month status

3-Month Responder Definition	9-Month Responder Definition*
Improved = Responder	Improved/Unchanged = Responder
	Worsened = Non-responder
Unchanged/Worsened = Non-responder	Improved = Responder
	Unchanged/Worsened = Non-responder

multicenter, prospective observational trial that enrolled a total of 584 patients at 52 centers in the United States. SMART MSP focused on evaluating the safety and effectiveness of LV MSP specifically in nonresponders to 6 months of conventional CRT. Patients were evaluated after 6 months of CRT pacing using the CCS. Responders exited the trial and nonresponders had their MSP feature turned on. Patients were evaluated at 12 months for the safety and effectiveness of the MSP feature. As shown in **Fig. 3**, after accounting for attrition, 102 patients who had their LV MSP feature turned on were examined for the safety end point. Of those, 78 patients who completed the 12-month follow-up visit and who had greater than 93% rate of LV MSP were examined for the effectiveness end point. The rate of freedom from MSP-related complications

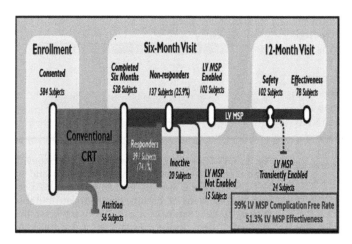

Fig. 3. SMART-MSP trial design and enrollment. (*From* Saba S, Nair D, Ellis C et al. Usefulness of Multisite Ventricular Pacing in Nonresponders to Cardiac Resynchronization Therapy. Am J Cardiol. 2021. https://doi.org/10.1016/j.amjcard.2021.10.027; with permission).

LV MSP Response by Subgroup at 12 Months

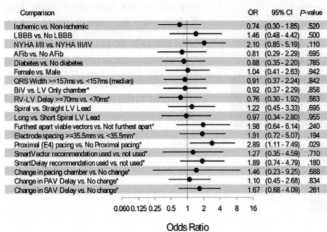

Comparison	OR	95% CI	P-value
Ischemic vs. Non-ischemic	0.74	(0.30 - 1.85)	.520
LBBB vs. No LBBB	1.46	(0.48 - 4.42)	.500
NYHA I/II vs. NYHA III/IV	2.10	(0.85 - 5.19)	.110
AFib vs. No AFib	0.81	(0.29 - 2.29)	.695
Diabetes vs. No diabetes	0.88	(0.35 - 2.20)	.785
Female vs. Male	1.04	(0.41 - 2.63)	.942
QRS Width >=157ms vs. <157ms (median)	0.91	(0.37 - 2.24)	.842
BiV vs. LV Only chamber*	0.92	(0.37 - 2.29)	.858
RV-LV Delay >=70ms vs. <70ms*	0.76	(0.30 - 1.92)	.563
Spiral vs. Straight LV Lead	1.22	(0.45 - 3.33)	.695
Long vs. Short Spiral LV Lead	0.97	(0.34 - 2.80)	.955
Furthest apart viable vectors vs. Not furthest apart*	1.98	(0.64 - 6.14)	.240
Electrode spacing >=35.5mm vs. <35.5mm*	1.91	(0.72 - 5.07)	.194
Proximal (E4) pacing vs. No Proximal pacing*	2.89	(1.11 - 7.49)	.029
SmartVector recommendation used vs. not used*	1.27	(0.35 - 4.59)	.710
SmartDelay recommendation used vs. not used*	1.89	(0.74 - 4.79)	.180
Change in pacing chamber vs. No change*	1.46	(0.23 - 9.25)	.688
Change in PAV Delay vs. No change*	1.10	(0.45 - 2.68)	.834
Change in SAV Delay vs. No change*	1.67	(0.68 - 4.09)	.261

0.060 0.125 0.25 0.5 1 2 4 8 16

Odds Ratio

*Value from 6 month visit   Decreased Odds of Response   Increased Odds of Response

Fig. 4. Forest plot examining the predictors of response in the SMART-MSP trial to LV MSP between the 6-month and 12-month visits in nonresponders to conventional CRT. Note that the only predictor of response was the use of the proximal-most electrode (E4) of the quadripolar LV lead in the LV MSP pacing. AFib, atrial fibrillation; BiV, biventricular; CI, confidence interval; LBBB, left bundle branch block; NYHA, New York Heart Association; OR, odds ratio; PAV, paced atrioventricular; RV, right ventricle; SAV, sensed atrioventricular. (*From* Saba S, Nair D, Ellis C et al. Usefulness of Multisite Ventricular Pacing in Nonresponders to Cardiac Resynchronization Therapy. Am J Cardiol. 2021. https://doi.org/10.1016/j.amjcard.2021.10.027; with permission)

was 99% with a lower boundary of the 95% confidence interval of 95%, clearing the predetermined performance goal of 90%. In terms of the effectiveness end point, 51.3% of patients who were nonresponders to conventional CRT by CCS became responders with the activation of MSP. This greater than 50% response rate was significantly higher than the predetermined performance goal of 5%, established after discussions with the Food and Drug Administration. Therefore, SMART MSP met its safety and effectiveness end points and outperformed its expected performance by wide margins. On subgroup analyses, SMART MSP demonstrated that the use of the proximal-most electrode on the quadripolar LV lead during MSP was associated with higher response rates (65% vs 39%; *P* = .029) **(Fig. 4)** suggesting that more basal pacing electrode positions are more likely to turn nonresponders to responders with MSP. Importantly, turning on the LV MSP feature had a small impact on the estimated battery longevity of the CRT-defibrillator device, projected to be between 3 and 4 months for the life of the device **(Fig. 5)**.

The More Response on Cardiac Resynchronization Therapy with MultiPoint Pacing (MORE-CRT MPP, NCT02006069) trial[40] is currently underway. This is a multicenter, international trial designed to enroll 6898 CRT recipients at 121 sites worldwide, examining the response rate after 6 months of MPP among nonresponders to conventional CRT. Enrolled subjects are assessed by echocardiography 6 months after enrollment and those who achieve at least 15% reduction in LV end-systolic volume are considered responders and exit the trial. Nonresponders are then randomized

to MPP on or off and followed for another 6 months. The primary outcome of this trial is the proportion of patients who convert from nonresponder to responder status. The MORE CRT MPP trial was designed in two phases. In phase I, patients randomized to MPP on had the feature turned on at the discretion of the treating physician, whereas in phase II, patients randomized to MPP had the feature turned on as mandated by the protocol. Although the final results of the MORE CRT MPP trial are expected to be available after September of 2021, the results of phase I were published[41] and showed no difference in conversion rates between MPP and conventional CRT (31.8% vs 33.9%; *P* = .72). As previously shown in the original MPP trial[39] published in 2017, subgroup analyses of the MORE CRT MPP

Device Estimate of Remaining Battery Longevity

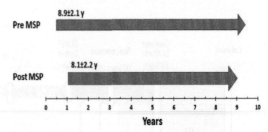

8.9±2.1y
Pre MSP

8.1±2.2 y
Post MSP

0 1 2 3 4 5 6 7 8 9 10

Years

Fig. 5. CRT-D device estimation of battery longevity after 6 months of conventional CRT pacing and at 12 months, after 6 months of additional LV MSP pacing. The estimate of battery depletion attributable to the LVMSP feature is about 3–4 months for the life of the device. Estimates presented as mean ± standard deviation.

trial demonstrated a better conversion rate with wider electrode separation in the MPP group (45.6% vs 26.2%; $P = .006$) but only a trend for higher conversion with MPP compared with conventional CRT (45.6% vs 33.8%; $P = .10$).

Although the population of patients enrolled in SMART MSP was not too dissimilar from that of the MPP[39] and MORE CRT MPP[41] trials, the conclusions of these studies are divergent, possibly reflecting differences in study design, types of patients considered in the primary end point, and in the definition of response. For instance, although the MPP trial studied all CRT recipients, SMART MSP and MORE CRT MPP focused only on nonresponders to conventional CRT, thus avoiding diluting the impact of MSP by including all patients. However, MPP and SMART MSP used the CCS to define response as opposed to echocardiographic measures in MORE CRT MPP. It is well known that even in the same patient, clinical and echocardiographic responses to CRT can be discordant.[42] It is hoped that the results of the larger phase II of the MORE CRT MPP trial add clarity to these issues.

FUTURE DIRECTIONS

Despite the extensive current literature on LV MSP there remains many questions that are unanswered. Who are the patients who most benefit from MSP? Why do some nonresponders not benefit from it? Are there groups of patients in whom MSP should be turned on early, such as at the time of initial device implantation? What are the pacing vectors that are most likely to convert a nonresponder to a responder? Is the impact of MSP on battery longevity equal among the various device manufacturers and models? The answers to these questions will likely trickle through from future analyses of data from the large clinical trials and from real-world experience captured through patient and device registries.

CLINICS CARE POINTS

- When your heart failure patient fails to respond to conventional CRT, consider turning on the MSP feature on their device.
- If they extract benefit from the MSP feature, you can keep it on for the long term.
- If a patient does not response to MSP, the feature could be turned off to save the device battery.

DISCLOSURE

Dr S. Saba reports receiving research support from Abbott and Boston Scientific and serving on advisory boards for Boston Scientific and Medtronic.

REFERENCES

1. Tracy CM, Epstein AE, Darbar D, et al. 2012 ACCF/AHA/HRS Focused Update Incorporated Into the ACCF/AHA/HRS 2008 Guidelines for Device-Based Therapy of Cardiac Rhythm Abnormalities. J Am Coll Cardiol 2013;61(3). https://doi.org/10.1016/j.jacc.2012.11.007.
2. Bristow MR, Saxon LA, Boehmer J, et al. Cardiac-resynchronization therapy with or without an implantable defibrillator in advanced chronic heart failure. N Engl J Med 2004;350(21):2140–50.
3. Cleland JGF, Daubert J-C, Erdmann E, et al. The effect of cardiac resynchronization on morbidity and mortality in heart failure. N Engl J Med 2005;352(15):1539–49.
4. Moss AJ, Hall WJ, Cannom DS, et al. Cardiac-resynchronization therapy for the prevention of heart-failure events. N Engl J Med 2009;361:1329–38.
5. Young JB, Abraham WT, Smith AL, et al. Combined cardiac resynchronization and implantable cardioversion defibrillation in advanced chronic heart failure: the MIRACLE ICD Trial. JAMA 2003;289:2685–94.
6. Tanaka H, Hara H, Saba S, et al. Prediction of response to cardiac resynchronization therapy by speckle tracking echocardiography using different software approaches. J Am Soc Echocardiogr 2009;22(6):677–84.
7. Tanaka H, Nesser H-J, Buck T, et al. Dyssynchrony by speckle-tracking echocardiography and response to cardiac resynchronization therapy: results of the Speckle Tracking and Resynchronization (STAR) study. Eur Heart J 2010;31(14):1690–700.
8. Adelstein EC, Saba S. Baseline scintigraphic abnormalities by myocardial perfusion imaging predict echocardiographic response to cardiac resynchronization therapy in nonischemic cardiomyopathy. Clin Cardiol 2008;31(5):217–24.
9. Varma N, Auricchio A, Connolly AT, et al. The cost of non-response to cardiac resynchronization therapy: characterizing heart failure events following cardiac resynchronization therapy. Europace 2021;00:1–10.
10. Bertini M, Höke U, van Bommel RJ, et al. Impact of clinical and echocardiographic response to cardiac resynchronization therapy on long-term survival. Eur Heart J Cardiovasc Imaging 2013;14(8). https://doi.org/10.1093/ehjci/jes290.
11. Gold MR, Thébault C, Linde C, et al. Effect of QRS duration and morphology on cardiac

resynchronization therapy outcomes in mild heart failure: results from the resynchronization reverses remodeling in systolic left ventricular dysfunction (REVERSE) study. Circulation 2012;126(7). https://doi.org/10.1161/CIRCULATIONAHA.112.097709.

12. Abraham WT, Fisher WG, Smith AL, et al. Cardiac resynchronization in chronic heart failure. N Engl J Med 2002;346(24):1845–53.

13. Rickard J, Bassiouny M, Cronin EM, et al. Predictors of response to cardiac resynchronization therapy in patients with a non-left bundle branch block morphology. Am J Cardiol 2011;108(11). https://doi.org/10.1016/j.amjcard.2011.07.017.

14. Saba S, Marek J, Alam MB, et al. Influence of QRS duration on outcome of death or appropriate defibrillator therapy by strategy of left ventricular lead placement in cardiac resynchronization therapy recipients. J Interv Card Electrophysiol 2014;41(3):211–5.

15. Barsheshet A, Goldenberg I, Moss AJ, et al. Response to preventive cardiac resynchronization therapy in patients with ischaemic and nonischaemic cardiomyopathy in MADIT-CRT. Eur Heart J 2011; 32(13). https://doi.org/10.1093/eurheartj/ehq407.

16. Daya HA, Alam MB, Adelstein E, et al. Echocardiography-guided left ventricular lead placement for cardiac resynchronization therapy in ischemic vs nonischemic cardiomyopathy patients. Hear Rhythm 2014;11(4). https://doi.org/10.1016/j.hrthm.2014.01.023.

17. Adelstein EC, Tanaka H, Soman P, et al. Impact of scar burden by single-photon emission computed tomography myocardial perfusion imaging on patient outcomes following cardiac resynchronization therapy. Eur Heart J 2011;32(1):93–103.

18. Beela AS, Duchenne J, Petrescu A, et al. Sex-specific difference in outcome after cardiac resynchronization therapy. Eur Heart J Cardiovasc Imaging 2019;20(5). https://doi.org/10.1093/ehjci/jey231.

19. Herz ND, Engeda J, Zusterzeel R, et al. Sex differences in device therapy for heart failure: utilization, outcomes, and adverse events. J Womens Health 2015;24(4). https://doi.org/10.1089/jwh.2014.4980.

20. Varma N, Lappe J, He J, et al. Sex-Specific response to cardiac resynchronization therapy: effect of left ventricular size and QRS duration in left bundle branch block. JACC Clin Electrophysiol 2017;3(8). https://doi.org/10.1016/j.jacep.2017.02.021.

21. Khan FZ, Virdee MS, Palmer CR, et al. Targeted left ventricular lead placement to guide cardiac resynchronization therapy: the TARGET study: a randomized, controlled trial. J Am Coll Cardiol 2012; 59(17). https://doi.org/10.1016/j.jacc.2011.12.030.

22. Saba S, Marek J, Schwartzman D, et al. Echocardiography-guided left ventricular lead placement for cardiac resynchronization therapy: results of the Speckle Tracking assisted resynchronization therapy for electrode region trial. Circ Heart Fail 2013; 6(3):427–34.

23. Marek JJ, Saba S, Onishi T, et al. Usefulness of echocardiographically guided left ventricular lead placement for cardiac resynchronization therapy in patients with intermediate QRS width and non-left bundle branch block morphology. Am J Cardiol 2014;113(1):107–16.

24. Gold MR, Birgersdotter-Green U, Singh JP, et al. The relationship between ventricular electrical delay and left ventricular remodelling with cardiac resynchronization therapy. Eur Heart J 2011;32(20). https://doi.org/10.1093/eurheartj/ehr329.

25. Cazeau S, Ritter P, Lazarus A, et al. Multisite pacing for end-stage heart failure: early experience. Pacing Clin Electrophysiol 1996;19(11 II). https://doi.org/10.1111/j.1540-8159.1996.tb03218.x.

26. Cazeau S, Leclercq C, Lavergne T, et al. Effects of multisite biventricular pacing in patients with heart failure and intraventricular conduction delay. N Engl J Med 2001;344(12):873–80.

27. Sohal M, Shetty A, Niederer S, et al. Mechanistic insights into the benefits of multisite pacing in cardiac resynchronization therapy: the importance of electrical substrate and rate of left ventricular activation. Hear Rhythm 2015;12(12). https://doi.org/10.1016/j.hrthm.2015.07.012.

28. Thibault B, Dubuc M, Khairy P, et al. Acute haemodynamic comparison of multisite and biventricular pacing with a quadripolar left ventricular lead. Europace 2013;15(7). https://doi.org/10.1093/europace/eus435.

29. Netzler P, Cuoco F, George A, et al. The effect of left ventricular sensing electrode position on electrical delay in cardiac resynchronization therapy. J Am Coll Cardiol 2014;63(12). https://doi.org/10.1016/s0735-1097(14)60448-4.

30. Heckman LIB, Kuiper M, Anselme F, et al. Evaluating multisite pacing strategies in cardiac resynchronization therapy in the preclinical setting. Hear Rhythm O2 2020;1(2). https://doi.org/10.1016/j.hroo.2020.03.003.

31. Siciliano M, Migliore F, Badano L, et al. Cardiac resynchronization therapy by multipoint pacing improves response of left ventricular mechanics and fluid dynamics: a three-dimensional and particle image velocimetry echo study. Europace 2017;19(11). https://doi.org/10.1093/europace/euw331.

32. Osca J, Alonso P, Cano O, et al. The use of multisite left ventricular pacing via quadripolar lead improves acute haemodynamics and mechanical dyssynchrony assessed by radial strain speckle tracking: initial results. Europace 2016;18(4). https://doi.org/10.1093/europace/euv211.

33. Zanon F, Marcantoni L, Baracca E, et al. Hemodynamic comparison of different multisites and multipoint pacing strategies in cardiac resynchronization therapies. J Interv Card Electrophysiol 2018;53(1). https://doi.org/10.1007/s10840-018-0362-y.

34. Ricciardi D, Giacomo DG, Antonio B, et al. 169-04: non invasive hemodynamic optimization of multisite left ventricular pacing: a multicenter pilot study. EP Eur 2016;18(Suppl_1). https://doi.org/10.1093/europace/18.suppl_1.i115c.

35. Rinaldi CA, Leclercq C, Kranig W, et al. Improvement in acute contractility and hemodynamics with multipoint pacing via a left ventricular quadripolar pacing lead. J Interv Card Electrophysiol 2014;40(1). https://doi.org/10.1007/s10840-014-9891-1.

36. Akerström F, Narváez I, Puchol A, et al. Estimation of the effects of multipoint pacing on battery longevity in routine clinical practice. Europace 2018;20(7). https://doi.org/10.1093/europace/eux209.

37. Antoniou K, Chrysohoou C, Dilaveris P, et al. Optimization in cardiac resynchronization therapy with quadripolar leads offer improvement in cardiac energetics in heart failure patients compared with bipolar leads: HUMVEE Clinical Trial. Eur Heart J 2020;41(Supplement_2). https://doi.org/10.1093/ehjci/ehaa946.0888.

38. Sterliński M, Sokal A, Lenarczyk R, et al. In heart failure patients with left bundle branch block single lead multispot left ventricular pacing does not improve acute hemodynamic response to conventional biventricular pacing. A multicenter prospective, interventional, non-randomized study. PLoS One 2016;11(4). https://doi.org/10.1371/journal.pone.0154024.

39. Niazi I, Baker J, Corbisiero R, et al. Safety and efficacy of multipoint pacing in cardiac resynchronization therapy: the MultiPoint pacing trial. JACC Clin Electrophysiol 2017;3(13). https://doi.org/10.1016/j.jacep.2017.06.022.

40. Leclercq C, Burri H, Curnis A, et al. Rationale and design of a randomized clinical trial to assess the safety and efficacy of multipoint pacing therapy: MOre REsponse on cardiac resynchronization therapy with MultiPoint Pacing (MORE-CRT MPP–PHASE II). Am Heart J 2019;209. https://doi.org/10.1016/j.ahj.2018.12.004.

41. Leclercq C, Burri H, Curnis A, et al. Cardiac resynchronization therapy non-responder to responder conversion rate in the more response to cardiac resynchronization therapy with MultiPoint Pacing (MORE-CRT MPP) study: results from phase I. Eur Heart J 2019;40(35). https://doi.org/10.1093/eurheartj/ehz109.

42. Abdelhadi R, Adelstein E, Voigt A, et al. Measures of left ventricular dyssynchrony and the correlation to clinical and echocardiographic response after cardiac resynchronization therapy. Am J Cardiol 2008;102(5):598–601.

43. Zanon F, Marcantoni L, Baracca E, et al. Optimization of left ventricular pacing site plus multipoint pacing improves remodeling and clinical response to cardiac resynchronization therapy at 1 year. Heart Rhythm. 2016 Aug;13(8):1644–51.

44. Forleo GB, Santini L, Giammaria M, et al. Multipoint pacing via a quadripolar left-ventricular lead: preliminary results from the Italian registry on multipoint left-ventricular pacing in cardiac resynchronization therapy (IRON-MPP). Europace. 2017 Jul 1;19(7):1170–1177.

45. Antoniou CK, Dilaveris P, Chrysohoou C, et al. Multipoint left ventricular pacing effects on hemodynamic parameters and functional status: HUMVEE single-arm clinical trial (NCT03189368). Hellenic J Cardiol. 2021 Mar 4:S1109-9666(21)00049-X. doi: 10.1016/j.hjc.2021.02.012.

46. Saba S, Nair D, Ellis CR, et al. Strategic Management to Improve CRT Using Multi-Site Pacing (SMART-MSP) Investigators.Usefulness of Multisite Ventricular Pacing in Nonresponders to Cardiac Resynchronization Therapy. Am J Cardiol. 2022 Feb 1;164:86–92.

Left Ventricular Endocardial Pacing
Update and State of the Art

Pierre Bordachar, MD, PhD[a,b], Marc Strik, MD, PhD[a,b],*,
Sylvain Ploux, MD, PhD[a,b]

KEYWORDS

- Encocardium • Endocardial • CRT • Left ventricle • Pacing

KEY POINTS

- Despite promising initial results, endocardial left ventricular (LV) pacing by atrial transseptal and wireless approaches remains anecdotal in clinical practice.
- Possible advantages of endocardial LV pacing are a more physiologic activation, being less arrhythmogenic, more effective on the hemodynamic level, with better thresholds, and without the risk of phrenic stimulation.
- Coupling leadless right and left ventricular endocardial pacing may represent a promising future for cardiac resynchronization therapy.

INTRODUCTION

Cardiac resynchronization therapy (CRT) is a well-established treatment of heart failure patients with left ventricular (LV) systolic dysfunction and intraventricular conduction disturbances.[1] The most common implantation technique consists of percutaneously placing the LV lead in one of the coronary sinus tributaries, which enables epicardial pacing of the LV. This approach is limited by unsuitable coronary venous anatomy in some patients and a relatively large proportion of unexpected nonresponders. These limitations have sparked the development of alternatives to pacing via the coronary sinus. Initially, LV endocardial pacing was performed as a bailout procedure after unsuccessful transvenous CRT implantation in the presence of surgical contraindications. In addition to being an alternative solution, LV pacing at the adjacent endocardial site allows for a more physiologic activation, restoring endocardial to epicardial transmural activation.[2] Favorable results observed on animals and then on a small number of patients suggesting superior hemodynamic benefit of endocardial over conventional epicardial LV stimulation generated further enthusiasm toward endocardial LV pacing.[2–4] Different techniques have been proposed to stimulate the LV endocardium in humans (Fig. 1), with feasibility and safety studies involving limited numbers of patients. There are 2 principle approaches that account for most of the implanted patients: atrial transseptal and wireless pacing.

A review we wrote in 2010 was in favor of extending the indications for LV endocardial pacing.[5] We outlined the advantages and disadvantages of the different options available, projected the potential future applications in light of the promising initial results, and emphasized the need for adequately powered randomized studies.[5] It is clear that after 10 years, the number of patients implanted worldwide with LV endocardial stimulation has remained anecdotal. The

Funding: This work received financial support from the French Government as part of the "Investments of the Future" program managed by the National Research Agency (ANR) [Grant number ANR-10-IAHU-04].
[a] Bordeaux University Hospital (CHU), Cardio-Thoracic Unit, Avenue Magellan, 33600 Pessac, France; [b] IHU Liryc, Electrophysiology and Heart Modeling Institute, Avenue Haut Lévêque, 33600 Pessac, France
* Corresponding author. Service Pr Haïssaguerre, Hôpital cardiologique du Haut-Lévêque, Avenue de Magellan, Pessac 33600, France.
E-mail address: marc.strik@chu-bordeaux.fr
Twitter: @StrikMarc (M.S.)

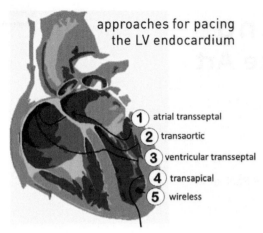

approaches for pacing
the LV endocardium

1. atrial transseptal
2. transaortic
3. ventricular transseptal
4. transapical
5. wireless

Fig. 1. Possible approaches for LV endocardial free wall pacing.

development of CRT alternatives has moved toward His bundle pacing and more recently, left bundle branch area pacing and LV septal pacing, the techniques of which are more elaborately described elsewhere. In this review, we will describe the different techniques proposed to allow LV endocardial pacing, the results observed, and then we will discuss the reasons why LV endocardial pacing seems to be out of fashion today and what are the possible perspectives for development.

RATIONALE FOR ENDOCARDIAL RATHER THAN EPICARDIAL LEFT VENTRICULAR PACING

Various theoretic advantages have generated the interest of the scientific community for endocardial rather than epicardial LV pacing. Endocardial pacing allows for a more physiologic activation, being less arrhythmogenic, more effective on the hemodynamic level, with better thresholds, and without the risk of phrenic stimulation.

Phrenic nerve stimulation is unlikely with endocardial pacing because the pacing electrode is separated from the nerve or the diaphragm by the myocardium. Moreover, endocardial LV pacing is not reliant on the coronary sinus anatomy and therefore allows for a wide choice of pacing sites. In the infrequent cases of phrenic nerve capture, operators can choose to deliver stimulation at any site within the LV cavity. This freedom of choice also allows an optimization of the capture threshold during the procedure, in contrary to when the lead is placed in a coronary sinus tributary. In case of high capture threshold, the lead can more easily be repositioned. Using active fixation LV leads, the incidence of lead dislodgement

should be lower than with a passive fixation lead positioned in a cardiac vein. These various elements should make it possible to significantly reduce the proportion of patients who are nonresponders because they have ineffective ventricular pacing.

More Physiologic Stimulation and Reduced Arrhythmogenic Risk

LV epicardial pacing reverses the normal depolarization sequence which is thought to also prolong the duration of the QT interval and to promote the occurrence of reentrant arrhythmias in vulnerable patients.[6] Endocardial LV pacing enables a more physiologic electrical activation of the left ventricle, with a near-normal transmural activation spreading from the endocardium to the epicardium. Animal and human experiments have shown that compared with LV epicardial pacing, endocardial LV pacing not only decreases the dispersion of depolarization but also repolarization.[2,7] This may potentially obviate the proarrhythmic effect and lower the risk of pacing-induced ventricular arrhythmia.

Faster Activation for Greater Hemodynamic Benefit

Pacing the endocardium may be hemodynamically more beneficial than epicardial pacing. Conduction velocities are higher at the endocardium, and wave-front propagation occurs along the smaller endocardial circumference of the heart explaining why endocardial stimulation allows for faster activation of the LV cavity. Invasive mapping studies in the canine heart show that a wavefront initiated by an LV endocardial electrode propagates faster through the LV than when initiated by an electrode across the wall on the LV epicardium.[2] **Fig. 2** shows that this difference in LV activation is more pronounced in concentric remodeling (myocardial infarction model) than in eccentric remodeling (dilated heart failure model).

The wall thickness is related to the amount of resynchronization amendable by endocardial pacing indicates that reversal of transmural conduction indeed plays an important role in why endocardial LV pacing delivers improved CRT. Hemodynamic studies performed in canine models of left bundle branch block with or without heart failure showed a highly significant hemodynamic superiority of LV endocardial over epicardial stimulation at the same LV site through the mitigation of ventricular dyssynchrony, shortening of QRS complex duration, improvement in maximum rate of increase of LV pressure, and stroke work.[2] Human data regarding the potential hemodynamic benefit of endocardial pacing are scarce and more

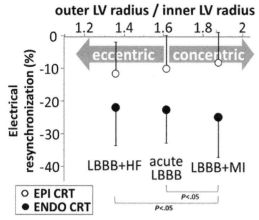

Fig. 2. Percent change in electrical resynchronization (LV activation time acquired by contact mapping) during epicardial (EPI) versus endocardial (ENDO) CRT as a function of the ratio of outer LV radius to inner LV radius in the 3 experimental groups. LBBB = left bundle branch block. HF = heart failure. MI = myocardial infarction. p-values signify the statistical difference between groups in effect size.

controversial.[3,4] In patients with nonischemic cardiomyopathy, the superiority of LV endocardial pacing over epicardial stimulation was not demonstrated when pacing was performed at the same site.[3] Similarly, in patients with ischemic heart failure, a first study did not demonstrate the superiority of endocardial pacing compared with a conventional lateral epicardial site.[4] In contrast, comparing multiple endocardial and epicardial pacing sites in 8 patients with ischemic heart disease, Behar and colleagues demonstrated a superior acute hemodynamic response to pacing from the LV endocardium compared with conventional epicardial CRT.[8]

Possibility to Choose the Pacing Site to Optimize Response

LV endocardial pacing offers greater choice of pacing site across the LV surface. It is, therefore, possible to screen at implant various pacing locations to determine the position which yields the greatest improvement in cardiac function. However, determining cardiac function acutely remains challenging, susceptible to noise,[9] and in addition, acute response does not necessarily guarantee chronic response.[10]

HOW TO PACE THE ENDOCARDIUM OF THE LEFT VENTRICLE?

Different techniques have been described for the permanent implantation of an endocardial LV lead, including transseptal, transapical, and transaortic endocardial stimulation. Within these approaches, there are multiple variations. The

various operators have shown great ingenuity in developing implantation kits, most of the time using equipment that was not initially designed for this type of intervention. Two techniques, atrial transseptal pacing and wireless LV endocardial pacing, represent most of the procedures performed and have benefited from the participation of 2 manufacturers (Medtronic and EBR Systems).

Transaortic, Transapical, and Transseptal Ventricular Approach

Although a study in pigs showed the safety of LV endocardial pacing by puncturing the carotid artery,[11] deliberate arterial access to the LV has not been yet investigated in human, and the clinical cases described in the literature correspond to inadvertent transarterial LV lead placement mostly diagnosed through thromboembolic complications.[12] Hungarian surgeons have described transapical LV endocardial stimulation through a mini-thoracotomy.[13] Using Seldinger's technique, an active fixation lead is introduced into the LV cavity by puncturing the apex, positioned and fixed at the endocardium under fluoroscopic guidance and tunneled up to the generator implanted in the conventional subclavicular position. To avoid the crossing of the mitral valve by the lead observed with atrial transseptal pacing, permanent transventricular endocardial LV pacing has been proposed and reported in a few patients.[14,15] Using a subclavian vein access, interventricular septal puncture is performed with radiofrequency energy applied to a wire via a steerable catheter, and the lead is deployed inside the LV cavity. Transapical and ventricular transseptal approaches require permanent effective anticoagulation to avoid thromboembolic complications. A few clinical cases and studies on limited numbers have been described with these different techniques, limiting the possibility of evaluating the feasibility, and safety in acute situations. Similarly, the long-term safety and efficacy of these techniques have not been evaluated.

Atrial Transseptal Approach

There is a little more experience with atrial transseptal pacing that can be performed through a superior, inferior, or mixed approach with different variants described in the literature and multiple modifications of the technique over the past 20 years.[16–18] The placement of a transseptal LV endocardial lead requires the puncture of the interatrial septum with or without the guidance of transesophageal echocardiography. The lead is then advanced from the right to the left atrium before entering the left ventricle through the mitral valve. Initially, the procedures were challenging because the instrumentation used was not dedicated and operators adapted existing equipment to comply with individual anatomic specificities. Experience with these techniques has been reported in small single-center studies, generally focusing on acute technical, feasibility, and safety outcomes. To disseminate this strategy on a wider scale, technical improvement and dedicated instrumentation were required to allow a purely superior approach. Medtronic (MN, USA) has developed LV lead implant equipment specifically designed to allow puncture of the interatrial septum from the superior vena cava with radiofrequency energy under guidance by transesophageal echocardiography. A SelectSecure lead (4.2- French bipolar lumenless lead) is then fixed at the LV endocardium with access solely from the left subclavian vein. The industry-sponsored, noncontrolled, multicenter Alternate Site Cardiac Resynchronization (ALSYNC) study evaluated the feasibility and safety of this approach and material and included 138 patients recruited from 18 centers.[17] All patients were maintained on therapeutic oral anticoagulation (International Normalized Ratio target of 3 with a range of 2–4). Implant success rate was 89%, with 14 failed implant attempts, 11 of which were due to failure to cross the interatrial septum. Long-term assessment of the lead electrical performance revealed stable parameters over the study period. However, safety concerns were significant with a nonnegligible number of complications such as stroke in 5 patients and transient ischemic attack in 9 patients.

Leadless Left Ventricular Pacing

A disruptive pacing strategy, wireless cardiac resynchronization system (WiSE-CRT, EBR Systems, Sunnyvale, California), was developed to pace the LV endocardium without either requiring a thoracotomy, presence of a lead crossing the mitral valve, or even systemic anticoagulation. Wireless pacing is provided by transmitting acoustic energy from an ultrasound pulse generator, implanted subcutaneously over the ribcage, to a small receiver electrode implanted in the LV which converts it to electrical energy to activate the myocardium. The implantation procedure is a 2-step process and takes place over consecutive days. In the first procedure, the battery and transmitter are implanted to locate the appropriate implanting site for the LV electrode. The pulse generator location is guided by preimplant screening through transthoracic echocardiography. The battery is placed near the pulse generator along the midaxillary line. A subcutaneous channel

is needed between the 2 pockets to pass a 30 cm cable connecting battery and transmitter. During the second procedure, an endocardial electrode is implanted under fluoroscopic guidance using either a retrograde transaortic approach via the femoral artery or a transseptal approach via the femoral vein (according to the operator preference taking into account known peripheral artery disease or a prosthetic aortic valve). The pacing site is selected through the use of echo evaluation for the acoustic window, electrical delay measurement (between onset QRS and electrode), and pacing thresholds. The components of the Wise-CRT system are shown in **Fig. 3**. The system uses the right ventricular pacing signal from a previously implanted pacemaker or implantable cardioverter-defibrillator to trigger LV stimulation. Following the implantation, aspirin and clopidogrel are usually prescribed for 3 to 6 months, while anticoagulation is not mandatory. Early clinical studies evaluating this system confirmed that implantation was feasible. However, the first version of the delivery system for the endocardial electrode was limited by prohibitive safety concerns, specifically the high incidence of pericardial tamponade which could be fatal. The company has subsequently redesigned the implanted equipment to reduce the risk of LV perforation. The prospective, multicenter, nonrandomized trial SELECT-LV study enrolled 39 for whom a "conventional" strategy to achieve resynchronization had previously failed.[19] Of the 39 patients initially enrolled, 3 were excluded because of the inadequate acoustic window and 1 dropped out before the planned intervention. Implantation was successful in 97% of the patients. After 6 months of follow-up, 94% of patients continued to correctly receive biventricular pacing. However, there was one occurrence of ventricular fibrillation due to delivery catheter-induced ventricular ectopy (before extrusion of the pacing electrode), which resulted in a prolonged resuscitation and death. Furthermore, there were 2 confirmed infections related to the subcutaneous pulse generator. Overall, 8 patients (22%) had adverse events over 6 months. The WICS-LV Post-Market Surveillance Registry is the largest experience with this technology with 90 patients from 14 European centers.[20] The procedural success was 94%. Implantation of the system was associated with a nonnegligible complication rate: 3 procedural deaths, 4 patients had a complication within 24 hours of the procedure, and 25.5% had a complication between 24 hours and 6 months after the procedure. During the roll-in phase of the recent prospective open-label single-arm multicenter SOLVE-CRT trial performed in centers with no prior implanting

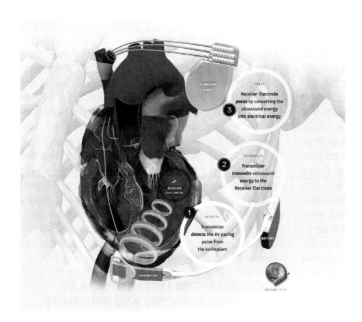

experience, efficacy and primary safety endpoints safety outcomes of 31 patients treated with the WiSE-CRT system were evaluated.[21] A high success rate of LV endocardial electrode placement was observed with no deaths or LV perforations associated with the procedure. Three complications were observed: one case of superficial infection treated with antibiotics, one case of electrode dislodgement which was successfully snared, and one case of poor LV capture.

TECHNICAL, TECHNOLOGICAL, AND SAFETY ISSUES

Currently, the most important approaches to pace the LV endocardial free wall (wireless system and atrial transseptal pacing) are limited by technical, technological, and safety issues.

Atrial Transseptal Approach

The development of material allowing implantation through the usual routes (subclavian or left axillary vein) represented an important step with satisfactory feasibility. On the other hand, there are a certain number of limitations, sometimes only theoretic but also sometimes demonstrated in the various studies carried out. During the procedure, the operation is systematically performed under heparin therapy, which may increase the risk of bleeding, hematoma, and tamponade. Similarly, the need to perform a transseptal puncture increases the risks associated with this procedure. The ALSYNC study carried out in experienced centers did not find any major intraoperative

complications.[17] An LV lead implanted through the interatrial septum crosses the mitral valve and theoretically increases the risks for adverse interaction, insufficiency, or endocarditis. The performed studies have not yet demonstrated pacing lead-induced mitral valve damage or increased mitral regurgitation. The use of thin, floppy leads and the minimal scar tissue reaction in the left heart may contribute to prevent valve dysfunction. Considering the risk of systemic embolization, percutaneous extraction of old leads in the case of lead infection may be too risky and open chest surgical intervention may be required. Few case reports have described safe extraction using standard percutaneous instrumentation when the LV endocardial lead had not been in place for a long time. The risk of thrombus formation on the lead is a major concern and a permanent fear with LV endocardial leads. Indeed, even small emboli may cause major systemic complications including cerebrovascular accidents. This thrombogenic risk has been described in cases of inadvertent implantation of a lead into the left ventricle through a patent foramen ovale.[22] Furthermore, the presence of an atrial septal orifice may be the source of paradoxical embolization.[23] All the patients who have had transseptal endocardial LV leads implanted received heparin during the procedure and anticoagulation therapy in the long term with its risks of inappropriate discontinuation or excessive doses and hemorrhagic complications. The level of anticoagulation representing an optimal compromise between hemorrhagic and thrombogenic risk remains to be defined. Even if small numbers of events are reported overall, despite the introduction of lifelong anticoagulation, thromboembolic complications were reported in many published experiences.[18] The results of the ALSYNC study, the study with the largest number of participants, are of concern with stroke in 5 patients and transient ischemic attack in 9 patients. These results have surely inhibited further development of this technique. The utilization of new anticoagulants may be proposed in these patients, after validation in a clinical study, to reduce the risk of thromboembolic complications by offering a steady state of anticoagulation. In fact, most of the cerebral accidents were related to periods of inappropriate discontinuation of anticoagulation therapy and of difficulty in maintaining a consistent INR level. The thrombotic risk may also be lower with ventricular transseptal implantation because the lead does not pass through the left atrium whereby the flow is reduced.

Leadless Left Ventricular Pacing

Leadless pacing has the major advantage to alleviate or to suppress some of the complications associated with lead presence inside the LV. There is no lead interaction with the mitral valve, the thromboembolic, and infection risks are largely decreased because the endocardial electrode is endothelialized after a few weeks, and therefore, there is no need for lifelong anticoagulation with its associated risks. However, the technical challenges confronting the implanting physicians are significant, and the system has several major limitations. A preprocedural screening is required, and a limited proportion of patients (<10%) are not suitable for implantation because they do not have an adequate acoustic window for the transmitter. In our opinion, the major limitations are the complexity of the implant procedure and the high acute complication rate. The intervention is carried out over consecutive days, requires different incisions, and either retrograde femoral artery or transseptal access. The quantity of implanted material is significant (transmitter, battery, endocardial electrode, and coimplanted transvenous right ventricular pacemaker or defibrillator) increasing the long-term risk of infection. In the initial evaluations, acute and short-term serious adverse effects were significant and severe including death, perforation, electrode embolization to lower extremities, and pocket infections. The initial evaluation of WiSE-CRT had to be stopped for safety reasons (high number of patients with pericardial tamponade after electrode delivery). To reduce this serious complication, the delivery system has been modified to be less traumatic. However, even if the recent results of the SOLVE-CRT study in terms of feasibility and safety carried out in centers with no previous experience are rather reassuring, the severe complications observed in the first evaluations have left their mark on a significant part of the scientific community which considers this option to be very invasive, risky, and reserved for highly experienced operators in high-volume centers experiencing in treating vascular and cardiothoracic complications. There are also some significant technological issues. Some cases of defective transmitter circuitry within the first months after implant have been described, and transmission via ultrasound requires additional energy leading to higher frequency of battery replacements.

CANDIDATES FOR LEFT VENTRICULAR ENDOCARDIAL PACING AND PROSPECTS

It appears that the number of patients currently implanted with transseptal or leadless pacing systems is limited. Moreover, at this time, there are few actively recruiting randomized trials evaluating LV endocardial pacing using these methods. The objectives of the SOLVE-CRT study have been considerably reduced with apparent difficulty in enrolling patients.[24] This strategy, regardless of the technical means, is therefore only rarely used in clinical practice and does not constitute an active research field. Different categories of patients can be considered for LV endocardial pacing.

Alternative Solution for Conventional Cardiac Resynchronization Therapy Implant

LV endocardial pacing has initially been proposed as an alternative option for the patients that failed a standard transvenous resynchronization and who were at prohibitive surgical risk. Most of the patients included in the studies fit this profile. The ALSYNC and SELECT-LV study recruited "complex and high risk" patients for whom conventional CRT had failed or was unsuitable. Although these studies were mainly designed to evaluate the feasibility and safety of these approaches, clinical and echocardiographic endpoints were also analyzed. Briefly, the outcomes seemed comparable with those observed in conventional CRT trials. Wireless CRT resulted in significant improvement in LV ejection fraction, end-diastolic volume, end-systolic volume, NYHA Class, and clinical composite score.[19] Additionally, only 56% of patients had a decrease in LVESV by $\geq$ 15%. In patients with intrinsic QRS data at baseline and 6 months, there were significant reductions in the intrinsic QRS and 55% of the patients were noted to have a shortening of the QRS duration by at least 20 ms. Similarly, ALSYNC reported in patients with failed implants, a response rate of 60% and identified improvement in functional class and LV function. Despite these positive results, there are 2 main reasons for the low number of patients implanted in this setting. (1) With current improvements in "conventional" CRT technology and development of dedicated instrumentation (improvement in delivery kit, greater operator experience, new generation quadripolar leads…), the procedure remains sometimes challenging, but the rate of failed CRT has steadily improved over time and occurs now in less than 5% of cases. Similarly, with the widespread utilization of quadripolar LV leads, which can reduce the risk of phrenic nerve stimulation, low pacing thresholds, and the need for lead reposition, the proportion of interrupted CRT for ineffective LV pacing is gradually declining. The need for an alternative strategy is, therefore, less important today than it was at the beginning of resynchronization and could decrease in the future with further technological progress. (2) For the rare patients with implantation failure, is the endocardial route, whether transseptal or wireless, the alternative reference technique? While the use of surgical epicardial electrodes placed has been an option since the advent of CRT, this option is now infrequently used. Surgical techniques are invasive requiring at least a mini-thoracotomy, can be challenging in patients with prior cardiac surgery, and the long-term performance and durability of surgically placed epicardial leads are poor. Alternative pacing techniques have recently been developed aiming to directly capture the ventricular conduction system (His bundle pacing, left bundle branch area pacing) and are now increasingly proposed as alternative solutions or even as first-line solutions. It must be stated that a significant amount of patients implanted with a left bundle branch area pacing lead actually receive LV septal endocardial pacing. This is the case for noncapture (approximately a quarter of patients) or nonselective capture (approximately half of patients) of the left bundle branch.[25,26] LV septal endocardial pacing has similar electrical and hemodynamic results as conventional CRT and can be performed by advancing a commercially available lead through the septum until the endocardial side of the LV is reached.[27–29]

Rescue Solution for Nonresponders

This category of patients represents one of the original targets of these different approaches.

Although there are no controlled studies and the numbers are small, the results in ALSYNC in this subgroup of patients were promising, the investigators reporting a significant clinical and echocardiographic improvement of 59% and 55%, respectively, in a group with prior nonresponse. In refractory heart failure and in a therapeutic dead-end, we consider that the safety and technological issues described with the different endocardial approaches may be acceptable as the expected benefit is substantial. However, the number of patients implanted in this setting is currently modest for much the same reasons. The main limitation of conventional CRT is often stated to be between 30% and 40% of patients receiving CRT. This figure no longer seems to reflect the current reality. The percentage of nonresponders has probably decreased significantly with current improvements in CRT technology and with the tightening of indications to patients with left bundle branch block, wide QRS, or right ventricular pacing. Similarly, in a nonresponder, left bundle branch area pacing rather than conventional transseptal or wireless pacing may now be preferred by a growing number of operators.

Implantation as First Intention

Conventional CRT pacing is a mature therapy, having demonstrated its efficacy with a limited risk of adverse events. In view of the safety and technological issues, there seems to be no justification today for choosing transseptal or wireless pacing as a first-line option in patients requiring CRT. No comparative study has been able to demonstrate that endocardial pacing actually provides a superior clinical benefit to conventional pacing. Although some results, mainly in animals, are promising, the superiority of endocardial pacing on the arrhythmogenic effect or on the response to resynchronization remains more theoretic than demonstrated. The ability to freely choose the LV pacing site for optimal response has often been presented as a strong argument for the development of these strategies. The problem is that there has been little progress on the question of which intraoperative measurement might best predict patient benefit and outcome after CRT.[30] Acute hemodynamic response may not necessarily indicate long-term outcome.[10] In the vast majority of transseptal device implantations, the lead is directly implanted in the lateral or posterolateral LV wall without the possibility of further optimization. The potential theoretical hemodynamic benefits of LV endocardial pacing cannot compensate today for the potential for harm by delivering stimulation within the LV cavity.

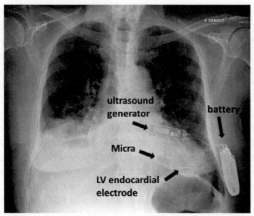

Fig. 4. A patient chest X-ray shows both Micra and WiSE-CRT systems. Green: Micra leadless pacemaker; blue: WiSE-CRT system LV endocardial electrode; and red: WiSE-CRT system subcutaneous battery and ultrasound generator. CRT, cardiac resynchronization therapy (*Adapted from* Carabelli A, Jabeur M, Jacon P, et al. European experience with a first totally leadless cardiac resynchronization therapy pacemaker system. Eur Eur Pacing Arrhythm Card Electrophysiol J Work Groups Card Pacing Arrhythm Card Cell Electrophysiol Eur Soc Cardiol. 2021;23(5):740-747. https://doi.org/10.1093/europace/euaa342; with permission).

Upgrading of a Leadless Pacemaker

Leadless technology and the use of leadless pacemakers, which are transvenously implanted in the right ventricle, are being more and more adapted. The Wise-CRT system may be a suitable indication here as it is the only option available if an upgrade to biventricular pacing is required in a patient implanted with a Micra leadless RV pacemaker. A study has shown that the Micra and the WiSE-CRT systems can successfully operate together to deliver total leadless CRT to a patient.[31] This combined solution (see example in **Fig. 4**) could also be proposed as a first line solution for a patient requiring resynchronization but with impossible access to the heart chambers by the upper route (venous stenosis or thrombosis) preventing the implantation of transvenous leads.

SUMMARY

Despite promising initial results, several factors have prevented the broad dissemination of transseptal and wireless stimulation strategies and it is reasonable to postulate that this is unlikely to change in the near future. However, there is probably a promising avenue for development as the future of antibradycardia cardiac pacing is going in the direction of leadless technology and

solutions coupling leadless right and LV pacing might also represent a promising future for CRT.

FUNDING

This work received financial support from the French Government as part of the "Investments of the Future" program managed by the National Research Agency (ANR) [Grant number ANR-10-IAHU-04].

CONFLICT OF INTEREST

The authors declare no conflict of interest.

REFERENCES

1. Vernooy K, van Deursen CJM, Strik M, et al. Strategies to improve cardiac resynchronization therapy. Nat Rev Cardiol 2014;11(8):481–93.
2. Strik M, Rademakers LM, van Deursen CJM, et al. Endocardial left ventricular pacing improves cardiac resynchronization therapy in chronic asynchronous infarction and heart failure models. Circ Arrhythm Electrophysiol 2012;5(1):191–200.
3. Derval N, Steendijk P, Gula LJ, et al. Optimizing hemodynamics in heart failure patients by systematic screening of left ventricular pacing sites: the lateral left ventricular wall and the coronary sinus are rarely the best sites. J Am Coll Cardiol 2010;55(6):566–75.
4. Spragg DD, Dong J, Fetics BJ, et al. Optimal left ventricular endocardial pacing sites for cardiac resynchronization therapy in patients with ischemic cardiomyopathy. J Am Coll Cardiol 2010;56(10):774–81.
5. Bordachar P, Derval N, Ploux S, et al. Left ventricular endocardial stimulation for severe heart failure. J Am Coll Cardiol 2010;56(10):747–53.
6. Deif B, Ballantyne B, Almehmadi F, et al. Cardiac resynchronization is pro-arrhythmic in the absence of reverse ventricular remodelling: a systematic review and meta-analysis. Cardiovasc Res 2018;114(11):1435–44.
7. Yamin M, Yuniadi Y, Alwi I, et al. Endocardial biventricular pacing for chronic heart failure patients: effect on transmural dispersion of repolarization. J Arrhythmia 2019;35(4):664–9.
8. Behar JM, Jackson T, Hyde E, et al. Optimized left ventricular endocardial stimulation is superior to optimized epicardial stimulation in ischemic patients with poor response to cardiac resynchronization therapy. Jacc Clin Electrophysiol 2016;2(7):799–809.
9. Pabari PA, Willson K, Stegemann B, et al. When is an optimization not an optimization? Evaluation of clinical implications of information content (signal-to-noise ratio) in optimization of cardiac resynchronization

therapy, and how to measure and maximize it. Heart Fail Rev 2011;16(3):277–90.

10. Prinzen FW, Houthuizen P, Bogaard MD, et al. Is acute hemodynamic response a predictor of long-term outcome in cardiac resynchronization therapy? J Am Coll Cardiol 2012;59(13):1198.

11. Reinig M, White M, Levine M, et al. Left ventricular endocardial pacing: a transarterial approach. Pacing Clin Electrophysiol PACE 2007;30(12):1464–8.

12. Reising S, Safford R, Castello R, et al. A stroke of bad luck: left ventricular pacemaker malposition. J Am Soc Echocardiogr Off Publ Am Soc Echocardiogr 2007;20(11):1316.e1–3.

13. Kassai I, Foldesi C, Szekely A, et al. New method for cardiac resynchronization therapy: transapical endocardial lead implantation for left ventricular free wall pacing. Eur Eur Pacing Arrhythm Card Electrophysiol J Work Groups Card Pacing Arrhythm Card Cell Electrophysiol Eur Soc Cardiol 2008;10(7): 882–3.

14. Gamble JHP, Herring N, Ginks MR, et al. Endocardial left ventricular pacing across the interventricular septum for cardiac resynchronization therapy: clinical results of a pilot study. Heart Rhythm 2018; 15(7):1017–22.

15. Betts TR, Gamble JHP, Khiani R, et al. Development of a technique for left ventricular endocardial pacing via puncture of the interventricular septum. Circ Arrhythm Electrophysiol 2014;7(1):17–22.

16. Morgan JM, Scott PA, Turner NG, et al. Targeted left ventricular endocardial pacing using a steerable introducing guide catheter and active fixation pacing lead. EP Eur 2009;11(4):502–6.

17. Morgan JM, Biffi M, Gellér L, et al. ALternate Site Cardiac ResYNChronization (ALSYNC): a prospective and multicentre study of left ventricular endocardial pacing for cardiac resynchronization therapy. Eur Heart J 2016;37(27):2118–27.

18. Gamble JHP, Herring N, Ginks M, et al. Endocardial left ventricular pacing for cardiac resynchronization: systematic review and meta-analysis. Eur Eur Pacing Arrhythm Card Electrophysiol J Work Groups Card Pacing Arrhythm Card Cell Electrophysiol Eur Soc Cardiol 2018;20(1):73–81.

19. Reddy VY, Miller MA, Neuzil P, et al. Cardiac resynchronization therapy with wireless left ventricular endocardial pacing: the SELECT-LV study. J Am Coll Cardiol 2017;69(17):2119–29.

20. Sieniewicz BJ, Betts TR, James S, et al. Real-world experience of leadless left ventricular endocardial cardiac resynchronization therapy: a multicenter international registry of the WiSE-CRT pacing system. Heart Rhythm 2020;17(8):1291–7.

21. Okabe T, Hummel JD, Bank AJ, et al. Leadless left ventricular stimulation with WiSE-CRT System - initial experience and results from phase I of SOLVE-CRT Study (nonrandomized, roll-in phase). Heart Rhythm 2021. https://doi.org/10.1016/j.hrthm.2021.06.1195. S1547-5271(21)01808-7.

22. Bologne JC, Garweg C, Lancellotti P, et al. [Inadvertent implantation of a defibrillation lead in the left ventricle through a patent foramen ovale]. Rev Med Liege 2012;67(2):58–60.

23. Webb G, Gatzoulis MA. Atrial septal defects in the adult. Circulation 2006;114(15):1645–53.

24. Singh JP, Walsh MN, Kubo SH, et al. Modified design of stimulation of the left ventricular endocardium for cardiac resynchronization therapy in nonresponders, previously untreatable and high-risk upgrade patients (SOLVE-CRT) trial. Am Heart J 2021;235:158–62.

25. Zhang J, Sheng X, Pan Y, et al. Electrophysiological insights into three modalities of left bundle branch area pacing in patients indicated for pacing therapy. Int Heart J 2021;62(1):78–86.

26. Heckman LIB, Luermans JGLM, Curila K, et al. Comparing ventricular synchrony in left bundle branch and left ventricular septal pacing in pacemaker patients. J Clin Med 2021;10(4):822.

27. Salden FCWM, Luermans JGLM, Westra SW, et al. Short-term hemodynamic and electrophysiological effects of cardiac resynchronization by left ventricular septal pacing. J Am Coll Cardiol 2020;75(4): 347–59.

28. Mills RW, Cornelussen RN, Mulligan LJ, et al. Left ventricular septal and left ventricular apical pacing chronically maintain cardiac contractile coordination, pump function and efficiency. Circ Arrhythm Electrophysiol 2009;2(5):571–9.

29. Strik M, van Deursen CJM, van Middendorp LB, et al. Transseptal conduction as an important determinant for cardiac resynchronization therapy, as revealed by extensive electrical mapping in the dyssynchronous canine heart. Circ Arrhythm Electrophysiol 2013;6(4):682–9.

30. Strik M, Ploux S, Huntjens PR, et al. Response to cardiac resynchronization therapy is determined by intrinsic electrical substrate rather than by its modification. Int J Cardiol 2018;270:143–8.

31. Carabelli A, Jabeur M, Jacon P, et al. European experience with a first totally leadless cardiac resynchronization therapy pacemaker system. Eur Eur Pacing Arrhythm Card Electrophysiol J Work Groups Card Pacing Arrhythm Card Cell Electrophysiol Eur Soc Cardiol 2021;23(5):740–7.

Case Studies of Cardiac Resynchronization Therapy "Nonresponders"

John Rickard, MD, MPH

KEYWORDS

• Cardiac resynchronization therapy • Nonresponder • Optimization clinic

KEY POINTS

• Upitration of medical therapies for heart failure in the psot CRT follow up period is important to optimizing outcomes.
• Suppression of atrial fibrillation and PVC's is important in promoting effective CRT.
• Dedicated CRT clinics offer an opportunity to standardize followup and promote cooperation amongst cardiovascular specialties.

 Video content accompanies this article at http://www.cardiacep.theclinics.com.

Cardiac resynchronization therapy (CRT) represents one of the biggest advances in the treatment of patients with systolic heart failure over the last 20 years. Multiple well-conducted large-scale clinical trials have shown that in select patients, CRT can induce a myriad of favorable effects including symptomatic improvement, reverse ventricular remodeling, reduction in heart failure hospitalizations, and improved survival.[1–4] From early on, however, it was noticed that many patients failed to derive meaningful improvement from CRT. A large body of literature evolved over the past 2 decades seeking to elucidate the reasons behind this. At first, CRT response was described as a dichotomous outcome, namely a patient either was a "responder "or a "nonresponder." Several issues have plagued this simplistic categorization. For one, there has been a lack of uniformity of what is meant by a "responder." The medical literature has well more than 20 definitions of response ranging from definitions focused on quality-of-life metrics to others with harder endpoints such as heart failure hospitalizations and/or mortality.[5] Secondly, it has become evident that the phenotypic response to CRT may be more complex

than the simple "responder"/"nonresponder" dichotomy, as such definitions fail to take into account the natural history of disease in any individual patient. The terms "super-responder," "responder," "nonprogressor," "true nonresponder," and "negative responder" have evolved to encapsulate the myriad of outcomes in patients receiving CRT.[6] Gold and colleagues recently looked at outcomes in CRT "nonprogressors" and demonstrated that patients who "stabilized" with CRT had similar positive outcomes to those who improved and superior outcomes to those who worsened following device implant.[7]

What is clear is that patients receiving CRT devices are among the most comorbid subsets of patients cared for in any cardiology practice. Such patients often necessitate care from multiple different cardiovascular subspecialists namely heart failure experts, electrophysiologists, and occasionally imaging experts. What is known is that patients whose left ventricular ejection fraction (LVEF) continues to decline despite CRT have very poor outcomes.[8] Nevertheless, patients noted to be doing poorly despite CRT have been shown to receive no further specialized care than

Section of Cardiac Electrophysiology, Department of Cardiovascular Medicine, Heart, and Vascular Institute, Cleveland Clinic, 9500 Euclid Avenue/J2-2, Cleveland, OH 44195, USA
E-mail address: Rickarj2@ccf.org

Card Electrophysiol Clin 14 (2022) 273–282
https://doi.org/10.1016/j.ccep.2021.12.014
1877-9182/22/© 2022 Elsevier Inc. All rights reserved.

patients who have responded.[8] In the ADVANCE CRT registry, 44% of CRT recipients who were deemed to be nonresponders received no intensification of treatment.[9] In response to this, there has been a concerted effort to intensify resources for CRT patients via specialized CRT clinics, which seek to break down the silo effect between cardiovascular subspecialists and promote cooperation and coordination of care.[10–12] The first clinics of this type was reported on by Mullens and colleagues in 2010.[10] The investigators found that in patients in whom a major intervention was possible had better outcomes than these patients in whom no intervention was performed.[10] In 2012 Altman and colleagues published results from a CRT optimization program.[11] In this program all patients receiving CRT regardless of response status were followed with intensification of care directed to nonresponders. The investigators showed that compared with a historical control, CRT patients going through a structured CRT clinic had improved event-free survival.[11]

Over the last decade, a handful of other structured CRT optimization programs have been started with varying levels of intensity in follow-up.[12] A common misconception about CRT optimization clinics is that they are dedicated to echocardiographic optimization of the atrioventricular (AV) and interventricular (VV) intervals. In general, AV and VV optimization has been disappointing in terms of changing outcomes following CRT implant. In the SMART AV trial echocardiographic optimization of the AV delays using both a device-mediated algorithm and echocardiographic guidance was not superior to a fixed AV delay of 120 ms in terms of reverse ventricular remodeling.[13] In the FREEDM trial, optimizing both AV and VV delays using a device-based algorithm failed to improve patient outcomes based on the clinical composite score.[14] Whether patients deemed to be nonresponders to CRT benefit from AV and VV optimization remains unknown. In the very small RESPONSE HF trial, there was a statistically significant improvement in patient symptoms and 6-minute hall walk distance among nonresponders to CRT with VV optimization.[15] If there is a benefit of AV and VV optimization among CRT nonresponders, the effect is likely to be small, as there is no universally accepted method for AV-VV optimization, all methods optimize relatively small changes, it is not achievable in many patients, and the optimal timing differs during various physiologic conditions.[16,17]

The reasons for CRT nonresponse have been widely studied and debated. Mullens and colleagues reported reasons for nonresponse, including suboptimal AV timing, arrhythmias, poor left ventricular lead position, anemia, and suboptimal medical therapy being the most common.[10] More recently the impact of comorbidities and frailty on CRT outcomes has come to the forefront.[18,19] Kubala and colleagues noted that frail patients experienced significantly less improvement in LVEF with CRT compared with nonfrail patients.[19] In general, many believe that poor electrical substrate, poor LV lead position, and arrhythmia burden leading to a low percentage of nonfused biventricular pacing are among the most common reasons for CRT nonresponse. In addition, the impact of scar burden and severity of myocardial dysfunction on the chances for meaningful improvement with CRT have been increasingly recognized.[20,21] In the following case vignettes, cases from a dedicated CRT optimization clinic are reviewed, highlighting common management scenarios for CRT nonresponders.

CASE #1

A 48-year-old man with nonischemic cardiomyopathy with an LVEF of 25%, obstructive sleep apnea, and diabetes mellitus underwent an attempt at CRT implant. The patient had New York Heart Association (NYHA) class III symptoms and could no longer work due to dyspnea. He had never been hospitalized for congestive heart failure. His baseline electrocardiogram (ECG) is shown in **Fig. 1**. At the time of implant he had 2 suitable

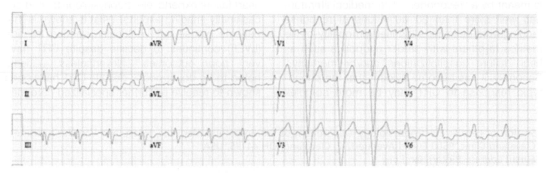

Fig. 1. Baseline 12-lead ECG. Wide left bundle branch meeting all widely accepted definitions of LBBB.

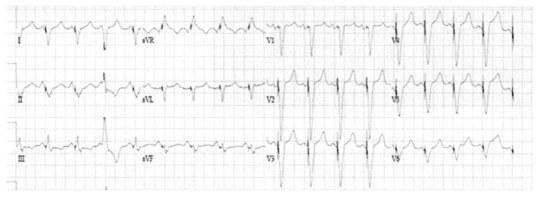

Fig. 2. Presenting paced ECG.

lateral branches (Video 1). The higher of the 2 branches could not be cannulated despite prolonged efforts due to a tortuous initial takeoff. The lower of the 2 branches could be cannulated; however, there was a midvessel stenosis that precluded the wire from passing. As such a left ventricular lead was not placed. Conduction system pacing was attempted; however, a satisfactory result could not be obtained due to significant septal scarring/fibrosis and difficulty advancing the lead despite prolonged efforts. The patient was then sent for a surgical LV lead, which was placed 2 weeks later. Six months later the patient was seen in the CRT clinic at which time he was found to be feeling poorly. He had been hospitalized for heart failure twice since implant of the surgical LV lead. His presenting ECG to the clinic is shown in **Fig. 2**. His medications were reviewed, and he was found to be on maximized doses of carvedilol, sacubitril-valsartan, and Aldactone. A device check showed normal device function. A posteroanterior (PA) and lateral chest radiography was performed and is shown in **Fig. 3**. Repeat echocardiography revealed LVEF of 25%. Longitudinal strain was −2.7% with pacing on and

−4.7% with pacing off, suggesting better cardiac function with pacing turned off. Ultimately computed tomography surgery was reconsulted and, due to body habitus, the patient was deemed not a candidate for a repeat surgical procedure to place another epicardial LV lead more laterally. As a result, the decision was made to take the patient back to the electrophysiology laboratory and attempt to balloon the small stenosis in the lower coronary sinus tributary, try to gain access to the upper branch, or to again revisit conduction system pacing. Ultimately the upper of the 2 branches were cannulated and a lead delivered. The differences in QLV between the anterior surgically placed lead and the new posterolateral percutaneously placed lead are shown in **Fig. 4**. The position of the new coronary sinus lead is shown in **Fig. 5**. The patient was discharged and seen in clinic 2 weeks later still doing very poorly. Device check showed new-onset persistent atrial flutter with very little biventricular pacing. The patient underwent successful ablation for typical atrial flutter. He was seen in follow-up 4 months thereafter, at which time he had a repeat echocardiogram showing his LVEF to have improved to 45%. A

Fig. 3. PA and lateral chest radiograph.

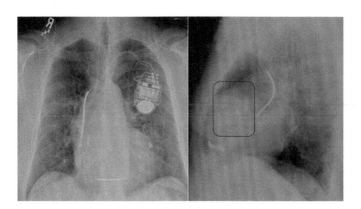

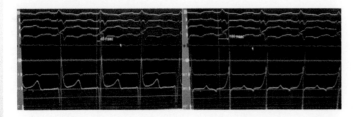

Fig. 4. QLV measurements with anterior surgically placed lead and endocardial posterolateral lead.

device check showed no arrhythmias, and he was noted to be biventricular pacing 99% of the time. He was noted to have NYHA class II symptoms and had returned to work.

Overview

This case highlights 2 important management strategies in managing CRT nonresponders. First, lead position is a key factor in CRT response. Dong and colleagues showed that lateral lead positions significantly outperformed nonlateral positions in terms of reverse ventricular remodeling.[22] Left ventricular leads placed in the great cardiac vein anteriorly or in the middle cardiac vein posteriorly are unlikely to be of benefit, as they are unlikely to course laterally and hence are not able to preexcite the lateral wall of the left ventricle and correct dyssynchrony. In addition, apically placed LV leads seem to be of lesser benefit than nonapical leads, although further study on this is needed.[23] Secondly, atrial arrhythmias such as atrial fibrillation and flutter are the most common reason for a significant drop in biventricular pacing percentage.[24] Atrial fibrillation commonly results in fused and ineffective paced beats, further limiting the effects of CRT. Typically achieving as close to 100% biventricular pacing is the goal, as even small decrements less than this level are associated with poorer outcomes.[25]

CASE #2

A 32-year-old woman presents to clinic with shortness of breath and recurrent heart failure hospitalizations. She has a history of nonischemic cardiomyopathy with an LVEF of 15% and underwent CRT with defibrillator (CRT-D) implant 3 years ago at an outside facility. Since CRT was implanted she has had 6 heart failure hospitalizations. She can walk one block before stopping due to dyspnea. She presents to clinic moderately volume overloaded. A device check showed normal device function with 99% biventricular pacing and no arrhythmias. A PA and lateral chest radiograph is shown in **Fig. 6**, demonstrating a midventricular laterally placed coronary sinus lead. She is noted to be on carvedilol and sacubitril-valsartan, and her blood pressure will not tolerate dose escalation. An echocardiogram in the clinic demonstrated an LVEF of 15% with mild-to-moderate mitral regurgitation. Biventricular pacing was suppressed, and an ECG was performed of the underlying rhythm shown in **Fig. 7**. The difference in aortic velocity time integral is shown in **Fig. 8** with biventricular pacing on versus off. The decision was made to suppress biventricular pacing and let the patient conduct on her own. Her LVEF increased to 30% over the course of 6 months, her symptoms improved, and she had no heart failure hospitalizations at 1-year follow-up.

Overview

Although biventricular pacing has resulted in tremendous benefit for many patients with systolic heart failure, multiple studies have shown no benefit in patients with a narrow QRS.[26,27] In the ECHO–CRT trial, patients with a narrow QRS

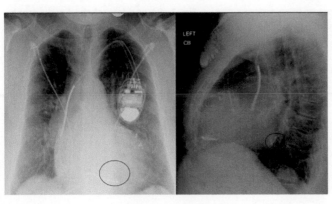

Fig. 5. PA and lateral chest radiograph (CXR). PA and lateral CXR highlighting the placement of a new percutaneous posterolateral left ventricular pacing lead.

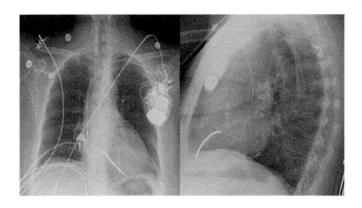

Fig. 6. PA and lateral chest radiograph.

who received CRT had an increase in mortality compared with a non-CRT control.[27] In patients with a CRT device in whom the original indication for device implant is unclear, it is imperative to obtain an ECG of the underlying rhythm. In patients with a robust remodeling response to CRT, resolution of left bundle branch block (LBBB) has been reported; this is not the case clinically in the current situation. Patients with intermittent LBBB pose a clinical conundrum for device implanters, as the incidence of narrow QRS conduction versus conduction with LBBB is difficult to measure. Whether this was the case in this patient is unknown but taking the step to suppress CRT when harm is suspected is important.

CASE #3

A 51-year-old man with severe coronary artery disease, ischemic cardiomyopathy with an LVEF of 20%, severe mitral regurgitation, NYHA class III symptoms, peripheral neuropathy, and hypertension underwent CRT-D implant 6 months before and presents to clinic complaining of shortness of breath and lack of improvement since device implant. He has had 2 heart failure hospitalizations in the past year, one 3 weeks before the clinic visit. On examination he seems slightly volume overloaded. He is on lisinopril, 20 mg, daily and carvedilol, 12.5 mg, twice daily. A PA and lateral chest radiograph revealed the left ventricular lead to be in a midventricular and lateral position. His device check shows normal device function with a QLV of 75% and 99% biventricular pacing. A repeat echocardiogram 6 months later revealed no change in his LVEF with ongoing severe functional mitral regurgitation. His device was suppressed and his underlying ECG is shown in **Fig. 9**. The patient was ultimately sent for a percutaneous mitral valve clip, and lisinopril was replaced by sacubitril-

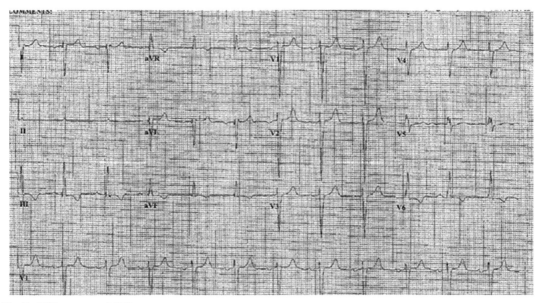

Fig. 7. CRT suppressed ECG.

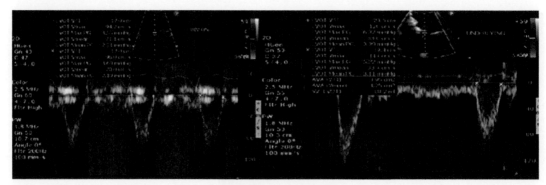

Fig. 8. Aortic VTI with pacing on versus off. VTI, velocity time integral.

valsartan. He was significantly better after these 2 interventions with no heart failure hospitalizations at follow-up and improvement in his functional status to NYHA class II.

Overview

In this case, the patient seemingly failed to develop meaningful clinical improvement with CRT. There was no sense that CRT was causing harm, rather it did not seem to be providing significant benefit. The most likely reason was the electrical substrate. In this case the patient's ECG meets most standard definitions for LBBB but not all. Van Stipdonk and colleagues report that the 3 LBBB signs associated with improved outcomes from CRT are a QS or rS in V1, lack of Q wav in V5 and v6, and notching in V5,V6, I, or AVI.[28] In this case the notching pattern in V5 and v6 is atypical and may be more of a nonspecific intraventricular conduction delay (NSIVCD). There seem to be 3 variants of NSIVCD: atypical LBBB, intraventricular parietal block, and periinfract block.[29] In this case, there is a qR pattern in lead I, and the R wave in V5 and V6 is not broad and has highly atypical notching potentially consistent with intraventricular parietal block where the block is in the Purkinje fiber network or diseased myocardium rather than the His bundle branches and main subdivisions.[29] Strik and colleagues performed ECG mapping in a cohort of patients with left ventricular systolic dysfunction and QRS widening.[30] Patients with NSVICD had more electrical dyssynchrony as measured by total activation times compared with those with an RBBB but significantly less than those with a typical LBBB.[30] What is apparent is that patients with an NSVICD tend to have more advanced myocardial disease and have a poorer prognosis than those with LBBB regardless of CRT.[29]

In this patient there is a QLV of only 76 ms despite a laterally placed lead, which argues that although some electrical dyssynchony may be present, it may not be the driver of the cardiomyopathy. As such, other interventions were sought to help this patient. In a substudy of the COAPT trial, which evaluated 224 patients with systolic heart failure and severe mitral regurgitation (MR) with prior CRT, patients undergoing percutaneous mitral valve intervention had improved heart failure–free survival compared with a control group.[31] In a smaller nonrandomized study of 42 patients with systolic heart failure, prior CRT, and severe MR, Seifert and colleagues reported significant reductions in NT-proBNP levels and reductions in left ventricular end-diastolic volume.[32]

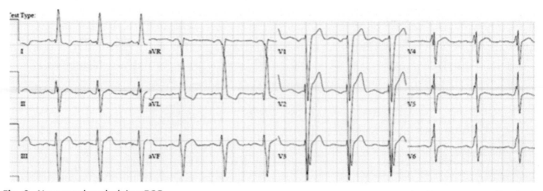

Fig. 9. Nonpaced underlying ECG.

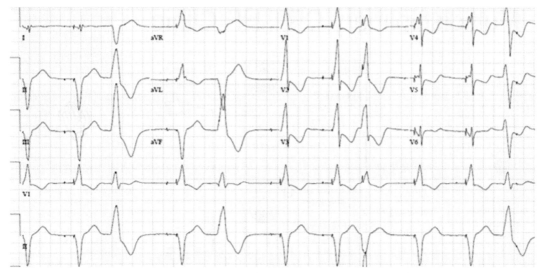

Fig. 10. ECG demonstrating biventricular pacing with frequent premature ventricular contractions.

Small nonrandomized studies have suggested that exchanging an ace inhibitor for sacubitril-valsartan in CRT nonresponders may be useful. In 40 nonresponders to CRT K-H Chun and colleagues showed that patients put on sacubitril-valsartan tended to have improved heart failure–free survival.[33]

CASE #4

A 68-year-old man with coronary artery disease s/p percutaneous coronary intervention and coronary artery bypass graft surgery, ischemic cardiomyopathy with an LVEF of 35%, NYHA class III symptoms, and complete heart block s/p dual chamber pacemaker 3 years before underwent an upgrade to a CRT-D device, given he was pacing unavoidably in the right ventricle constantly. At 6 months postimplant he felt no better. A repeat echocardiogram showed his LVEF to be 30%. His presenting 12-lead ECG is shown in **Fig. 10.**

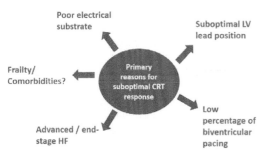

Fig. 11. Common reasons for suboptimal CRT response.

He was noted to be biventricular pacing 86% on device check. The cause of CRT nonresponse was noted to be a heavy premature ventricular contraction (PVC) burden, which accounted for 21% of his total beats. A discussion was had with the patient about ablation or starting an antiarrhythmic medication such as amiodarone. Ultimately the patient underwent successful ablation of a PVC arising from the anterolateral papillary muscle. At 3-month follow-up his PVC burden was negligible. His LVEF increased to 50%, and his symptoms had improved dramatically.

Overview

PVCs are an often overlooked reason why some patients failed to respond to CRT. Many CRT devices have algorithms by which a biventricular paced stimulus is delivered to try to fuse with PVCs. Such fused beats are exceptionally unlikely to produce synchronous LV contraction. As such in nonresponders to CRT, PVC suppression may be indicated. In a multicenter registry of 65 nonresponders to CRT with a daily PVC burden greater than 10,000, PVC ablation was associated with significant reverse ventricular remodeling and symptomatic improvement.[34] Long-term suppression of PVCs in this study was 88%. Ablation of PVCs may not be the right choice for all CRT nonresponders. Antiarrhythmics such as amiodarone or mexiletine may also have a role especially in instances with multiple PVC morphologies or in patients not suitable to undergo an ablation procedure. The decision to ablate, treat with antiarrhythmics, or simply observe is made on an individualized basis.

Multidisciplinary CRT-HF Clinic

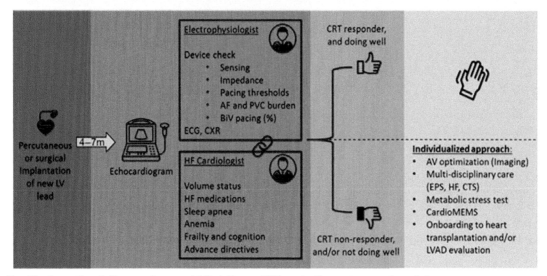

Fig. 12. Operational diagram for a multidisciplinary CRT/conduction system pacing clinic.

SUMMARY

Patients receiving CRT devices represent a challenging patient population, as inputs from multiple cardiac subspecialties are required for optimal care. Multiple studies have sought to define predictors of supoptimal outcomes following CRT. **Fig. 11** depicts the common reasons behind suboptimal CRT response. Dedicated CRT/conduction system pacing clinic offers a mechanism to foster collaboration among different cardiac subspecialties with the goals of device troubleshooting and resource intensification for what is a very comorbid population. In addition, identifying patients at high risk for decompensation earlier in their disease course is imperative if improved long-term outcomes are to be achieved. **Fig. 12** shows one such algorithm for multidisciplinary care of CRT/conduction system pacing patients.[12]

CLINICS CARE POINTS

- A PA and lateral chest X-ray is a useful tool to screen for poorly placed left ventricular leads.
- Biventricular pacing may cause harm in patients with left ventricular systolic dysfunction and a narrow QRS complex.
- Patients with non-left bundle branch block morhologies on a 12 lead ECG have poorer outcomes with CRT compared to those with a traditional left bundle branch block.

DISCLOSURE

Research support: abbott major; speaking minor medtronic consulting minor.

SUPPLEMENTARY DATA

Supplementary data related to this article can be found online at https://doi.org/10.1016/j.ccep.2021.12.014.

REFERENCES

1. Young JB, Abraham WT, Smith AL, et al. Combined cardiac resynchronization and implantable cardioversion defibrillation in advanced chronic heart failure: the MIRACLE ICD trial. JAMA 2003;289: 2685–94.
2. Linde C, Abraham WT, Gold MR, et al. Randomized trial of resynchronization in mildly symptomatic heart failure patients and in asymptomatic patients with left ventricular dysfunction and previous heart failure symptoms. J Am Coll Cardiol 2008;52:1834–43.
3. Moss AJ, Hall WJ, Cannom DS, et al. Cardiac-resynchronization therapy for the prevention of heart-failure events. N Engl J Med 2009;361: 1329–38.
4. Tang A, Wells GA, Talajic M, et al. Cardiac -resynchronization therapy for mild-to- moderate heart failure. N Engl J Med 2010;363:2385–95.
5. Rickard J, Michtalik H, Sharma R, et al. Predictors of response to cardiac resynchronization therapy: a systematic review. Int J Cardiol 2016;225:345–52.

6. Steffel J, Ruschitzka f. Superresponse to cardiac resynchronization therapy. Circulation 2014;130: 87–90.

7. Gold M, Rickard J, Daubert JC, et al. Redefining the classification of response to cardiac resynchronization therapy: results from the REVERSE study. JACC Clin Electrophysiol 2021;7:871–80.

8. Rickard J, Chang A, Spragg DD, et al. Durability of the survival effect of cardiac resynchronization therapy by level of left ventricular functional improvement: fate of "nonresponders. Heart Rhythm 2014; 11:412–6.

9. Varma N, Boehmer J, Bhargava K, et al. Evaluation, management, and outcomes of patients poorly responsive to cardiac resynchronization device therapy. J Am Coll Cardiol 2019;21:2588–603.

10. Mullens W, Grimm RA, Verga T, et al. Insights from a cardiac resynchronization optimization clinic as part of a heart failure disease management program. J Am Coll Cardiol 2009;53(9):765–73.

11. Altman RK, Parks KA, Schlett CL, et al. Multidisciplinary care of patients receiving cardiac resynchronization therapy is associated with improved clinical outcomes. Eur Heart J 2012;17:2181–8.

12. Gorodeski EZ, Magnelli-Reyes C, Moennich LA, et al. Cardiac resynchronization therapy-heart failure (CRT-HF) clinic: a novel model of care. PLoS One 2019;14:e0222610.

13. Ellenbogen KA, Gold MR, Meyer TE, et al. Primary results from the smartdelay determined AV optimization: a comparison to other AV delay methods used in cardiac resynchronization therapy (SMART-AV) trial: a randomized trial comparing empirical, echocardiography- guided, and algorithmic atrioventricular delay programming in cardiac resynchronization therapy. Circulation 2010;122:2660–8.

14. Abraham WT. Frequent optimization study using the QuickOpt method. Am Heart J 2010;159: 944–8.

15. Weiss R. V-V Optimization in cardiac resynchronization therapy non-responders: RESPONSE-HF trial results. Abstract AB12-5, HRS 2010, Denver, Colorado.

16. Jones S, Shun-Shin MJ, Cole GD, et al. Applicability of the iterative technique for cardiac resynchronization therapy optimization: full-disclosure, 50-sequential-patient dataset of transmitral Doppler traces, with implications for future research design and guidelines. Europace 2014;16:541–50.

17. Sun JP, Lee AP, Grimm RA, et al. Optimization of atrioventricular delay during exercise improves cardiac output in patients stabilized with cardiac resynchronization therapy. Heart 2012;98(1): 54–9.

18. Vergrugge FH, Dubont MH, Rivero-Ayerz M, et al. Comorbidity significantly affects clinical outcome after cardiac resynchronization therapy regardless of ventricular remodeling. J Card Fail 2012;18(11): 845–53.

19. Kubala M, Guedon-Moreau L, Snelme F, et al. Utility of frailty assessment for elderly patients undergoing cardiac resynchronization therapy. JACC Clin Electrophysiol 2017;13:1523–33.

20. Rickard J, Brennan DO, Martin DO, et al. The impact of left ventricular size on response to cardiac resynchronization therapy. Am Heart J 2011;162: 646–53.

21. Rickard J, Patel D, ParkC, et al. Long-term outcomes in patients with a left ejection fraction ≤15% undergoing cardiac resynchronization therapy. JACC Clin Electrophysiol 2021;7:36–46.

22. Dong YX, Powell BD, Asirvatham SJ, et al. Left ventricular lead position for cardiac resynchronization: a comprehensive cinegraphic, echocardiographic, clinical, and survival analysis. Europace 2012;14: 1139–47.

23. Singh JP, Klein HU, Huang DT, et al. Left ventricular lead position and clinical outcome in the multicenter automatic defibrillator implantation trial-cardiac resynchronization therapy (MADIT-CRT) trial. Circulation 2011;123:1159–66.

24. Cheng A, Landman SR, Stadler RW. Reasons for loss of cardiac resynchronization therapy pacing insights from 32 844 patient. Circ Arrythm Electrophysiol 2012;5:885–8.

25. Hayes D, Boehmer JP, Day JD, et al. Cardiac resynchronization therapy and the relationship of percent biventricular pacing to survival. Heart Rhythm 2011;8:1469–75.

26. Beshai JF, Grimm RA, Nagueh SF, et al. Cardiac-resynchronization therapy in heart failure with narrow QRS complexes. N Engl J Med 2007;357: 2461–71.

27. Ruschitzka F, Abraham WT, Singh JP, et al. Cardiac-resynchronization therapy in heart failure with a narrow QRS complex. N Engl J Med 2013;369: 1395–405.

28. Van Stipdonk, Hoogland R, Ter Horst I, et al. Evaluating electrocardiography-based identification of cardiac resynchronization therapy responders beyond current left bundle branch block definitions. J Am Coll Cardiol 2020;6: 193–203.

29. Escahlier R, Ploux S, Ritter P, et al. Nonspecific intraventrciualr conduction delay: definitions, prognosis, and implictions for cardiac resynchronization therapy. Heart Rhythm 2015;12:1071–9.

30. Strik M, Ploux S, Huntjens PR, et al. Response to cardiac resynchronization therapy is determined by intrinsic electrical substrate rather then by its modifications. Int J Cardiol 2018;270: 143–8.

31. Kosmidou I, Lindenfeld J, Abraham WT, et al. Transcatheter mitral valve repair in patients with and

without cardiac resynchronization therapy. Circ Heart Fail 2020;13(11):e007293.

32. Seifert M, Schau T, Schoepp M, et al. MitraClip in CRT non-responders with severe mitral regurgitation. Int J Cardiol 2014;177(1):79–85.

33. Chun K-H, Oh J, Yu HT, et al. The role of sacubitril/valsartan in the management of cardiac resynchronization therapy non-responders: a retrospective analysis. ESC Heart Fail 2020;11:4404–7.

34. Lakireddy D, Di Biase L, Ryschon K, et al. Radiofrequency ablation of premature ventricular ectopy improves the efficacy of cardiac resynchronization therapy in nonresponders. J Am Coll Cardiol 2012;60:1531–9.

What Have We Learned in the Last 20 Years About CRT Non-Responders?

Peregrine G. Green, BMBCh[a,b,c], Neil Herring, DPhil[a,c],
Timothy R. Betts, MD[c,d],*

KEYWORDS

- Cardiac resynchronization therapy • Biventricular pacing • Heart failure • Optimization
- Non-Responders

KEY POINTS

- There are many criteria used to measure response to cardiac resynchronization therapy. Response is a continuous variable, both in degree and over time.
- Women, absence of diabetes, true left bundle branch block, QRS greater than 150 ms and less than 200 ms plus fewer additional comorbidities all predict a good response. Preassessment can exclude those with very unfavorable characteristics.
- Medical optimization post-CRT implant, including addition of Sacubitril/Valsartan, can benefit non-responders.
- If non-response is due to suboptimal lead placement, alternatives include left ventricular endocardial pacing, His bundle and left bundle branch area pacing.
- AV interval optimization to facilitate fusion pacing produces greater QRS narrowing.

INTRODUCTION

Over the past 20 years, cardiac resynchronization therapy (CRT) has become a key therapy for the treatment of severe heart failure with reduced ejection fraction (HFrEF) with left bundle branch block (LBBB)[1] or particularly prolonged (>150 msec) QRS duration on the ECG. Randomized controlled clinical trials have demonstrated clear improvements in both morbidity and mortality, giving it an established position in heart failure guidelines.[2] However, improvement in both cardiac function and symptoms in response to CRT can be variable and difficult to predict, with 30% to 50% of patients not experiencing benefit (termed "non-responders").[3,4] The importance of this can be seen by the much better prognosis of responders compared with non-responders at long-term follow-up.[5,6]

Not only would improved response rates reduce morbidity and mortality, but the ability to better predict response may allow more targeted patient selection and so prevent potentially futile invasive procedures in those patients who are unlikely to receive a benefit. This would have important clinical implications by removing unnecessary periprocedural risk, and also provide economic savings at a time when health care systems are under unprecedented financial strain.

The ability to predict and improve patient response has therefore been a cornerstone of CRT research. This review will discuss how

[a] Department of Physiology, Anatomy and Genetics, University of Oxford, Sherrington Building, Parks Road, Oxford, OX1 3PT, UK; [b] Oxford Centre for Clinical Magnetic Resonance Research (OCMR), University of Oxford, Level 0 John Radcliffe Hospital, Oxford, OX3 9DU, UK; [c] Oxford Heart Centre, John Radcliffe Hospital, Oxford University Hospitals NHS Foundation Trust, Oxford, OX3 9DU, UK; [d] Oxford Biomedical Research Centre, Oxford University Hospitals NHS Foundation Trust, Oxford, UK
* Corresponding author. Oxford Heart Centre, John Radcliffe Hospital, Oxford University Hospitals NHS Foundation Trust, Oxford, OX3 9DU, UK.
E-mail address: tim.betts@ouh.nhs.uk

Card Electrophysiol Clin 14 (2022) 283–296
https://doi.org/10.1016/j.ccep.2021.12.019
1877-9182/22/© 2022 Elsevier Inc. All rights reserved.

response is defined, those factors which have been found to influence response rates, and the ways in which these can be optimized to improve non-responder rates.

WHAT IS "RESPONSE"?

To be able to define non-responders, it is first necessary to consider the criteria used to define response to CRT. Although this is generally taken to mean an improvement in cardiac function and/or symptoms, the measures used have varied between studies and there is no consensus as to an overall definition. The outcomes used have included clinical measures such as symptom scores and quality of life (QoL) assessments, functional assessments of exercise capacity such as the 6-minute walk test (6MWT), measures of left ventricular (LV) reverse remodeling, and rates of death or hospitalization from either all-causes, major adverse cardiovascular events or heart failure[7–12] (summarized in **Table 1**). With such a broad range of criteria, it is therefore important to consider which were used when discussing response rates reported in clinical trials. The importance of this is shown by the study by Fornwalt and colleagues, which found up to 17 different criteria being used in 26 studies, with agreement between these

criteria being poor 75% of the time and strong only 4% of the time.[13] Furthermore, non-responder rates tend to be higher when more subjective symptom measurements are used as opposed to "harder" measures such as LV reverse remodeling or mortality/hospitalization[14,15] and one international registry has found that local site-defined non-response tends to underestimate non-responder rates, compared with if the clinical composite score is used.[16] This then has the potential for impact on patient outcomes if those missed patients are not followed up appropriately for further optimization.

Another factor to consider along with the measure used to define response is the range of response. Although some patients experience only a modest improvement in a few criteria, some can have an excellent response. Such patients have been termed "super-responders" and although there is again no consensus as to the definition of super-response, in general, it encompasses a marked improvement or even near-normalization in LV volumes and systolic function,[17] and is associated with improved clinical outcomes.[18] Although the factors associated with super-response have not been as well characterized as those with non-response, it would appear that, as would be expected, they are often the same factors but exist at the opposite end of the spectrum.[18] Super-responders may therefore reflect a population who have none of the factors (or the opposite factors) associated with non-responders. In addition, a minority of patients may only respond briefly, with one study finding that 15% of responders (based on reduction in LV end-systolic volume) did not actually have long-lasting response at 1 to 2 years.[19] Although all-cause mortality was still better in these patients than in non-responders, it was worse than in long-term responders.

Finally, it is important to consider that the term "response" may be misleading. Although some patients may not experience an actual improvement in function or symptoms, CRT may still prevent or slow the rate of any deterioration which would otherwise be expected to occur as part of the HFrEF disease process. These patients have been termed "non-progressors."[18] Strictly relying on rates of improvement alone is therefore likely to lead to an overestimation of non-responder rates. Accordingly, the recent REVERSE study found that patients who were classified as "stabilized" in response to CRT had a better prognosis than those who worsened.[20] The authors propose that the term "non-responder" is therefore actually obsolete, and they suggest classifying patients instead as improved, stabilized, or worsened.

Table 1 Measurements of CRT response	
Clinical/Functional	NYHA Class QoL measures (eg, Minnesota Living with Heart Failure Questionnaire) 6MWT Exercise duration CPET
LV Reverse Remodeling	Acute hemodynamic measurements Increase in LVEF Reduction in LVESV and LVEDV
Outcomes	Reduction in HF hospitalization Reduction in cardiac mortality Reduction in all-cause mortality

Abbreviations: 6MWT, 6-minute walk test; CPET, cardiopulmonary exercise testing; HF, heart failure; LVEDV, left ventricular end-diastolic volume; LVEF, left ventricular ejection fraction; LVESV, left ventricular end-systolic volume; NYHA, New York Heart Association; QoL; quality of life.

FACTORS AFFECTING RESPONSE AND THEIR OPTIMIZATION

Multiple studies, reviews, and post-hoc analyses have investigated those factors which are correlated to the degree of response, with the aim of identifying either better patient selection, optimal implant characteristics, optimal post-implant CRT settings, or developing novel technology. In general and as would be expected, the degree of resynchronization as reflected by the extent of QRS duration narrowing with biventricular pacing (BiVP) is associated with response,[21–23] as are other electrocardiographic (ECG) markers of appropriate resynchronization, such as a dominant S wave in lead I and large R wave in V1.[24,25]

Those factors which influence non-responder rates will be discussed in turn, along with current recommendations for their optimization.

Patient Selection

Although under-represented in CRT studies,[26] multiple studies have indicated that women have better outcomes in response to CRT, with lower all-cause mortality,[27,28] including in large real-world registry data,[29] with some evidence in addition that women receive benefit at a shorter pre-implant QRS duration.[30] Comorbidity also influences CRT response, with diabetes mellitus (DM), chronic kidney disease, and chronic obstructive pulmonary disease being associated with either increased all-cause mortality or heart failure admissions.[31,32] In particular, although patients with DM do still receive benefit from CRT,[33,34] a meta-analysis has shown a higher mortality in diabetic patients.[35] This has also been observed in large real-world registry studies[31,36] which have shown that HbA1c, as an expression of poor glycaemic control, is predictive of a worse CRT outcome.[37] Similar studies also suggest a reduction in reverse remodeling following CRT in patients with DM despite similar levels of resynchronization.[38,39] In addition, iron deficiency is well recognized as a comorbidity in the heart failure population, as are the benefits of iron replacement,[2] and this appears to extend to the CRT population. A retrospective study of 541 CRT patients showed that iron deficiency was not only correlated with worse symptomatic outcomes but also with increased all-cause mortality, heart failure admissions, and LV reverse remodeling,[40] with the latter hypothesized to be related to the role of iron as a cofactor metabolism.[41] The recently published IRON-CRT trial has shown a n improvement in LV function in those patients with a persitsstently reduced LVEF after CRT and iron deficiencyency, treated with ferric carboxymaltose.[42] Finally, the etiology of heart failure is also important, with those with ischemic cardiomyopathy having worse outcomes[43] and rates of reverse remodeling.[44]

True LBBB morphology is also associated with response,[45] with 2 meta-analyses indicating that CRT only improves clinical outcomes in those with LBBB and not in those with other conduction abnormalities.[46,47] Finally, QRS duration is also key, with those with a broader QRS having a greater response in the RAFT study[48] and in a meta-analysis.[49] Current guidelines, therefore, recommend CRT in patients with non-LBBB only if QRS duration is more than 150 msec. Although those with a very wide QRS duration more than 200 ms seem to have worse survival rates after CRT[50] (possibly due to it being a marker of disease severity), there is some evidence that in patients with non-LBBB QRS widening, benefit is only in those with QRS durations more than 180 ms, even though this may be due to the electrical uncoupling which can be seen in advanced heart failure.[51]

Although these factors cannot normally be modified or altered (if patients are already on optimal medical therapy, as discussed in the following section), their use does allow for potentially better patient selection, reducing the potential number of futile implant procedures and so unnecessary periprocedural risk.

Medical Optimization

The importance of maintaining optimal medical therapy after CRT should not be understated. Although the importance of medical therapy in heart failure and compliance is well known, one center found that nearly a third of non-responders referred to a CRT optimization clinic had suboptimal medical treatment.[52] Patients who have a protocol-driven approach to optimization following implant, including optimization of medical therapy and heart failure education, have better rates of reverse remodeling and adverse events.[53] Similarly, those with optimal medical therapy at 1-year post-implant had a reduced risk of heart failure and death compared with those who did not[54] Indeed, one study specifically looking at the use of Sacubitril/Valsartan in non-responders showed that its use was associated with better outcomes in this population, including lower rates of cardiac death,[55] and higher dosages of neurohormonal blockade and beta-blockers following CRT implantation are also associated with lower morbidity and mortality.[56,57]

Lead Positioning

Given the latent contraction of the lateral LV wall which is associated with LBBB dyssynchrony, it is perhaps not surprising that optimal CRT necessitates placement of the LV lead at this site. Subgroup analyses of the Madit-CRT[58] and REVERSE[59] trials demonstrated improved outcomes when the LV lead is placed at the lateral wall and also away from the apex of the heart, with a recent retrospective analysis of more than 2000 patients confirming a long-term mortality benefit of lateral placement even after adjustment for other variables known to influence reponse.[60] Furthermore, pacing at site of latest activation as measured by the time from the onset of the surface ECG to the LV electrogram (QLV) has been shown to be associated both with improved reverse remodeling and QoL[61] and with improved heart failure hospitalization and mortality.[62] Tying these 2 factors together, if the longest QLV is at the lateral wall then it implies that the dyssynchrony is due to an LBBB pattern. Longer interventricular conduction delay (RV-LV conduction time based on intracardiac electrograms [IEGMs]) also correlates not only with response as defined by reverse remodeling and QoL[63] but also with heart failure outcome measures.[64]

Both the TARGET[65] and STARTER[66] trials took this concept further and suggested that the use of speckle tracking echocardiography to place leads away from myocardial scar or at the latest site of mechanical activation improves response rates. There has also been some success with doing this using cardiac MRI (CMR) to assess the extent and location of myocardial scar and so guide lead placement, with focal scar burden as assessed by late gadolinium enhancement on CMR correlating with degree of response.[67] Furthermore, a meta-analysis of CRT in patients with posterolateral scar showed that there was a 46% lower chance of echocardiographic response and 67% lower chance of clinical response to CRT compared with those with non-significant scar pacing.[68] Finally, using multimodality imaging to target lead position closest to the latest mechanically activated non-scarred LV segment appears to reduce the non-responder rate in a randomized controlled trial of 182 patients.[69]

However, echocardiographic measures of dyssynchrony alone in the absence of QRS prolongation do not seem to predict response to CRT. The RETHINQ,[70] ESTEEM-CRT,[71] and then ECHO-CRT[72] studies all showed that echo measures of dyssynchrony in narrow QRS patients did not identify responders, whereas the PROSPECT[73] study showed that even in patients with a QRS duration more than 130 ms, use of additional echo measures of dyssynchrony did not improve outcomes. It is worth noting, however, that these echo-derived parameters are likely to have been limited by significant intra-observer and inter-observer variability.[74]

In those patients for whom optimal LV lead placement is not possible either due to a lack of suitable target veins, phrenic nerve capture or myocardial scar, newer developments for lead placement have also emerged, including LV endocardial pacing and conduction system pacing (His-bundle pacing [HBP] and left bundle branch area pacing).[75] LV endocardial pacing is promising in those with poor CRT response,[76] with a recent meta-analysis finding comparable response rates to conventional CRT,[77] whereas the His-SYNC[78] study was the first randomized pilot trial of HBP versus conventional CRT and demonstrated similar primary outcomes, albeit with the caveat of a high cross-over rate. Left bundle branch area pacing, first described by Huang and colleagues,[79] may also be promising, with a recent non-randomized study showing similar response rates in terms of symptoms and LV function compared with both conventional BiVP and HBP,[80] and a meta-analysis of 4 non-randomized studies even potentially demonstrating better echocardiographic response and symptom improvement compared with BiVP.[81] LBB area pacing may be useful if there is area of block higher in the His system, but in that scenario will not excite the right bundle branch physiologically to produce physiologic RV activation. Both HBP and LBB area pacing also suffer from the need for higher pacing outputs, increased thresholds over time and potentially higher lead displacement rates.[82,83] Finally, leadless LV endocardial pacing using the WiSE-CRT system (EBR systems, Sunnyvale, CA, USA) has also shown promise in non-responders to conventional CRT, with improvement in patient symptoms and LV reverse remodeling.[84]

Programming

The importance of optimizing both atrioventricular (AV) delay (AVD) and interventricular delay (VVD) to maximize CRT effectiveness is well recognized.[85] Indeed, the importance of frequent AVD and VVD optimization at follow-up and not just at implant has been suggested.[86] Multiple methods have been described to assess AV optimization, including echocardiographic measurement of the mitral valve inflow pattern, and invasive and non-invasive hemodynamic measurements.[85] However, echo-based methods are labor-intensive, and their value is uncertain.[87] Device algorithms using analysis of the IEGM have become an attractive alternative because of their rapid and automated nature, although evidence suggests that they may not have clinical benefit over using fixed AV delays.[88] In addition, the physiologic changing of intrinsic AV conduction with exercise[89] has led to methods that allow for adjustment of AVD. Rate-adaptive AVD algorithms adjust delays as heart rate changes, with their use shown to increase exercise capacity.[90] The SonR lead (Sorin CRM SAS, Clamart, France) has a peak endocardial acceleration (PEA) sensor embedded in its tip. As PEA correlates with LV contractility, this can be assessed at a range of AV and VV delays to find the optimal settings at repeated intervals including during exercise.[91] The RESPOND-CRT trial has demonstrated non-inferiority in responder rates with the use of the SonR sensor compared with echo-optimisation.[92]

More recently, adaptive AVD optimization has also become important to allow fusion between intrinsic conduction and LV pacing ± RV pacing wavefronts (so-called fusion pacing).[93] SmartDelay from Boston Scientific (300 Boston Scientific Way, Marlborough, MA, USA) allows automatic AVD optimization and LV-only pacing but does not dynamically reassess this outside of follow-up visits. AdaptivCRT from Medtronic (710 Medtronic Parkway Minneapolis, USA) and SyncAV or SyncAV+ from Abbott (Abbott Medical Inc., Abbott Park, Illinois, USA) allow continuous reassessment of intrinsic AV conduction at set intervals to allow dynamic adjustment of the AVD, maintaining fusion. This not only may result in greater QRS narrowing and more efficient LV activation,[94–96] but also lengthens battery life if RV pacing is not required.[93] Although the AdaptivCRT Trial showed non-inferiority to echo-based optimization overall, there were improved outcomes in the subset with LBBB, and additionally RV pacing was reduced.[97] One potential limitation is the ability of these algorithms to maintain fusion on exercise if there are rapid or non-linear changes in intrinsic AV conduction, with the potential for loss of effective resynchronization. The ongoing AdaptResponse[98] and SyncAV Post-Market trials will hopefully give more evidence as to the effectiveness of fusion pacing in improving CRT response.

Finally, the advent of multipoint (MPP, Abbott) or multisite (Boston Scientific) pacing may also help response[99] and reduce mortality.[100] By pacing at multiple sites in the LV using a quadripolar lead, there is more rapid and uniform activation and additionally it may help overcome local areas of conduction block in the presence of myocardial scar.[101] There is also evidence that combining multisite pacing with optimized LV lead positioning further enhances reverse remodeling and outcomes.[102,103]

Arrhythmia

Patients with atrial fibrillation (AF) and CRT have worse prognosis, in part due to the loss of AV synchrony and high ventricular rates.[104] In addition, the atrial arrhythmia burden and inhibition of pacing can result in lower BiVP percentages. The degree of BiVP achieved with CRT has been shown to be key to response, with even a small reduction in percentage adversely affecting outcomes, and better survival rates are seen with BiVP greater than 98%[105–107]; those with persistent or permanent AF have lower BiVP percentages and increased mortality.[108] Using device counters as a marker of BIVP percentage can be misleading, with overestimation caused by fusion and pseudo-fusion beats meaning that perhaps less than half of patients receive greater than 90% effective BiVP when assessed by Holter monitoring.[109] To this end, effective rate control of atrial arrhythmia should be aggressively pursued, using either medical therapy or AV node (AVN) ablation,[110] Indeed, the CERTIFY study found that use of AVN ablation in these patients led to lower mortality rates which were similar to patients in sinus rhythm, and higher than those treated with rate-limiting medication alone.[111] Similarly, high rates of ventricular extrasystoles can inhibit effective CRT,[52] with evidence that reducing the burden with radiofrequency ablation in non-responders improves the degree of reverse remodeling.[112]

Metabolic Limitations

The metabolic hypothesis of heart failure pathogenesis is gaining increasing interest, with emerging evidence that reduced metabolic flux and flexibility may drive decreased contractility.[113,114] There is evidence using ^{18}F-fluorodeoxyglucose (FDG) and positron emission tomograph (PET) that the mechanical dyssynchrony seen in LBBB results in differential myocardial glucose uptake,[115,116] and that this is rebalanced by CRT.[117] Indeed, CRT can influence the mitochondrial proteome[118] and improve cardiac efficiency, increasing cardiac work without increasing myocardial oxygen consumption.[119,120] As efficiency is linked to metabolic substrate usage, there is some evidence that the baseline substrate used is correlated to CRT response rate.[121] This raises the intriguing potential that poor response to CRT in terms of reverse remodeling may be linked to decreased cardiac metabolic flexibility and flux, which may in part explain the worse response rates seen in DM.

Use of Non-CRT Adjuncts

In addition to new CRT technology to improve responder rates, novel non-CRT technologies are also showing promise in improving heart failure outcomes and can be used as adjuncts to CRT.

The CardioMEMS HF System (Micro-Electro-Mechanical HF System, Abbott Medical Inc., Abbott Park, IL, USA), provides pulmonary artery hemodynamic measurements to enable optimization of heart failure treatment before symptom exacerbation.[122] There is increasing evidence that it reduces the number of heart failure hospitalizations,[123,124] and its use in combination with CRT may improve responder rates, although trial data with this specific combination is currently lacking.

Cardiac contractility modulation (CCM) delivers electrical impulses to the RV wall during the refractory period and results in improved contractility and remodeling.[125] There is some evidence of modest improvements in symptoms, QoL, and reverse remodeling,[126,127] and possibly in survival[128,129] although randomized control trial data is lacking and it is not currently supported in the European Society of Cardiology (ESC) guidelines.[2] Importantly, however, there may be some evidence that addition of CCM in CRT non-responders may improve reverse remodeling and symptoms, although only in a very limited number of patients so far.[130,131]

Baroreflex activation therapy (BAT) aims to reduce sympathetic outflow and increase parasympathetic activity and so improve symptoms in HFrEF patients. There is some trial evidence that it succeeds, with better QoL and functional scores,[132,133] although again it is not currently included in the ESC guidelines.[2] Vagal nerve stimulation trials such as NECTAR-HF[134] and INOVATE-HF[135] have also shown no improvement in functional capacity, remodeling, heart failure events or death, although again some improvement in QoL measures. The ANTHEM-HF[136] trial did show some improvements in reverse remodeling, although did not include a control group.[137] Finally, spinal cord neuromodulation has also had similarly disappointing results.[138]

A Synthesized Approach

Although patients are often classified as "responders" or "non-responders," changes brought about by CRT are not dichotomous but instead represent a continuous spectrum.[139] This is reflected by the range of subjective and objective measures which can be used to measure response, with many patients exhibiting improvement in only some of these. Of the patient factors discussed earlier, a systematic review identified LBBB, female gender, non-ischemic cardiomyopathy, sinus rhythm, and a wider QRS duration as being the criteria that were most associated with response.[140] Use of these factors can then therefore aid patient selection and help guide patients during the consent process as to the likely benefit. Use of a synthesized and logical approach to identify suitable patients pre-implant and then to follow-up, fully evaluate and optimize all possible modifiable factors post-implant is key and can be aided by use of a sequential approach.[141] A model approach to this is the advent of specialist CRT clinics. The use of a CRT preassessment clinic to assess those patients already being considered for CRT led to 20% not being implanted as they did not meet guideline criteria.[142] The authors calculate that use of this approach across the National Health Service would lead to potential savings of £39 million per year. In addition, use of specialist follow-up clinics to take a multi-disciplinary approach to CRT management and treatment of non-responders is also likely to be increasingly seen as the best model of care.[52,143]

SUMMARY

CRT has established a key role in the treatment of HFrEF over the last 20 years, but persistent non-responder rates remain problematic. However, dedicated research has identified several factors associated with non-response. Use of these has led to a continuous evolution of practice, with patient selection, implant techniques, device programming, and novel technologies all being advanced to help improve response. A key challenge remains the identification and optimization of non-responders and the increasing role of dedicated clinics which can take a synthesized, multidisciplinary approach to their management. Continuing advances in practice and technology will hopefully continue to improve non-responder rates.

CLINICS CARE POINTS

- Patient selection is key. Non-LBBB patients and those with QRS less than 150 ms are unlikely to respond well to CRT.

- Target LV lead position based on the longest Q-LV interval achievable avoiding scar and phrenic nerve stimulation.

- Optimize the AV interval. Fusion pacing with intrinsic RBB conduction produces the narrowest QRS duration.

- Multipoint LV pacing, providing there is wide separation and simultaneous stimulation, improves response and may turn non-responders into responders
- If adequate epicardial LV lead positioning cannot be achieved, consider LV endocardial or conduction system pacing.

DISCLOSURE

Prof T.R. Betts has received honoraria for speaking, proctoring, and product development plus unrestricted research grants from Abbott.

REFERENCES

1. Glikson M, Nielsen JC, Kronborg MB, et al. 2021 ESC Guidelines on cardiac pacing and cardiac resynchronization therapy: Developed by the Task Force on cardiac pacing and cardiac resynchronization therapy of the European Society of Cardiology (ESC) with the special contribution of the European Heart Rhythm Association (EHRA). Eur Heart J 2021. https://doi.org/10.1093/eurheartj/ehab364.

2. Mcdonagh TA, Metra M, Adamo M, et al. 2021 ESC Guidelines for the diagnosis and treatment of acute and chronic heart failure: Developed by the Task Force for the diagnosis and treatment of acute and chronic heart failure of the European Society of Cardiology (ESC) with the special contribution of the Heart Failure Association (HFA) of the ESC. Eur Heart J 2021. https://doi.org/10.1093/eurheartj/ehab368.

3. Sohaib SM, Chen Z, Whinnett ZI, et al. Meta-analysis of symptomatic response attributable to the pacing component of cardiac resynchronization therapy. Eur J Heart Fail 2013;15(12):1419–28. ISSN 1879-0844 (Electronic) 1388-9842 (Linking). Disponível em: Available at: https://www.ncbi.nlm.nih.gov/pubmed/24259043.

4. Daubert, C., Behar N., Martins R.P. et al. Avoiding non-responders to cardiac resynchronization therapy: a practical guide. European Heart Journal, Volume 38, Issue 19, 2017, Pages 1463–1472.

5. Rickard J, Cheng A, Spragg D, et al. Durability of the survival effect of cardiac resynchronization therapy by level of left ventricular functional improvement: fate of "nonresponders". Heart Rhythm 2014. 1556-3871 (Electronic).

6. Ypenburg C, van Bommel RJ, Borleffs JW, et al. Long-term prognosis after cardiac resynchronization therapy is related to the extent of left ventricular reverse remodeling at midterm follow-up. J Am Coll Cadiol 2009. 1558-3597 (Electronic).

7. Bristow MR, Saxon LA, Boehmer J, et al. Cardiac-resynchronization therapy with or without an implantable defibrillator in advanced chronic heart failure. N Engl J Med 2004;350(21):2140–50. ISSN 1533-4406 (Electronic) 0028-4793 (Linking). Disponível em: Available at: https://www.ncbi.nlm.nih.gov/pubmed/15152059. >Disponível em. https://www.nejm.org/doi/pdf/10.1056/NEJMoa032423?articleTools=true.

8. Moss AJ, Hall WJ, Cannom DS, et al. Cardiac-resynchronization therapy for the prevention of heart-failure events. N Engl J Med 2009;361(14):1329–38. ISSN 1533-4406 (Electronic) 0028-4793 (Linking). Disponível em: Available at: https://www.ncbi.nlm.nih.gov/pubmed/19723701.

9. Cleland JG, Daubert JC, Erdmann E, et al. The effect of cardiac resynchronization on morbidity and mortality in heart failure. N Engl J Med 2005;352(15):1539–49. ISSN 1533-4406 (Electronic) 0028-4793 (Linking). Disponível em: Available at: https://www.ncbi.nlm.nih.gov/pubmed/15753115.

10. Cazeau S, Leclercq C, Lavergne T, et al. Effects of multisite biventricular pacing in patients with heart failure and intraventricular conduction delay. N Engl J Med 2001;344(12):873–80. n. 0028-4793.

11. Tang AS, Wells GA, Talajic M, et al. Cardiac-resynchronization therapy for mild-to-moderate heart failure. N Engl J Med 2010;363(25):2385–95. ISSN 1533-4406 (Electronic)0028-4793 (Linking). Disponível em: Available at: https://www.ncbi.nlm.nih.gov/pubmed/21073365.

12. Abraham WT, Fisher WG, Smith AL, et al. Cardiac resynchronization in chronic heart failure. N Engl J Med 2002;346(24):1845–53, 1533-4406.

13. Fornwalt BK, Sprague WW, BeDell P, et al. Agreement is poor among current criteria used to define response to cardiac resynchronization therapy. Circulation 2010;121(18):1985–91, 1524-4539 (Electronic).

14. Sieniewicz BJ, Gould J, Porter B, et al. Understanding non-response to cardiac resynchronisation therapy: common problems and potential solutions. Heart Fail Rev 2019;24(1):41–54, 1573-7322 (Electronic).

15. Daubert JC FAU - SAXON L, au fnm, au fnm, et al. Heart Rhythm 2012;9(9):1524–76.

16. Varma N, Boehmer J, Bhargava K, et al. Evaluation, management, and outcomes of patients poorly responsive to cardiac resynchronization device therapy. J Am Coll Cardiol 2019;74(21):2588–603. ISSN 0735-1097. Disponível em: Available at: https://www.sciencedirect.com/science/article/pii/S0735109719378039.

17. Steffel J, Milosevic G, Hurlimann A, et al. Characteristics and long-term outcome of echocardiographic super-responders to cardiac resynchronisation therapy: 'real world' experience from a single tertiary

care centre. n. 1468-201X (Electronic). Heart 2011; 97(20):1668–74.

18. Steffel J, Ruschitzka F. Superresponse to cardiac resynchronization therapy. Circulation 2014; 130(1):87–90, 1524-4539 (Electronic).

19. Oka T, Inoue K, Tanaka K, et al. Duration of reverse remodeling response to cardiac resynchronization therapy: rates, predictors, and clinical outcomes. n. 1874-1754 (Electronic). Int J Cardiol 2017;243: 340–6.

20. Gold MR, Rickard J, Daubert JC, et al. Redefining the Classifications of response to cardiac resynchronization therapy: results from the REVERSE study. JACC Clin Electrophysiol 2021;7(7):871–80, 2405-5018 (Electronic).

21. Coppola G, Ciaramitaro G, Stabile G, et al. Magnitude of QRS duration reduction after biventricular pacing identifies responders to cardiac resynchronization therapy. Int J Cardiol 2016;221:450–5, 1874-1754 (Electronic).

22. Bazoukis G, Naka KK, Alsheikh-Ali A, et al. Association of QRS narrowing with response to cardiac resynchronization therapy-a systematic review and meta-analysis of observational studies. Heart Fail Rev 2020;25(5):745–56.

23. Rickard J, Popovic Z, Verhaert D, et al. The QRS narrowing index predicts reverse left ventricular remodeling following cardiac resynchronization therapy. Pacing Clin Electrophysiol 2011;34(5): 604–11. n. 1540-8159 (Electronic).

24. Coverstone E, Sheehy J, Kleiger RE, et al. The postimplantation electrocardiogram predicts clinical response to cardiac resynchronization therapy. Pacing Clin Electrophysiol 2015;38(5):572–80, 1540-8159 (Electronic).

25. Bode WD, Bode MF, Gettes L, et al. Prominent R wave in ECG lead V1 predicts improvement of left ventricular ejection fraction after cardiac resynchronization therapy in patients with or without left bundle branch block. Heart Rhythm 2015 Oct; 12(10):2141–7.

26. Zusterzeel R, Selzman KA, Sanders WE, et al. Toward Sex-specific guidelines for cardiac resynchronization therapy? J Cardiovasc Transl Res 2016; 9(1):12–22. n. 1937-5395 (Electronic).

27. Zabarovskaja S, Gadler F, Braunschweig F, et al. Women have better long-term prognosis than men after cardiac resynchronization therapy. Europace 2012;14(8):1148–55, 1532-2092 (Electronic).

28. Zusterzeel R, Curtis JP, Caños DA, et al. Sex-specific mortality risk by QRS morphology and duration in patients receiving CRT: results from the NCDR. J Am Coll Cardiol 2014;64(9):887–94. ISSN 0735-1097. Disponível em: Available at: https:// www.sciencedirect.com/science/article/pii/ S0735109714042612.

29. Zusterzeel R, Spatz ES, Curtis JP, et al. Cardiac resynchronization therapy in women versus men. Circ Cardiovasc Qual Outcomes 2015;8(2_suppl_ 1):S4–11. https://doi.org/10.1161/ CIRCOUTCOMES.114.001548 >. Acesso em: 2021/09/02.

30. Zusterzeel R, Selzman KA, Sanders WE, et al. Cardiac resynchronization therapy in women: US Food and Drug Administration meta-analysis of patient-level data. JAMA Intern Med 2014;174(8):1340–8. Available at: https://doi.org/10.1001/ jamainternmed.2014.2717>. Acesso em: 9/2/ 2021. ISSN 2168-6106. Disponível em:.

31. Verbrugge FH, Dupont M, Rivero-Ayerza M, et al. Comorbidity significantly affects clinical outcome after cardiac resynchronization therapy regardless of ventricular remodeling. J Card Fail 2012;18(11): 845–53, 1532-8414 (Electronic).

32. Bazoukis G, Letsas KP, Korantzopoulos P, et al. Impact of baseline renal function on all-cause mortality in patients who underwent cardiac resynchronization therapy: a systematic review and meta-analysis. J Arrhythm 2017;33(5):417–23. Available at: https://doi.org/10.1016/j.joa.2017.04.005>. Acesso em: 2021/09/28. ISSN 1880-4276. Disponível em:.

33. Ghali JK, Boehmer J, Feldman AM, et al. Influence of diabetes on cardiac resynchronization therapy with or without defibrillator in patients with advanced heart failure. J Card Fail 2007;13(9): 769–73. ISSN 1532-8414 (Electronic) 1071-9164 (Linking). Disponível em: Available at: https:// www.ncbi.nlm.nih.gov/pubmed/17996827.

34. George J, Barsheshet A, Moss AJ, et al. Effectiveness of cardiac resynchronization therapy in diabetic patients with ischemic and nonischemic cardiomyopathy. Ann Noninvasive Electrocardiol 2012;17(1):14–21. . ISSN 1542-474X (Electronic) 1082-720X (Linking). Disponível em: Available at: https://www.ncbi.nlm.nih.gov/pubmed/22276624.

35. Sun H, Guan Y, Wang L, et al. 2015 Influence of diabetes on cardiac resynchronization therapy in heart failure patients: a meta-analysis. BMC Cardiovasc Disord 2015;15(25):25. ISSN 1471-2261 (Electronic) 1471-2261 (Linking). Disponível em: Available at: https://www.ncbi.nlm.nih.gov/ pubmed/25880202.

36. Echouffo-tcheugui JB, Masoudi FA, Bao H, et al. Diabetes mellitus and outcomes of cardiac resynchronization with implantable Cardioverter-defibrillator therapy in Older patients with heart failure. Circ Arrhythm Electrophysiol 2016;9:8. ISSN 1941-3084 (Electronic) 1941-3084 (Linking). Disponível em: Available at: https://www.ncbi.nlm.nih. gov/pubmed/27489243.

37. SHAH RV, Altman RK, Park MY, et al. Usefulness of hemoglobin A(1c) to predict outcome after cardiac

resynchronization therapy in patients with diabetes mellitus and heart failure. Am J Cardiol 2012; 110(5):683–8. ISSN 1879-1913 (Electronic) 0002-9149 (Linking). Disponível em: Available at: https://www.ncbi.nlm.nih.gov/pubmed/22632827.

38. Mangiavacchi M, Gasparini M, Genovese S, et al. Insulin-treated type 2 diabetes is associated with a decreased survival in heart failure patients after cardiac resynchronization therapy. Pacing Clin Electrophysiol 2008;31(11):1425–32. ISSN 1540-8159 (Electronic) 0147-8389 (Linking). Disponível em: Available at: https://www.ncbi.nlm.nih.gov/pubmed/18950300.

39. Hoke U, Thijssen J, van Bommel RJ, et al. Influence of diabetes on left ventricular systolic and diastolic function and on long-term outcome after cardiac resynchronization therapy. Diabetes Care 2013; 36(4):985–91. ISSN 1935-5548 (Electronic) 0149-5992 (Linking). Disponível em: Available at: https://www.ncbi.nlm.nih.gov/pubmed/23223348.

40. Martens P, Verbrugge F, Nijst P, et al. Impact of iron deficiency on response to and remodeling after cardiac resynchronization therapy. Am J Cardiol 2017;119:65–70. Available at: https://doi.org/10.1016/j.amjcard.2016.09.017>. Acesso em: 2021/09/28. ISSN 0002-9149. Disponível em:.

41. Dauw J, Martens P, Mullens W. CRT optimization: what is new? What is necessary? Curr Treat Options Cardiovasc Med 2019;21(9):45. https://doi.org/10.1007/s11936-019-0751-2. Available at: ISSN 1534-3189. Disponível em.

42. Martens P, Dupont M, Dauw J, et al. The effect of intravenous ferric carboxymaltose on cardiac reverse remodelling following cardiac resynchronization therapy—the IRON-CRT trial. European Heart Journal 2021;42(48):4905–14.

43. Cleland, J. Freemantel N., Ghio S., et al. Predicting the long-term effects of cardiac resynchronization therapy on mortality from baseline variables and the early response a Report from the CARE-HF (Cardiac Resynchronization in Heart Failure) Trial. J Am Coll Cardiol. 2008 Aug 5;52(6):438-45

44. Goldenberg I, Moss AJ, Jackson Hall W, et al. Predictors of response to cardiac resynchronization therapy in the Multicenter automatic defibrillator implantation trial with cardiac resynchronization therapy (MADIT-CRT). Circulation 2011;124(14): 1527–36, 1524-4539 (Electronic).

45. Tian Y, Zhang P, Li X, et al. True complete left bundle branch block morphology strongly predicts good response to cardiac resynchronization therapy. Europace 2013;15(10):1499–506, 1532-2092 (Electronic).

46. Cunnington C, Kwok CS, Satchithananda DK, et al. Cardiac resynchronisation therapy is not associated with a reduction in mortality or heart failure hospitalisation in patients with non-left bundle branch block QRS morphology: meta-analysis of randomised controlled trials. PLoS One 2019; 14(1):e0206611, 1468-201X (Electronic).

47. Sipahi I, Chou JC, Hyden M, et al. Effect of QRS morphology on clinical event reduction with cardiac resynchronization therapy: meta-analysis of randomized controlled trials. Am Heart J 2012; 163(2):260–7.e3, 1097-6744 (Electronic).

48. Birnie DH, Ha A, Higginson L, et al. Impact of QRS morphology and duration on outcomes after cardiac resynchronization therapy: results from the resynchronization-Defibrillation for ambulatory heart failure trial (RAFT). Circ Heart Fail 2013;6(6): 1190–8, 1941-3297 (Electronic).

49. Sipahi I, Carrigan TP, Rowland DY, et al. Impact of QRS duration on clinical event reduction with cardiac resynchronization therapy: meta-analysis of randomized controlled trials. Arch Intern Med 2011;171(16):1454–62, 1538-3679 (Electronic).

50. Gasparini M, Leclercq C, Yu CM, et al. Absolute survival after cardiac resynchronization therapy according to baseline QRS duration: a multinational 10-year experience: data from the Multicenter International CRT Study. Am Heart J 2014; 167(2):203-e1. Disponível em: Available at: https://www.sciencedirect.com/science/article/pii/S0002870313007266.

51. Sundaram V, Sahadevan J, Waldo AL, et al. Implantable Cardioverter-Defibrillators with versus without resynchronization therapy in patients with a QRS duration >180 ms. J Am Coll Cardiol 2017; 69(16):2026–36. https://doi.org/10.1016/j.jacc.2017.02.042 >. Acesso em: 2021/10/07. Disponível em: Available at:.

52. Mullens, W., Grimm R.A., Verga T. et al. Insights from a cardiac resynchronization optimization clinic as part of a heart failure disease management program. J Am Coll Cardiol. 2009 Mar 3; 53(9):765-73

53. Mullens W, Kepa J, De Vusser P, et al. Importance of adjunctive heart failure optimization immediately after implantation to improve long-term outcomes with cardiac resynchronization therapy. Am J Cardiol 2011;108(3):409–15, 1879-1913 (Electronic).

54. Alvarez-alvarez B, García-Seara J, Martínez-Sande JL, et al. Cardiac resynchronization therapy outcomes in patients under nonoptimal medical therapy. J Arrhythm 2018;34(5):548–55. n. 1880-4276 (Print).

55. Chun KH, Oh J, Yu HT, et al. The role of sacubitril/valsartan in the management of cardiac resynchronization therapy non-responders: a retrospective analysis. ESC Heart Fail 2020;7(6):4404–7, 2055-5822 (Electronic).

56. Schmidt S, Hurlimann D, Starck CT, et al. Treatment with higher dosages of heart failure medication is associated with improved outcome following

cardiac resynchronization therapy. Eur Heart J 2014;35(16):1051–60, 1522-9645 (Electronic).

57. Witt CT, Kronborg MB, Nohr EA, et al. Optimization of heart failure medication after cardiac resynchronization therapy and the impact on long-term survival. Eur Heart J Cardiovasc Pharmacother 2015; 1(3):182–8, 2055-6845 (Electronic).

58. Kutyifa V, Kosztin A, Klein HU, et al. Left ventricular lead location and long-term outcomes in cardiac resynchronization therapy patients. JACC Clin Electrophysiol 2018;4(11):1410–20. ISSN 2405-500X. Disponível em: Available at: https://www.sciencedirect.com/science/article/pii/S2405500X18305991.

59. Thébault C, Donal E, Meunier C, et al. Sites of left and right ventricular lead implantation and response to cardiac resynchronization therapy observations from the REVERSE trial. Eur Heart J 2012;33(21):2662–71. Available at: https://doi.org/10.1093/eurheartj/ehr505>. Acesso em: 9/28/2021. ISSN 0195-668X. Disponível em:.

60. Behon A, Schwertner WR, Merkel ED, et al. Lateral left ventricular lead position is superior to posterior position in long-term outcome of patients who underwent cardiac resynchronization therapy. ESC Heart Fail 2020;7(6):3374–82. https://doi.org/10.1002/ehf2.13066 >. Acesso em: 2021/09/28. Available at: ISSN 2055-5822. Disponível em:.

61. Gold MR, Birgersdotter-Green U, Singh JP, et al. The relationship between ventricular electrical delay and left ventricular remodelling with cardiac resynchronization therapy. Eur Heart J 2011; 32(20):2516–24, 1522-9645 (Electronic).

62. Roubicek T, Wichterle D, Kucera P, et al. Left ventricular lead electrical delay is a predictor of mortality in patients with cardiac resynchronization therapy. Circ Arrhythm Electrophysiol 2015;8(5):1113–21, 1941-3084 (Electronic).

63. Gold MR, Singh JP, Ellenbogen KA, et al. Interventricular electrical delay is predictive of response to cardiac resynchronization therapy. JACC Clin Electrophysiol 2016;2(4):438–47, 2405-5018 (Electronic).

64. Gold MR, Yu Y, Wold N, et al. The role of interventricular conduction delay to predict clinical response with cardiac resynchronization therapy. Heart Rhythm 2017;14(12):1748–55, 1556-3871 (Electronic).

65. Khan FZ, Virdee MS, Palmer CR, et al. Targeted left ventricular lead placement to guide cardiac resynchronization therapy: the TARGET study: a randomized, controlled trial. J Am Coll Cardiol 2012; 59(17):1509–18, 1558-3597 (Electronic).

66. Saba S, Marek J, Schwartzman D, et al. Echocardiography-guided left ventricular lead placement for cardiac resynchronization therapy: results of the Speckle Tracking Assisted Resynchronization Therapy for Electrode Region trial. Circ Heart Fail 2013;6(3):427–34, 1941-3297 (Electronic).

67. Chen Z, Sohal M, Sammut E, et al. Focal But Not Diffuse Myocardial Fibrosis Burden Quantification Using Cardiac Magnetic Resonance Imaging Predicts Left Ventricular Reverse Modeling Following Cardiac Resynchronization Therapy. J Cardiovasc Electrophysiol 2016 Feb;27(2):203–9.

68. Daoulah A, Alsheikh-Ali AA, Al-Faifi SM, et al. Cardiac resynchronization therapy in patients with postero-lateral scar by cardiac magnetic resonance: a systematic review and meta-analysis. J Electrocardiol 2015;48(5):783–90, 1532-8430 (Electronic).

69. Sommer A, Kronborg MB, Nørgaard BL, et al. Multimodality imaging-guided left ventricular lead placement in cardiac resynchronization therapy: a randomized controlled trial. n. 1879-0844 (Electronic). Eur J Heart Fail 2016;18(11):1365–74.

70. Beshai JF, Grimm RA, Nagueh SF, et al. Cardiac-resynchronization therapy in heart failure with narrow QRS complexes. N Engl J Med 2007; 357(24):2461–71. Available at: https://doi.org/10.1056/NEJMoa0706695 >. Acesso em: 2021/09/02. ISSN 0028-4793. Disponível em:.

71. Donahue T, Niazi I, Leon A, et al. Acute and chronic response to CRT in narrow QRS patients. J Cardiovasc Transl Res 2012;5(2):232–41, 1937-5395 (Electronic).

72. Ruschitzka F, Abraham WT, Singh JP, et al. Cardiac-resynchronization therapy in heart failure with a narrow QRS Complex. N Engl J Med 2013; 369(15):1395–405. Available at: https://doi.org/10.1056/NEJMoa1306687 >. Acesso em: 2021/09/02. ISSN 0028-4793. Disponível em:.

73. Chung ES, Leon AR, Tavazzi L, et al. Results of the predictors of response to CRT (PROSPECT) trial. Circulation 2008;117(20):2608–16, 1524-4539 (Electronic).

74. Yu CM, Sanderson JE, Gorcsan J III. Echocardiography, dyssynchrony, and the response to cardiac resynchronization therapy. Eur Heart J 2010; 31(19):2326–37. Available at: https://doi.org/10.1093/eurheartj/ehq263>. Acesso em: 10/7/2021. ISSN 0195-668X. Disponível em:.

75. Vijayaraman P, Subzposh FA. His-bundle pacing and LV endocardial pacing as alternatives to Traditional cardiac resynchronization therapy. Curr Cardiol Rep 2018;20(11):109, 1534-3170 (Electronic).

76. Behar JM, Jackson T, Hyde E, et al. Optimized left ventricular endocardial stimulation is superior to optimized epicardial stimulation in ischemic patients with poor response to cardiac resynchronization therapy: a combined magnetic resonance imaging, Electroanatomic Contact mapping, and Hemodynamic study to target endocardial lead

placement. JACC Clin Electrophysiol 2016;2(7): 799–809, 2405-500X (Print).

77. Gamble JHP, Herring N, Ginks M, et al. Endocardial left ventricular pacing for cardiac resynchronization: systematic review and meta-analysis. Europace 2018;20(1):73–81, 1532-2092 (Electronic).

78. Upadhyay GA, Vijayaraman P, Nayak HM, et al. His Corrective pacing or biventricular pacing for cardiac resynchronization in heart failure. J Am Coll Cardiol 2019;74(1):157–9, 1558-3597 (Electronic).

79. Huang W, Su L, Wu S, et al. A novel pacing Strategy with low and stable output: pacing the left bundle branch immediately beyond the conduction block. Can J Cardiol 2017;33(2):1736, e3. Available at: https://doi.org/10.1016/j.cjca.2017.09.013>. Acesso em: 2021/09/02. ISSN 0828-282X. Disponível em:.

80. Wu S, Su L, Vijayaraman P, et al. Left bundle branch pacing for cardiac resynchronization therapy: Nonrandomized on-treatment comparison with His bundle pacing and biventricular pacing. Can J Cardiol 2021;37(2):319–28, 1916-7075 (Electronic).

81. Liu J, Sun F, Wang Z, et al. Left bundle branch area pacing vs. Biventricular pacing for cardiac resynchronization therapy: a meta-analysis. Front Cardiovasc Med 2021;8:408. Available at: https://www.frontiersin.org/article/10.3389/fcvm.2021.669301.

82. Ravi V, Hanifin JL, Larsen T, et al. The Pros and Cons of left bundle branch pacing: a single center experience. Circ Arrhythm Electrophysiol 2020; 13(12):e008874. Available at: https://doi.org/10.1161/CIRCEP.120.008874>. Acesso em: 2021/09/28. Disponível em:.

83. Arora V, SURI P. Physiological pacing: a new Road to future. Indian J Clin Cardiol 2021;2(1):32–43. Available at: https://doi.org/10.1177/2632463620978045>. Acesso em: 2021/09/28. ISSN 2632-4636. Disponível em:.

84. Sidhu BS, Porter B, Gould J, et al. Leadless left ventricular endocardial pacing in nonresponders to conventional cardiac resynchronization therapy. Pacing Clin Electrophysiol 2020;43(9):966–73, 1540-8159 (Electronic).

85. Brabham WW, Gold MR. The role of AV and VV optimization for CRT. J Arrhythmia 2013;29(3):153–61. ISSN 18804276.

86. Delnoy PP, Ritter P, Naegele H, et al. Association between frequent cardiac resynchronization therapy optimization and long-term clinical response: a post hoc analysis of the Clinical Evaluation on Advanced Resynchronization (CLEAR) pilot study. Europace 2013;15(8):1174–81, 1532-2092 (Electronic).

87. Brignole M, Auricchio A, Baron-Esquivias G, et al. 2013 ESC guidelines on cardiac pacing and cardiac resynchronization therapy: the task force on cardiac pacing and resynchronization therapy of the European Society of Cardiology (ESC). Developed in collaboration with the European Heart Rhythm Association (EHRA). Europace 2013; 15(8):1070–118. ISSN 1532-2092 (Electronic) 1099-5129 (Linking). Disponível em: Available at: https://www.ncbi.nlm.nih.gov/pubmed/23801827.

88. Ellenbogen KA, Gold MR, Meyer TE, et al. Primary results from the SmartDelay determined AV optimization: a comparison to other AV delay methods used in cardiac resynchronization therapy (SMART-AV) trial: a randomized trial comparing empirical, echocardiography-guided, and algorithmic atrioventricular delay programming in cardiac resynchronization therapy. Circulation 2010;122(25): 2660–8. ISSN 1524-4539 (Electronic) 0009-7322 (Linking). Disponível em: Available at: https://www.ncbi.nlm.nih.gov/pubmed/21098426.

89. Luceri RM, Brownstein SL, Vardeman L, et al. PR interval behavior during exercise: implications for physiological pacemakers. Pacing Clin Electrophysiol 1990;13(n. 12 Pt 2):1719–23. ISSN 0147-8389 (Print) 0147-8389 (Linking). Disponível em: Available at: https://www.ncbi.nlm.nih.gov/pubmed/1704529.

90. Shanmugam N, Prada-Delgado O, Campos AG, et al. Rate-adaptive AV delay and exercise performance following cardiac resynchronization therapy. Heart Rhythm 2012;9(11):1815–21. ISSN 1556-3871 (Electronic) 1547-5271 (Linking). Disponível em: Available at: https://www.ncbi.nlm.nih.gov/pubmed/22772135.

91. Ritter P, Delnoy PP, Padeletti L, et al. A randomized pilot study of optimization of cardiac resynchronization therapy in sinus rhythm patients using a peak endocardial acceleration sensor vs. standard methods. Europace 2012;14(9):1324–33. Available at: https://doi.org/10.1093/europace/eus059 >. Acesso em: 9/28/2021. ISSN 1099-5129. Disponível em:.

92. Brugada J, Delnoy PP, Brachmann J, et al. Contractility sensor-guided optimization of cardiac resynchronization therapy: results from the RESPOND-CRT trial. Eur Heart J 2017;38(10):730–8. Available at: https://doi.org/10.1093/eurheartj/ehw526 >. Acesso em: 9/28/2021. ISSN 0195-668X. Disponível em:.

93. Burri H, Prinzen FW, Gasparini M, et al. Left univentricular pacing for cardiac resynchronization therapy. Europace 2017;19(6):912–9. ISSN 1532-2092 (Electronic) 1099-5129 (Linking). Disponível em: Available at: https://www.ncbi.nlm.nih.gov/pubmed/28339579.

94. Vatasescu R, Berruezo A, Mont L, et al. Midterm 'super-response' to cardiac resynchronization therapy by biventricular pacing with fusion: insights from electro-anatomical mapping. Europace 2009; 11(12):1675–82. ISSN 1532-2092 1099-5129.

Disponível em: Available at: https://pubmed.ncbi.nlm.nih.gov/19880850. >.Disponível em. https://www.ncbi.nlm.nih.gov/pmc/articles/PMC2780924/.

95. Strik M, van Middendorp LB, Houthuizen P, et al. Interplay of electrical wavefronts as Determinant of the response to cardiac resynchronization therapy in dyssynchronous canine hearts. Circ Arrhythm Electrophysiol 2013;6(5):924–31. Available at: https://doi.org/10.1161/CIRCEP.113.000753>. Acesso em: 2021/09/03. Disponível em:.

96. Arbelo E, Tolosana JM, Trucco E, et al. Fusion-optimized intervals (FOI): a new method to achieve the narrowest QRS for optimization of the AV and VV intervals in patients undergoing cardiac resynchronization therapy. J Cardiovasc Electrophysiol 2014; 25(3):283–92, 1540-8167 (Electronic).

97. Birnie D, Lemke B, Aonuma K, et al. Clinical outcomes with synchronized left ventricular pacing: analysis of the adaptive CRT trial. Heart Rhythm 2013;10(9):1368–74. ISSN 1547-5271. Disponível em: Available at: http://www.sciencedirect.com/science/article/pii/S1547527113007327. >.Disponível em. https://ac.els-cdn.com/S1547527113007327/1-s2.0-S1547527113007327-main.pdf?_tid=8ef4b5fb-ede8-4882-a36a-1891b0c787aa&acdnat=1531301441_a42cf252b1c6fc06063cbde225e38084.

98. Filippatos G, Birnie D, Gold MR, et al. Rationale and design of the AdaptResponse trial: a prospective randomized study of cardiac resynchronization therapy with preferential adaptive left ventricular-only pacing. Eur J Heart Fail 2017;19(7):950–7, 1879-0844 (Electronic).

99. Pappone C, Ćalović Z, Vicedomini G, et al. Improving cardiac resynchronization therapy response with multipoint left ventricular pacing: Twelve-month follow-up study. Heart Rhythm 2015; 12(6):1250–8, 1556-3871 (Electronic).

100. Behar JM, Bostock J, Li APZ, et al. Cardiac resynchronization therapy delivered via a Multipolar left ventricular lead is associated with reduced mortality and Elimination of phrenic nerve stimulation: long-term follow-up from a Multicenter registry. J Cardiovasc Electrophysiol 2015;26(5):540–6, 1540-8167 (Electronic).

101. Rinaldi CA, Burri H, Thibault B, et al. A review of multisite pacing to achieve cardiac resynchronization therapy. Europace 2015;17(1):7–17. Available at: https://doi.org/10.1093/europace/euu197 >. Acesso em: 9/3/2021. ISSN 1099-5129. Disponível em:.

102. Zanon F, Marcantoni L, Baracca E, et al. Optimization of left ventricular pacing site plus multipoint pacing improves remodeling and clinical response to cardiac resynchronization therapy at 1 year. Heart Rhythm 2016;13(8):1644–51, 1556-3871 (Electronic).

103. Forleo GB, Santini L, Giammaria M, et al. Multipoint pacing via a quadripolar left-ventricular lead: preliminary results from the Italian registry on multipoint left-ventricular pacing in cardiac resynchronization therapy (IRON-MPP). Europace 2017;19(7):1170–7, 1532-2092 (Electronic).

104. Barold SS, Herweg B. Cardiac resynchronization in patients with atrial fibrillation. J Atr Fibrillation 2015; 8(4):1383. ISSN 1941-6911. Disponível em: Available at: https://pubmed.ncbi.nlm.nih.gov/279572 35. >.Disponível em. https://www.ncbi.nlm.nih.gov/pmc/articles/PMC5135194/.

105. Koplan BA, Kaplan AJ, Weiner S, et al. Heart failure decompensation and all-cause mortality in relation to percent biventricular pacing in patients with heart failure: is a goal of 100% biventricular pacing necessary? J Am Coll Cardiol 2009;53(4):355–60, 1558-3597 (Electronic).

106. Lubitz SA, SINGH JP. Biventricular pacing: more is better! Eur Heart J 2015;36(7):407–9. Available at: https://doi.org/10.1093/eurheartj/ehu347>. Acesso em: 9/2/2021. ISSN 0195-668X. Disponível em:.

107. Hayes DL, Boehmer JP, Day JD, et al. Cardiac resynchronization therapy and the relationship of percent biventricular pacing to symptoms and survival. Heart Rhythm 2011;8(9):1469–75. Available at: https://doi.org/10.1016/j.hrthm.2011.04.015 >. Acesso em: 2021/09/07. ISSN 1547-5271. Disponível em:.

108. Ousdigian KT, Borek PP, Koehler JL, et al. The epidemic of inadequate biventricular pacing in patients with persistent or permanent atrial fibrillation and its association with mortality. Circ Arrhythm Electrophysiol 2014 Jun;7(3):370–6.

109. Kamath GS, Cotiga D, Koneru JN, et al. The utility of 12-lead Holter monitoring in patients with permanent atrial fibrillation for the identification of nonresponders after cardiac resynchronization therapy. J Am Coll Cardiol 2009;53(12):1050–5. ISSN 0735-1097. Disponível em: Available at: https://www.sciencedirect.com/science/article/pii/S0735109709000321.

110. Gasparini M, Galimberti P, Ceriotti C. The importance of increased percentage of biventricular pacing to improve clinical outcomes in patients receiving cardiac resynchronization therapy. Curr Opin Cardiol 2013;28(4):50. ISSN 0268-4705. Disponível em: Available at: https://journals.lww.com/co-cardiology/Fulltext/2013/01000/The_importance_of_increased_percentage_of.9.aspx.

111. Gasparini M, Leclercq C, Lunati M, et al. Cardiac resynchronization therapy in patients with atrial fibrillation: the CERTIFY study (cardiac resynchronization therapy in atrial fibrillation patients multinational registry). JACC Heart Fail 2013;1(6):500–7. ISSN 2213-1779. Disponível em: Available at: https://www.sciencedirect.com/science/article/pii/S2213177913003193.

112. Lakkireddy D, Di Biase L, Ryschon K, et al. Radiofrequency ablation of Premature ventricular ectopy improves the Efficacy of cardiac resynchronization therapy in nonresponders. J Am Coll Cardiol 2012; 60(16):1531–9. ISSN 0735-1097. Disponível em: Available at: https://www.sciencedirect.com/science/article/pii/S0735109712028033.

113. Neubauer S. The failing heart–an engine out of fuel. N Engl J Med 2007;356(11):1140–51. Available at: https://www.ncbi.nlm.nih.gov/pubmed/17360992 https://www.nejm.org/doi/full/10.1056/NEJMra063052?url_ver=Z39.88-2003&rfr_id=ori:rid:crossref.org&rfr_dat=cr_pub%3dpubmed.

114. Stanley WC, RECCHIA FA, LOPASCHUK GD. Myocardial substrate metabolism in the normal and failing heart. Physiol Rev 2005;85(3):1093–129. ISSN 0031-9333 (Print) 0031-9333 (Linking). Disponível em: Available at: https://www.ncbi.nlm.nih.gov/pubmed/15987803.

115. Zanco P, Desideri A, Mobilia G, et al. Effects of left bundle branch block on myocardial FDG PET in patients without significant coronary artery stenoses. J Nucl Med 2000;41(6):973–7. ISSN 0161-5505 (Print) 0161-5505 (Linking). Disponível em: Available at: https://www.ncbi.nlm.nih.gov/pubmed/10855620.

116.. Degtiarova G, Claus P, Duchenne J, et al. Low septal to lateral wall (18)F-FDG ratio is highly associated with mechanical dyssynchrony in non-ischemic CRT candidates. EJNMMI Res 2019;9: 105.

117. Nowak B, Sinha AM, Schaefer WM, et al. Cardiac resynchronization therapy homogenizes myocardial glucose metabolism and perfusion in dilated cardiomyopathy and left bundle branch block. J Am Coll Cardiol 2003;41(9):1523–8. ISSN 07351097.

118. Agnetti G, Kaludercic N, Kane LA, et al. Modulation of mitochondrial proteome and improved mitochondrial function by biventricular pacing of dyssynchronous failing hearts. Circ Cardiovasc Genet 2010;3(1):78–87. Available at: https://www.ncbi.nlm.nih.gov/pubmed/20160199.

119. UKKONEN H, et al. Effect of cardiac resynchronization on myocardial efficiency and regional oxidative metabolism. Circulation 2003;107:28–31.

120. Nelson GS, Berger RD, Fetics BJ, et al. Left ventricular or biventricular pacing improves cardiac function at diminished energy cost in patients with dilated cardiomyopathy and left bundle-branch block. Circulation 2000;102(25):3053–9. ISSN 1524-4539 (Electronic) 0009-7322 (Linking). Disponível em: Available at: https://www.ncbi.nlm.nih.gov/pubmed/11120694.

121. Obrzut S, Tiongson J, Jamshidi N, et al. Assessment of metabolic phenotypes in patients with non-ischemic dilated cardiomyopathy undergoing cardiac resynchronization therapy. J Cardiovasc Transl Res 2010;3(6):643–51. ISSN 1937-5395 (Electronic) 1937-5387 (Linking). Disponível em: Available at: https://www.ncbi.nlm.nih.gov/pubmed/20842468.

122. Ayyadurai P, Alkhawam H, Saad M, et al. An update on the CardioMEMS pulmonary artery pressure sensor. Ther Adv Cardiovasc Dis 2019;13. ISSN 1753-9455 1753-9447. Disponível em: Available at: https://pubmed.ncbi.nlm.nih.gov/30803405 https://www.ncbi.nlm.nih.gov/pmc/articles/PMC6376505/. 1753944719826826-1753944719826826.

123. Abraham WT, Adamson PB, Bourge RC, et al. Wireless pulmonary artery haemodynamic monitoring in chronic heart failure: a randomised controlled trial. Lancet 2011;377(9766):658–66. Available at: https://doi.org/10.1016/S0140-6736(11)60101-3 >. Acesso em: 2021/09/07. ISSN 0140-6736. Disponível em:.

124. Angermann CE, Assmus B, Anker SD, et al. Pulmonary artery pressure-guided therapy in ambulatory patients with symptomatic heart failure: the CardioMEMS European Monitoring Study for Heart Failure (MEMS-HF). Eur J Heart Fail 2020;22(10):1891–901. Available at: https://doi.org/10.1002/ejhf.1943 >. Acesso em: 2021/09/07. ISSN 1388-9842. Disponível em:.

125. Borggrefe M, MANN DL. Cardiac contractility modulation in 2018. Circulation 2018;138(24):2738–40. Available at: https://doi.org/10.1161/CIRCULATIONAHA.118.036460>. Acesso em: 2021/09/07. Disponível em:.

126. Giallauria F, Vigorito C, Piepoli MF, et al. Effects of cardiac contractility modulation by non-excitatory electrical stimulation on exercise capacity and quality of life: an individual patient's data meta-analysis of randomized controlled trials. Int J Cardiol 2014;175(2):352–7. Available at: https://doi.org/10.1016/j.ijcard.2014.06.005 >. Acesso em: 2021/09/07. ISSN 0167-5273. Disponível em:.

127. Yu CM, Chan JY, Zhang Q, et al. Impact of cardiac contractility modulation on left ventricular Global and Regional function and remodeling. JACC Cardiovasc Imaging 2009;2(12):1341–9. ISSN 1936-878X. Disponível em: Available at: https://www.sciencedirect.com/science/article/pii/S1936878X09006615.

128. Anker SD, Borggrefe M, Neuser H, et al. Cardiac contractility modulation improves long-term survival and hospitalizations in heart failure with reduced ejection fraction. Eur J Heart Fail 2019;21(9): 1103–13. Available at: https://doi.org/10.1002/ejhf.1374 >. Acesso em: 2021/09/07. ISSN 1388-9842. Disponível em:.

129. Kloppe A, Lawo T, Mijic D, et al. Long-term survival with Cardiac Contractility Modulation in patients with NYHA II or III symptoms and normal QRS duration. Int J Cardiol 2016;209:291–5. Available

at: https://doi.org/10.1016/j.ijcard.2016.02.001 >. Acesso em: 2021/09/07. ISSN 0167-5273. Disponível em:.

130. Tint D, FLOREA R, MICU S. New Generation cardiac contractility modulation device-Filling the Gap in heart failure treatment. J Clin Med 2019;8(5):588. ISSN 2077-0383. Disponível em: Available at: https://pubmed.ncbi.nlm.nih.gov/31035648. >.Disponível em. https://www.ncbi.nlm.nih.gov/pmc/articles/PMC6572164/.

131. Butter C, Meyhöfer J, Seifert M, et al. First use of cardiac contractility modulation (CCM) in a patient failing CRT therapy: clinical and technical aspects of combined therapies. Eur J Heart Fail 2007;9(9): 955–8. Available at: https://doi.org/10.1016/j.ejheart.2007.05.012 >. Acesso em: 2021/09/07. ISSN 1388-9842. Disponível em:.

132. Abraham WT, Zile MR, Weaver FA, et al. Baroreflex activation therapy for the treatment of heart failure with a reduced ejection fraction. JACC Heart Fail 2015;3(6):487–96. ISSN 2213-1779. Disponível em: Available at: https://www.sciencedirect.com/science/article/pii/S2213177915001250.

133. Zile MR, Lindenfeld J, Weaver FA, et al. Baroreflex activation therapy in patients with heart failure with reduced ejection fraction. J Am Coll Cardiol 2020; 76(1):1–13. ISSN 0735-1097. Disponível em: Available at: https://www.sciencedirect.com/science/article/pii/S0735109720352980.

134. Zannad F, De Ferrari GM, Tuinenburg AE, et al. Chronic vagal stimulation for the treatment of low ejection fraction heart failure: results of the NEural Cardiac TherApy foR Heart Failure (NECTAR-HF) randomized controlled trial. Eur Heart J 2015; 36(7):425–33. https://doi.org/10.1093/eurheartj/ehu345 >. Acesso em: 9/28/2021. ISSN 0195-668X. Disponível em: Available at:.

135. Gold MR, Van Veldhuisen DJ, Hauptman PJ, et al. Vagus nerve stimulation for the treatment of heart failure: the INOVATE-HF trial. J Am Coll Cardiol 2016;68(2):149–58. ISSN 0735-1097. Disponível em: Available at: https://www.sciencedirect.com/science/article/pii/S0735109716324044.

136. Premchand RK, Sharma K, Mittal S, et al. Autonomic Regulation therapy via left or right Cervical Vagus nerve stimulation in patients with chronic heart failure: results of the ANTHEM-HF trial. J Card Fail 2014;20(11):808–16. Available at: https://doi.org/10.1016/j.cardfail.2014.08.009>. Acesso em: 2021/09/28. ISSN 1071-9164. Disponível em:.

137. Herring N, Kalla M, Paterson DJ. The autonomic nervous system and cardiac arrhythmias: current concepts and emerging therapies. Nat Rev Cardiol 2019;16(12):707–26. Available at: https://doi.org/10.1038/s41569-019-0221-2. ISSN 1759-5010. Disponível em:.

138. Zipes DP, Neuzil P, Theres H, et al. Determining the Feasibility of spinal cord neuromodulation for the treatment of chronic systolic heart failure: the DEFEAT-HF study. JACC Heart Fail 2016;4(2): 129–36. ISSN 2213-1779. Disponível em: Available at: https://www.sciencedirect.com/science/article/pii/S2213177915006848.

139. Cavaco DM. Response to cardiac resynchronization therapy: dichotomous or continuous variable? Rev Port Cardiol 2017;36(12):893–4, 2174-2030 (Electronic).

140. Rickard J, Michtalik H, Sharma R, et al. Predictors of response to cardiac resynchronization therapy: a systematic review. Int J Cardiol 2016;225: 345–52, 1874-1754 (Electronic).

141. Curtis AB, POOLE JE. The right response to Nonresponse to cardiac resynchronization therapy. J Am Coll Cardiol 2019;74(21):2604–6, 1558-3597 (Electronic).

142. Sidhu BS, Rua T, Gould J, et al. Economic evaluation of a dedicated cardiac resynchronisation therapy preassessment clinic. Open Heart 2020; 7(2):e001249. Disponível em: Available at: http://openheart.bmj.com/content/7/2/e001249.abstract.

143. Gorodeski EZ, Magnelli-Reyes C, Moennich LA, et al. Cardiac resynchronization therapy-heart failure (CRT-HF) clinic: a novel model of care. PloS one 2019;14(9):e0222610. ISSN 1932-6203. Disponível em: Available at: https://pubmed.ncbi.nlm.nih.gov/31536565. >.Disponível em. https://www.ncbi.nlm.nih.gov/pmc/articles/PMC6752801/.

Conduction System Pacing for Cardiac Resynchronization Therapy

Bengt Herweg, MD, FHRS[a,b,*], Allan Welter-Frost, MD, MPH[a,b],
David R. Wilson II, MD[a,b], Pugazhendhi Vijayaraman, MD[c]

KEYWORDS

- His bundle pacing • Left bundle area pacing • Physiologic pacing
- Cardiac resynchronization therapy • Cardiomyopathy

KEY POINTS

- Acute hemodynamic and observational studies have shown more effective electrical and mechanical resynchronization with His-Purkinje conduction system pacing when compared with conventional BiV pacing.
- Conduction system pacing re-establishes physiologic ventricular activation and repolarization and, thus, may be less arrhythmogenic and may improve diastolic function more efficiently.
- Conduction system pacing can currently be viewed as a viable bailout strategy in patients with lack of access to the coronary venous system or intractable diaphragmatic pacing. It also can be considered as an alternative option in CRT nonresponders.
- However, CSP as the go-to resynchronization strategy is highly provocative in the absence of controlled randomized clinical trial data.

INTRODUCTION

Ventricular conduction disturbance, most commonly left bundle branch block (LBBB), is present in approximately one-third of patients with heart failure, leading to loss of synchronous ventricular contraction. Cardiac resynchronization therapy (CRT) by simultaneous biventricular (BiV) pacing was first conceptualized in 1990.[1] Currently, CRT by BiV pacing is the only heart failure therapy that improves cardiac function, functional capacity, and survival while decreasing cardiac workload and hospitalizations.[2–5] The response to BiV pacing is variable, ranging from complete normalization of cardiac function to lack of benefit. In 1978 El-Sherif and coworkers[6] described evidence of longitudinal dissociation in the His-Purkinje system and acute normalization of bundle branch block by distal His bundle pacing (HBP). Permanent conduction system pacing (CSP) in form of HBP was first achieved in 2000.[7] Correction of LBBB by permanent HBP was first reported by Barba-Pichardo and coworkers in 2013.[8] We present a systematic review of evolving CSP techniques (**Figs. 1** and **2**) as a more physiologic alternative to conventional CRT in patients with cardiomyopathy, bundle branch block, or intraventricular conduction defect (IVCD). Although still considered experimental, CSP is currently undergoing rigorous clinical investigation.

LIMITATIONS OF CONVENTIONAL CARDIAC RESYNCHRONIZATION THERAPY

Many challenges of conventional CRT have been improved with VV-interval programmability,

[a] Department of Cardiovascular Sciences, University of South Florida Morsani College of Medicine, South Tampa Center (3rd Floor), Tampa, FL 33606, USA; [b] Tampa General Hospital, 1 Tampa General Circle, Tampa, FL 33606, USA; [c] Geisinger Heart Institute, Geisinger Commonwealth School of Medicine, 1000 E. Mountain Blvd, Wilkes-Barre, PA 18711, USA
* Corresponding author. USF Health, South Tampa Center (3rd Floor),2 Tampa General Circle. Tampa, FL, 33606.
E-mail address: Bengt@usf.edu

Card Electrophysiol Clin 14 (2022) 297–310
https://doi.org/10.1016/j.ccep.2021.12.005
1877-9182/22/© 2021 Elsevier Inc. All rights reserved.

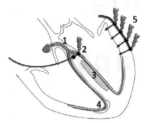

Possible CRT strategies:
• HBP-CRT = site 1
• LBBP-CRT = site 2
• BVP-CRT = site 4 and 5
• HOT-CRT = site 1 and 5
• LOT-CRT = site 2 and 5

Fig. 1. Sites for conduction system pacing and cardiac resynchronization therapy. Locations for permanent lead placement and possible cardiac resynchronization therapy strategies using conduction system pacing. BVP, biventricular pacing; HOT-CRT, His-optimized CRT; LBBP, left bundle branch pacing; LOT-CRT, left bundle branch optimized CRT.

device-based fusion optimization algorithms, quadripolar left ventricular (LV) leads allowing electronic repositioning, multipoint-stimulation, and targeted LV pacing from the LV lateral base.[9] However, the inability to stimulate severely diseased myocardium or myocardial scar without massive stimulus-to-QRS latency presents a major obstacle for effective CRT delivery.[10,11] Many patients have underlying atrioventricular (AV) block, omitting delivery of fused CRT, or advanced IVCD complicating CRT delivery. Furthermore, CRT requires LV pre-excitation, which often is in conflict with delivery of ventricular pacing at the optimal AV interval. These obstacles are further limited by suboptimal coronary venous anatomy and frequently cannot be solved by conventional CRT. CSP (alone or in conjunction with LV pacing) may yield a viable solution to some of these obstacles. The His-Purkinje system is an endocardial structure. Endocardial LV pacing may represent a form of distal CSP and is associated with improved hemodynamic response compared with epicardial LV pacing.[12,13]

CONDUCTION SYSTEM PACING

Observational studies have demonstrated HBP with recruitment of fibers predestined to become the left bundle or direct left bundle branch pacing (LBBP) can result in highly efficient resynchronization.[14–24] Acute hemodynamic studies have shown CSP may result in superior electrical and mechanical resynchronization when compared with BiV pacing.[25,26]

A compelling rationale for CSP is its ability to restore physiologic ventricular activation. Although classic CRT achieves a reduction in LV dyssynchrony, CSP may result in complete restoration of cardiac electrical depolarization and repolarization. Thus, it should result in improved LV systolic and diastolic performance. Classic CRT has a

proarrhythmic potential because of epicardial to endocardial activation resulting also in altered repolarization, and colliding activation wave fronts that can result in ventricular tachycardia. CSP is unlikely to pose proarrhythmic risk.[27,28] In fact, CSP has been reported to potentially abolish CRT-related proarrhythmia.[23]

Presently, CSP serves as an attractive bailout strategy in patients with lack of coronary venous access, diaphragmatic pacing, and/or failure to respond to classic CRT.[13] This pacing method should be strongly considered for the prevention of pacing-induced cardiomyopathy in patients with preserved LV systolic function requiring long-term ventricular pacing (class IIa indication).[24–26] Its role as a primary resynchronization therapy for patients with heart failure with bundle branch block remains to be elucidated by randomized clinical trials.

Fig. 3 shows correction of LBBB by HBP, correction of LBBB by LBBP, and His-optimized (HOT)-CRT, discussed in the following sections.

His Bundle Pacing with Left Bundle Recruitment

Cardiac resynchronization by HBP is highly effective in patients with AV block dependent on ventricular pacing. In a high percentage of these patients, complete electrical resynchronization and hemodynamic optimization of the AV interval is achieved. In patients with LBBB HBP has emerged as a viable CRT alternative. Based on observational studies left bundle recruitment is achieved in 75% to 90% of patients acutely with an implant success rate ranging from 56% to 90%.[12,13,29,30] Observational studies of HBP in patients with heart failure with LBBB have demonstrated excellent electrical resynchronization with marked QRS reduction, improved LV ejection fraction (LVEF), decreased LV dimensions, improved New York Heart Association (NYHA) functional class, 6-minute-walk tests, and quality of life.[16–20,25,31] Unfortunately, the pacing and left bundle recruitment thresholds are frequently high with HBP, and R-wave amplitudes in the His region are low, requiring lead revision in up to 7% to 10% of implants.[18] Currently, HBP in patients with LBBB is viewed as a backup option in patients with lack of coronary venous access and diaphragmatic pacing. Randomized controlled clinical trial data of HBP in LBBB are lacking.

Deep Septal Left Bundle Branch Pacing

The technique of deep septal LBBP was developed by Huang and coworkers in 2017.[21] The lead is advanced from the right ventricular (RV) septum

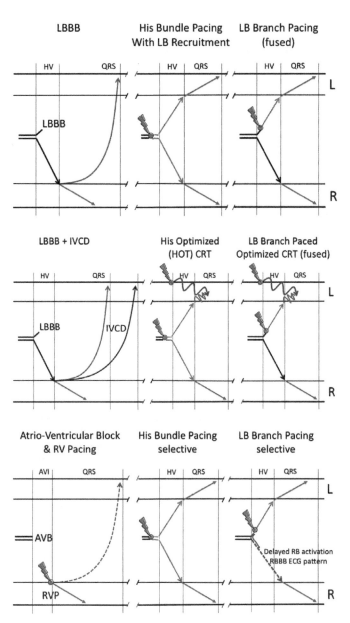

Fig. 2. Conduction system pacing in left bundle branch block, coexistent IVCD, and atrioventricular block. ECG, electrocardiogram; HV, His-ventricular; IVCD, intraventricular conduction defect; RBBB, right bundle branch block; AVB, atrio ventricular block; AVI, atrio ventricular interval; RVP, right ventricular pacing; RB, right bundle.

to the subendocardial LV septum to directly stimulate the left bundle branch region. The optimal site of fixation is approximately 1 to 1.5 cm distal to the His recording site on the RV septum. The paced QRS morphology before fixation usually demonstrates a "w" pattern with a notch at the nadir of the QRS in lead V1. As the lead is being advanced into the septum the paced QRS morphology changes from an LBBB to a right bundle branch block (RBBB) pattern and, frequently, RBBB fixation beats are observed.[32] In a series of 100 patients requiring pacing for bradycardia or heart failure with failed LV lead the implant success rate

was 93%.[22] The pacing threshold was 0.6 ± 0.4 V at 0.5 milliseconds and R waves were 10 ± 6 mV and remained stable at a median follow-up of 3 months. LBBP has been evaluated in patients with heart failure with persistent atrial fibrillation undergoing an AV junctional ablation, and was shown to decrease the combined end point of heart failure hospitalizations and death and inappropriate implantable cardioverter-defibrillator therapies.[33] Two recent observational studies of LBBP in patients with heart failure with LBBB demonstrated marked QRS reduction and shortened LV activation time, improved LVEF, diminished LV dimensions,

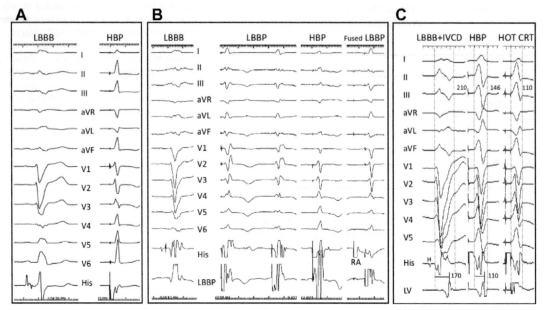

Fig. 3. (*A–C*) Examples of electrical resynchronization by conduction system pacing. HOT, His optimized.

and reduced NYHA functional class.[22,33] LBBB and large LV end-diastolic diameter were independent predictors of response.[34] In all observational studies mentioned here, the implant success rate varied from 85% to 97%. The left bundle stimulation threshold was consistently excellent with a large R-wave amplitude, indicating that LBBP may be a viable CRT alternative. Randomized controlled clinical trials are needed to firmly establish this novel pacing therapy as a primary resynchronization option.

Special Considerations in Conduction System Pacing to Correct Left Bundle Branch Block

The success of CSP depends on the location of disease within the His-Purkinje system. This was elegantly demonstrated in a study by Upadhyay and coworkers.[35] A total of 88 left septal conduction recordings were analyzed in 85 patients: 72 LBBB pattern and 16 control subjects (narrow QRS, n = 11; RBBB, n = 5). Among patients with LBBB pattern, complete conduction block within the proximal left conduction system was observed in 64% (n = 46) and intact Purkinje activation in the remaining 36% (n = 26), suggesting either distal first-degree LBBB or IVCD. Intact Purkinje activation was observed in all control subjects. The site of block in patients with complete conduction block was at the level of the left His bundle in 72% and in the proximal left bundle branch in 28%. HBP corrected wide QRS in 54% of all patients with LBBB pattern and 85% of those with complete conduction block (94% left

intrahisian, 62% proximal LBBB). No patients with intact Purkinje activation demonstrated correction of QRS with HBP.

In some patients with prolonged His-ventricular intervals, HBP may fail to shorten the left bundle conduction time because of more distal disease. This may be corrected by direct LBBP. During LBBP fusion optimization with the intrinsic right bundle conducted QRS complex yields maximal electric resynchronization and QRS narrowing. In contrast to classic CRT and LBBP, fusion with the conducted QRS complex is not of any benefit and not desirable with HBP. Therefore, in patients with AV block or atrial fibrillation undergoing AV junctional ablation, HBP may be the preferred pacing technique, because it grants complete control over the AV interval without requiring pre-excitation or fusion optimization. In patients with LBBB in absence of long first-degree AV block or higher degree AV block, LBBP has significant advantages because of markedly lower pacing thresholds and better local signal amplitude, which may result in superior outcomes when compared with BiV pacing.

Furthermore, in patients with LBBB and left axis deviation, LBBP can correct the electrical axis in 75% of patients by recruitment of fibers predestined to become the left anterior fascicle.[36] Whether this will translate into better clinical response is currently unclear. Patients with heart failure with LBBB and left axis deviation respond less well to conventional CRT when compared with patients with normal axis.

Conduction System Pacing in Patients with Right Bundle Branch Block

HBP was attempted as a primary or rescue strategy (failed LV lead implant) in patients with NYHA functional class II to IV heart failure, reduced LVEF, and RBBB with a QRS duration greater than or equal to 120 milliseconds.[37] HBP was successful in 37 of 39 patients (95%) with narrowing of RBBB in 78% of cases. His capture and bundle branch block correction thresholds were 1.1 ± 0.6 V and 1.4 ± 0.7 V at 1.0 milliseconds, respectively. During a mean follow-up of 15 ± 23 months, there was a significant narrowing of QRS from 158 ± 24 to 127 ± 17 milliseconds ($P = .0001$), increase in LVEF from 31 ± 10% to 39 ± 13% ($P = .004$), and improvement in NYHA functional class from 2.8 ± 0.6 to 2 ± 0.7 ($P = .0001$) with HBP.

In another multicenter observational study LBBP was attempted in 121 patients with RBBB, LVEF less than 50%, and indications for CRT/pacing and CRT was successfully achieved in 107 (88%).[38] LBBP resulted in some narrowing of the QRS from 156 ± 20 milliseconds to 150 ± 24 milliseconds ($P = .05$) with an LV activation time of 85 ± 16 milliseconds. Complete elimination of RBBB pattern was achieved in 35 (32%) patients, whereas significant attenuation of RBBB conduction delay pattern (reduction in R′ duration and amplitude) was accomplished in 68 patients (64%). Ejection fraction improved from 35 ± 9% to 43 ± 12% ($P < .01$). There was a significant improvement in overall NYHA functional class from 2.5 ± 0.8 at baseline to 1.7 ± 0.8 on follow-up ($P < .01$).

Conventional CRT in patients with non-LBBB (RBBB and IVCD) is currently recommended in patients with a QRS duration of greater than 150 milliseconds and less established in patients with RBBB and QRS less than 150 milliseconds. A meta-analysis of five randomized clinical trials has shown that QRS duration greater than 140 milliseconds is a powerful predictor of the effects of CRT on morbidity and mortality independent of QRS morphology in patients with heart failure with moderate to severe LV dysfunction.[39] Randomized controlled clinical trials are needed to evaluate if CSP is useful in patients with RBBB and which pacing modality at which QRS cutoff should be used.

His or Left Bundle Optimized Cardiac Resynchronization Therapy

In advanced cardiomyopathy, LBBB and IVCD may coexist. This may amplify LV dyssynchrony because LV activation in the setting of LBBB relies on long myocardial conduction pathways and thus, coexistent IVCD further delays activation of some myocardial segments. Therefore, CSP may paradoxically improve the impact of a coexistent IVCD. In these circumstances, resynchronization may be more complete when intervened on at the level of the specialized conduction system in conjunction with sequential LV pacing in myocardial areas activated late (**Fig. 2**B). In a small retrospective, observational multicenter study, HOT-CRT was performed in a series of 27 patients with LBBB/IVCD where partial or insignificant QRS narrowing was achieved by HBP alone compared with baseline.[40] All patients had therapy-refractory NYHA functional class III to IV heart failure symptoms and a baseline LVEF less than or equal to 35%. At the time of the device implantation, HOT-CRT resulted in improved electrical resynchronization when compared with conventional BiV pacing or HBP alone and was believed to be the best clinical option for these patients. The baseline QRS was reduced from 183 ± 27 to 120 ± 16 milliseconds (34%) by HOT-CRT compared with 162 ± 18 milliseconds (11%) by conventional BiV pacing and 151 ± 25 milliseconds (17%) with HBP alone ($P < .05$). The investigators observed significant echocardiographic and clinical improvement in patients with advanced heart failure treated with HOT-CRT.

A multicenter observational study reported 112 patients with CRT indication undergoing LBBP-optimized (LOT)-CRT.[41] The implant success rate was 81%. LOT-CRT resulted in improved electrical resynchronization when compared with conventional BiV pacing or LBBP alone. The baseline QRS was reduced to from 182 ± 267 to 144 ± 22 milliseconds (21%) by LOT-CRT compared with 170 ± 30 milliseconds (7%) by conventional BiV pacing and 162 ± 23 milliseconds (11%) by LBBP alone ($P < .001$). This resulted in an improvement of LVEF from 28.5 ± 9.9 to 37.2 ± 12.0 ($P < .001$) and improvement of NYHA functional class from 2.9 ± 0.6 to 1.9 ± 0.6 ($P < .0001$).

Left Ventricular Septal Pacing without Targeted Conduction System Capture

The electrocardiographic and hemodynamic effects of deep LV septal pacing without targeted conduction system capture have been studied in canine models with LBBB and in humans with LBBB and classic CRT indication by the Maastricht group.[26,42] Electrocardiography (QRS duration), vectorcardiography (QRS area), and multielectrode body surface mapping (standard deviation of activation times) were used to assess electrical resynchronization. Hemodynamic changes were assessed as the first derivative of LV pressure (LVdP/dtmax). LV septal pacing resulted in a larger reduction in QRS duration/area and LV activation time when compared with BiV pacing or combined LV septal and RV pacing.[26] The increase in LVdP/dtmax was similar during LV septal and BiV pacing and larger than during combined LV septal and RV pacing.[26] Basal, mid, and apical LV septal pacing positions resulted in similar results, indicating that within the LV, the position of the pacing electrode is not critical. Changes in QRS area, LV activation time, and LVdP/dtmax were comparable between LV septal and HBP. The authors concluded LV septal pacing results in short-term electrical resynchronization and hemodynamic improvement that may be as good as during BiV and HBP.[26]

LIMITATIONS OF CONDUCTION SYSTEM PACING
Technical Limitations

His bundle and deep septal LBBP require a highly motivated operator willing to overcome a steep learning curve to develop the necessary skill set to target the discrete structures of the specialized conduction system. In this respect the current experience is reminiscent of the early era of conventional CRT. Likely, advances in lead technology and delivery systems will streamline this process. In a multicenter registry of HBP, Keene and coworkers[43] report it takes approximately 40 cases to achieve improved implant success rates with acceptable capture thresholds, procedure, and fluoroscopy times. Even in the hands of experienced operators 7.5% of patients had to undergo lead revisions, which exceeds the reported incidence in recent conventional CRT trials.[43] Implantation success rates for HBP to correct LBBB ranged from 56% to 90% (mean, 72%) compared with 85% to 100% (mean, 94%) for LBBP (**Table 1**).[16–18,20,25,31,44] Longitudinal LBBB recruitment threshold stability was acceptable for HBP during a follow-up of 3 to 37 (mean, 19 ± 12) months and excellent for LBBP during a follow-up of 3 to 31 (mean, 13 ± 11) months (see **Table 1**).[22,33,34,45,46] Multiple observational studies have shown proximal HBP is associated with higher pacing thresholds, smaller R-wave amplitudes, and atrial and His potential oversensing when compared with more distal HBP or LBBP.[16,18–20,31] Although LBBP seems to deliver a more predictable result, its utility is limited in patients with a tricuspid valve prosthesis, and patients with a fibrosed septum precluding LBBP. On occasion, CSP can lead to AV block or bundle branch block. These injuries tend to be transient. The use of electroanatomic mapping systems during placement of conduction system leads has been reported and can omit the need for fluoroscopy, facilitate lead placement in patients with congenital heart disease, and seems attractive when AV junctional ablation is performed at the time of lead implantation.[37,40,47]

There is still uncertainty about the feasibility and safety of lead extraction from the His bundle region. Vijayaraman and coworkers[48] reported 30 patients who underwent extraction of HBP leads older than 6 (mean, 25 ± 18) months. Removal was successful in 97% of patients, with an 86% successful reimplantation rate in the His-Purkinje conduction system.[48]

Physiologic Limitations

Recruitment of bundle branch block is not guaranteed with proximal HBP because of disease in the more distal conduction system.[20] Recruitment of LBBB seems to be more successful with LBBP. Distal LBBB or coexistent IVCD is not expected to be corrected by LBBP. In a subset of patients, it is challenging to advance a pacing lead deep into the septum, which may be caused by local fibrosis and scarring. We rarely have observed an unexpectedly long stimulus to QRS interval with CSP, which could be explained by latency caused by myocardial fibrosis, scar, or infiltrative disease. Further investigation into the mechanism and frequency of these observations is required.

Lack of Evidence of Efficacy

Initial observational data of CSP seems encouraging with regard to more complete electrical resynchronization, improved LV dimensions and ejection fraction, and improved rates of heart failure rehospitalization when compared with baseline. Although there are two small single-center, prospective, randomized clinical trials comparing HBP with conventional CRT, there are currently no appropriately powered multicenter randomized controlled clinical trials comparing HBP or deep septal LBBP with conventional BiV pacing.

His-Sync (HBP vs Coronary Sinus Pacing for Cardiac Resynchronization Therapy) is a multicenter, randomized controlled trial comparing HBP with conventional BiV pacing. Forty-one patients were enrolled (88% with LBBB). Bidirectional crossover between study arms was a limitation of this study, occurring in more than one-third of study participants. Crossover was mandated per protocol because of insufficient narrowing of QRS narrowing with HBP (<130 milliseconds or 20% reduction) and unfavorable coronary venous anatomy in the BiV pacing arm. By intention-to-treat analysis, there was no significant difference in QRS narrowing between study arms.

Table 1

Investigations into the role of conduction system pacing in cardiac resynchronization therapy

Author, Year	Design	Indication	N	Success	Follow-Up (m)	Echocardiographic Hemodynamic	ECG/QRS-duration	Outcomes
Section A: HBP with LBB Recruitment								
Barba-Pichardo et al,[31] 2013	Single-center, prospective observational	HBP in CRT with dilated LV, LBBB, no coronary venous access	16	56%	31	LVEF 29→36% LVEDD 66→60 mm LVESD 55◇51 mm	QRS-duration 166◇97 ms	Improved NYHA functional class III◇II
Lustgarten et al,[16] 2015	Multicenter, prospective crossover of HBP vs BiV	HBP for CRT −97% LBBB	29	59%	6	LVEF: Baseline 26% HBP 32% BiV 31%	QRS-duration: Baseline 169 ms NSHBP 160 ms SHBP 131 ms BiV 165 ms	Improved NYHA functional class Improved 6-min-walk test Improved quality of life
Ajijola et al,[17] 2017	Single-center, prospective observational	HBP for CRT	21	76%	12	LVEF 27→41% LVEDD 54◇45 mm	QRS-duration 180◇129 ms	NYHA functional class III◇II
Sharma et al,[18] 2018	Multicenter, prospective observational	HBP for CRT after BiV failure or primary HBP 45% BBB 39% paced 16% AVB	106	90%	14	LVEF 30◇44% LVEF 25→40% (BL LVEF ≤35%) LVEDD 55→54 mm	QRS-duration 157◇118 ms	NYHA functional class 2.8→1.8 Demonstrates HBP feasibility, safety as alternative to CRT
Upadhyay et al,[20] 2019	Multicenter, prospective, randomized, crossover trial	HBP for CRT in LBBB	41	76%	12	LVEF 26→32%	QRS-duration 172◇144 ms	Demonstrated feasibility and safety of HBP as an alternative to CRT
Huang et al,[19] 2019	Single-center, prospective observational	HBP in LBBB, NYHA II-IV with CRT or pacing indication	74	76%	37	LVEF 31→57% LVESV 140◇65 mL	QRS-duration: Baseline 171 ms HBP 113 ms SHBP 173→105 ms NSHBP161◇140 ms	NYHA functional class 2.8→1.0 HBP corrected LBBB in most patients with HF and typical LBBB

(continued on next page)

Table 1
(continued)

Author, Year	Design	Indication	N	Success	Follow-Up (m)	Echocardiographic Hemodynamic	ECG/QRS-duration	Outcomes
Arnold et al,[25] 2018	Acute crossover study	Acute hemodynamic study of HBP in CRT patients with LBBB	18	n/a	n/a	Increased SBP with HBP compared with BiV	QRS-duration: Baseline 178 ms BiV 158 ms HBP 139 ms HBP resulted in shorter LV activation time compared with BiV	HBP delivers superior hemodynamic response compared with BiV pacing
Vinther et al,[49] 2021	Single-center, prospective, randomized controlled clinical trial	HBP for CRT in patients with LBBB	50	76%	6	BiV CRT: LVEF 30→43% HBP CRT: LVEF 30→46%	QRS duration BiV CRT 167→134 ms HBP CRT 165→131 ms	Δ NYHA functional class ≥1: BiV CRT, 40% HBP CRT, 48% HBP provided similar clinical and physical improvement compared with BiV pacing

Section B: HBP in RBBB

Author, Year	Design	Indication	N	Success	Follow-Up (m)	Echocardiographic Hemodynamic	ECG/QRS-duration	Outcomes
Sharma et al,[37] 2018	Retrospective, observational multicenter study	HBP in RBBB QRSd ≥120 ms NYHA class II to IV, LVEF ≤50%	39	95%	15	LVEF 31→39% LVEF 26→34% (BL LVEF≤35%) 19% superresponders	QRS-duration 158→127 ms	NYHA functional class 2.8→2.0 HBP seems to be a reasonable therapy for patients with RBBB and depressed LVEF

Section C: Deep Septal LBBP

Author, Year	Design	Indication	N	Success	Follow-Up (m)	Echocardiographic Hemodynamic	ECG/QRS-duration	Outcomes
Vijayaraman et al,[22] 2019	Single-center, prospective observational	LBBP for bradycardia or CRT (11%) if CS lead or HBP failed LBBB 24% RBBB 25% IVCD 8% AV block 61%	100	93%	3	n/a	QRS-duration 133→136 ms QRS-duration 162→137 ms for LBBB subgroup	LBBP feasible Low thresholds observed

Study	Design	Population/Indication	N	Success	Follow-up	Echo outcomes	QRS-duration	Conclusions
Wang et al,[33] 2019	Retrospective, single-center case control	LBBP after AV junctional ablation in persistent AF and HF	83	95%	31	LVEF 35→49% LVESV 161◇96 mL	QRS-duration 95 ms (baseline)	NYHA functional class 2.6→1.7 Lower rate of inappropriate ICD shocks, death, HF hospitalizations
Huang et al,[45] 2020	Prospective multicenter observational	Nonischemic cardiomyopathy LBBB LVEF <50%	63	97%	12	LVEF 33→55% LVESV 123→67 mL	QRS-duration Baseline 169 ms LBBP 118 ms	NYHA functional class 2.8→1.4 LBBP may be a reasonable therapy for patients with LBBB and nonischemic cardiomyopathy
Wu et al,[46] 2020	Prospective, observations, case-control	CRT with BVP, HBP or LBBP in LVEF <40%, LBBB	137	100%	12	ΔLVEF 24%	QRS-duration Baseline 166 ms LBBP 111 ms	Echo outcomes were similar to HBP and significantly greater than BVP
Vijayaraman et al,[34] 2020	Retrospective multicenter observational	CRT/pacing LVEF <50%	325	85%	6	LVEF 33→44% LVEDD 56→54 mm LVESV 114→83 mL LVEF 27→40% (BL LVEF ≤35%) Response 73% Superresponse 31%	QRS-duration 152→137 ms LBBB subgroup 162→133 ms	NYHA functional class 2.7→1.8 LBBB (odds ratio, 3.96; $P < .01$) LVEDD (odds ratio, 0.62; $P < .01$) were independent predictors of response LBBP may be a reasonable CRT alternative
Section D: Septal Pacing Without Targeted Conduction System Capture								
Rademakers et al,[42] 2016	Canine HF model with LBBB	Nonresponders to conventional CRT, inaccessible coronary venous system, phrenic nerve capture, or LV lead dislodgement	12	n/a	n/a	LV septal pacing improved LVdP/dtmax in ischemic and nonischemic LBBB LV septal pacing improved LVEF similar to BiV	QRS-duration LBBB 108→102 ms LBBB + MI 106→84 ms	LV septal pacing resulted in electrical and hemodynamic benefits similar to BiV LV septal pacing may be a reasonable CRT alternative

(continued on next page)

Table 1
(continued)

Author, Year	Design	Indication	N	Success	Follow-Up (m)	Echocardiographic Hemodynamic	ECG/QRS-duration	Outcomes
Salden et al,[26] 2020	Multicenter retrospective	CRT indication LBBB 89% IVCD 11%	27	100%	36	LV septal, LV septal + RV, BiV, and HBP all increased LVdP/dtmax (although LV septal + RV was inferior)	QRS-duration Baseline 151 ms LV septal 135 ms LV septal + RV 134 ms BiV 136 ms HBP 110 ms	LV septal pacing resulted in electric resynchronization and hemodynamic improvement similar to BiV pacing LV septal pacing may be a reasonable CRT alternative

Section E: Deep Septal LBBP in RBBB

Author, Year	Design	Indication	N	Success	Follow-Up (m)	Echocardiographic Hemodynamic	ECG/QRS-duration	Outcomes
Vijayaraman et al,[38] 2021	Retrospective multicenter observational	CRT indication, LVEF <50%, RBBB	121	88%		LVEF 35→43% (P < .01)	156→150 ms (P = .05)	LBBP is feasible, safe, and provides alternative option for CRT in patients with RBBB

Section F: HOT-CRT

Author, Year	Design	Indication	N	Success	Follow-Up (m)	Echocardiographic Hemodynamic	ECG/QRS-duration	Outcomes
Vijayaraman et al,[40] 2019	Retrospective multicenter observational	HOT-CRT in LBBB and IVCD with QRS ≥140 ms or AV block with LBBB type escape	27	93%	12	LVEF 24→38% LVEDD 65→59 mm LVEDV 225→200 mL LVESV 171→138 mL Superresponse 28%	QRS-duration Baseline 183 ms BiV 162 ms HBP 151 ms HOT-CRT 120 ms	NYHA functional class 3.3→2.0 Reduced HF hospitalizations Reduced loop diuretic and aldosterone antagonist doses
Zweerink et al,[52] 2021	Prospective single-center observational	CRT	19	n/a		Baseline LVEF 31%	QRS-duration Baseline 142 ms HBP 142 ms BiV 154 ms HOT-CRT 126 ms	HOT-CRT acutely improves ventricular electrical synchrony compared with BiV and HBP HOT-CRT reduced LV activation time by 21% compared with HBP

Study	Design	Indication					QRS-duration	Outcome
Deshmukh et al,[53] 2020	Retrospective single center	CRT indication in whom His pacing did not result in resynchronization	21	100%	32	LVEF 27→41%	Baseline 170 ms, HBP 157 ms, BiV 141 ms, HOT-CRT 110 ms	NYHA functional class 3→2. HOT-CRT resulted in superior acute electrical synchrony in this population
Section G: LOT-CRT								
Vijayaraman et al,[38] 2021	Prospective multicenter observational	CRT indication or nonresponders to BiV CRT	112	81%	≥3	LVEF 29→37% (P < .0001), LVEDD 62→59 mm, Superresponse 24%	Baseline 181 ms, LOT-CRT 144 ms, LBBP 162 ms, BiV 170 ms	LOT-CRT provides significantly greater resynchronization than LBBP or BiV CRT. NYHA functional class 2.9→1.9

Abbreviations: AF, atrial fibrillation; BBB, bundle branch block; BL, baseline; CS, coronary sinus; ECG, electrocardiogram; HF, heart failure; ICD, implantable cardioverter-defibrillator; LBBP, left bundle branch pacing; LVEDD, left ventricular end-diastolic diameter; LVESD, left ventricular end-systolic diameter; MI, myocardial infarction; n/a, not applicable; NSHBP, nonselective HBP; SBP, systolic blood pressure; SHBP, selective HBP.

However, by per-protocol analysis, QRS narrowing was more pronounced with HBP compared with conventional BiV pacing (124 ± 19 milliseconds vs 162 ± 24 milliseconds; $P < .001$).[16]

His-Alternative is a single-center, prospective randomized trial of HBP versus BiV pacing in 50 patients with cardiomyopathy (nonischemic 78%), congestive heart failure, and LBBB (QRS >130 milliseconds for women and >140 milliseconds for men; ejection fraction ≤35%, congestive heart failure NYHA functional class II to IV).[49] This study differed from His-Sync because only patient's with an LBBB by Strauss' criteria were included.[50] Procedural success for HBP with left bundle capture was 72%. Similar to His-Sync, a high rate of crossover from HBP to the BiV pacing occurred because of lack of left bundle capture or high left bundle recruitment threshold (7/25 [28%] with HBP vs 1/25 [4%] with BiV pacing). Intention-to-treat analysis showed no significant difference in QRS duration or echocardiographic response. Per-protocol analysis showed no significant difference in QRS duration, but LVEF was higher in the HBP group (48 ± 8% vs 42 ± 8%; $P < .05$). Pacing thresholds were higher in the HBP group.

Using hard end points, such as mortality, or soft end points, such as LV dimensions and ejection fraction, we have not proven noninferiority nor superiority for CSP compared with conventional CRT. In contrary, there is level I evidence from multiple randomized controlled trials to support BiV pacing in patients with LVEF less than or equal to 35% and LBBB (level IIa evidence for non-LBBB with a QRS ≥150 milliseconds).[2–5,51]

CSP can currently be viewed as a viable bailout strategy in patients with lack of access to the coronary venous system or intractable diaphragmatic pacing. It also can be considered as an alternative option in CRT nonresponders.[18] CSP as a primary resynchronization strategy is currently experimental (class IIb, level of evidence B).

SUMMARY

Although conventional CRT has evolved into a highly effective therapy for patients with heart failure with LBBB, it does not produce a satisfactory clinical response in a substantial subset of patients. Acute hemodynamic and observational studies have shown more effective electrical and mechanical resynchronization with His-Purkinje CSP when compared with conventional BiV pacing. Furthermore, CSP re-establishes physiologic ventricular activation and repolarization and, thus, may be less arrhythmogenic and may improve diastolic function more efficiently. Therefore, CSP is appealing and should be embraced with enthusiasm. However, CSP as the go-to

resynchronization strategy is highly provocative in the absence of controlled randomized clinical trial data.

Preliminary observational studies justify rigorous controlled randomized clinical trials investigating CSP as a primary resynchronization therapy in patients with CRT indications, such as bundle branch block, and AV block with need for long-term ventricular pacing.

Patients with RBBB or primary IVCD deserve separate more individualized investigation. In patients with RBBB, HBP can be attempted first and if complete correction of RBBB is achieved with a capture/correction threshold of less than 1.5 V, it should be accepted. In the absence of right bundle recruitment, nonselective HBP or LBBP with fusion correction of RBBB pattern (either by local septal capture or RV apical pacing) may be considered.

With increasing evidence from controlled clinical trials and technical improvements in lead and delivery systems, His-Purkinje CSP is likely to become a viable resynchronization strategy in the toolbox of CRT.

CLINICS CARE POINTS

- His-Purkinje conduction system pacing may yield more effective electrical and mechanical resynchronization when compared to conventional biventricular pacing.

- Conduction system pacing re-establishes physiologic ventricular depolarization and repolarization.

- Conduction system pacing can currently be viewed as a viable bailout strategy in patients with lack of access to the coronary venous system or intractable diaphragmatic pacing. It can also be considered in CRT nonresponders.

- Conduction system pacing as the primary, go-to resynchronization strategy cannot be accepted without controlled randomized clinical trial data.

REFERENCES

1. Mower M. Method and apparatus for treating hemodynamic dysfunction by simultaneous pacing of both ventricles. US patent 1990. #4,928,688.
2. Auricchio A, Stellbrink C, Sack S, et al. Long-term clinical effect of hemodynamically optimized cardiac resynchronization therapy in patients with heart

failure and ventricular conduction delay. J Am Coll Cardiol 2002;39(12):2026–33.

3. Linde C, Gold MR, Abraham WT, et al. Long-term impact of cardiac resynchronization therapy in mild heart failure: 5-year results from the REsynchronization reVErses Remodeling in Systolic left vEntricular dysfunction (REVERSE) study. Eur Heart J 2013; 34(33):2592–9.

4. Moss AJ, Hall WJ, Cannom DS, et al. Cardiac-resynchronization therapy for the prevention of heart-failure events. N Engl J Med 2009;361(14):1329–38.

5. Tang AS, Wells GA, Talajic M, et al. Cardiac-resynchronization therapy for mild-to-moderate heart failure. N Engl J Med 2010;363(25):2385–95.

6. El-Sherif N, Amay YLF, Schonfield C, et al. Normalization of bundle branch block patterns by distal His bundle pacing. Clinical and experimental evidence of longitudinal dissociation in the pathologic His bundle. Circulation 1978;57(3):473–83.

7. Deshmukh P, Casavant DA, Romanyshyn M, et al. Permanent, direct His-bundle pacing: a novel approach to cardiac pacing in patients with normal His-Purkinje activation. Circulation 2000;101(8):869–77.

8. Barba-Pichardo R, Manovel Sánchez A, Fernández-Gómez JM, et al. Ventricular resynchronization therapy by direct His-bundle pacing using an internal cardioverter defibrillator. Europace 2013;15(1):83–8.

9. Herweg B, Welter-Frost A, Vijayaraman P. The evolution of cardiac resynchronization therapy and an introduction to conduction system pacing: a conceptual review. Europace 2021;23(4):496–510.

10. Herweg B, Ali R, Ilercil A, et al. Site-specific differences in latency intervals during biventricular pacing: impact on paced QRS morphology and echo-optimized V-V interval. Pacing Clin Electrophysiol 2010;33(11):1382–91.

11. Herweg B, Ilercil A, Madramootoo C, et al. Latency during left ventricular pacing from the lateral cardiac veins: a cause of ineffectual biventricular pacing. Pacing Clin Electrophysiol 2006;29(6):574–81.

12. van Deursen C, van Geldorp IE, Rademakers LM, et al. Left ventricular endocardial pacing improves resynchronization therapy in canine left bundle-branch hearts. Circ Arrhythm Electrophysiol 2009; 2(5):580–7.

13. Derval N, Steendijk P, Gula LJ, et al. Optimizing hemodynamics in heart failure patients by systematic screening of left ventricular pacing sites: the lateral left ventricular wall and the coronary sinus are rarely the best sites. J Am Coll Cardiol 2010;55(6):566–75.

14. Mills RW, Cornelussen RN, Mulligan LJ, et al. Left ventricular septal and left ventricular apical pacing chronically maintain cardiac contractile coordination, pump function and efficiency. Circ Arrhythm Electrophysiol 2009;2(5):571–9.

15. Mafi-Rad M, Luermans JG, Blaauw Y, et al. Feasibility and acute hemodynamic effect of left ventricular septal pacing by transvenous approach through the interventricular septum. Circ Arrhythm Electrophysiol 2016;9(3):e003344.

16. Lustgarten DL, Crespo EM, Arkhipova-Jenkins I, et al. His-bundle pacing versus biventricular pacing in cardiac resynchronization therapy patients: a crossover design comparison. Heart Rhythm 2015; 12(7):1548–57.

17. Ajijola OA, Upadhyay GA, Macias C, et al. Permanent His-bundle pacing for cardiac resynchronization therapy: initial feasibility study in lieu of left ventricular lead. Heart Rhythm 2017;14(9):1353–61.

18. Sharma PS, Dandamudi G, Herweg B, et al. Permanent His-bundle pacing as an alternative to biventricular pacing for cardiac resynchronization therapy: a multicenter experience. Heart Rhythm 2018;15(3):413–20.

19. Huang W, Su L, Wu S, et al. Long-term outcomes of His bundle pacing in patients with heart failure with left bundle branch block. Heart 2019;105(2):137–43.

20. Upadhyay GA, Vijayaraman P, Nayak HM, et al. His corrective pacing or biventricular pacing for cardiac resynchronization in heart failure. J Am Coll Cardiol 2019;74(1):157–9.

21. Huang W, Su L, Wu S, et al. A novel pacing strategy with low and stable output: pacing the left bundle branch immediately beyond the conduction block. Can J Cardiol 2017;33(12):1736. e1731-1736.e1733.

22. Vijayaraman P, Subzposh FA, Naperkowski A, et al. Prospective evaluation of feasibility and electrophysiologic and echocardiographic characteristics of left bundle branch area pacing. Heart Rhythm 2019;16(12):1774–82.

23. Zhang S, Zhou X, Gold MR. Left bundle branch pacing: JACC review Topic of the Week. J Am Coll Cardiol 2019;74(24):3039–49.

24. Hou X, Qian Z, Wang Y, et al. Feasibility and cardiac synchrony of permanent left bundle branch pacing through the interventricular septum. Europace 2019;21(11):1694–702.

25. Arnold AD, Shun-Shin MJ, Keene D, et al. His resynchronization versus biventricular pacing in patients with heart failure and left bundle branch block. J Am Coll Cardiol 2018;72(24):3112–22.

26. Salden F, Luermans J, Westra SW, et al. Short-term hemodynamic and electrophysiological effects of cardiac resynchronization by left ventricular septal pacing. J Am Coll Cardiol 2020;75(4):347–59.

27. Sofi A, Vijayaraman P, Barold SS, et al. Utilization of permanent His-bundle pacing for management of proarrhythmia related to biventricular pacing. Pacing Clin Electrophysiol 2017;40(4):451–4.

28. Logue JVP, Pavri B. Could cardiac resynchronization via His bundle pacing reduce arrhythmic risk? Circulation 2018;136:A16112.

29. Jais P, Douard H, Shah DC, et al. Endocardial biventricular pacing. Pacing Clin Electrophysiol 1998; 21(11 Pt 1):2128–31.

30. Bordachar P, Derval N, Ploux S, et al. Left ventricular endocardial stimulation for severe heart failure. J Am Coll Cardiol 2010;56(10):747–53.

31. Barba-Pichardo R, Manovel Sanchez A, Fernandez-Gomez JM, et al. Ventricular resynchronization therapy by direct His-bundle pacing using an internal cardioverter defibrillator. Europace 2013;15(1):83–8.

32. Jastrzębski M, Kiełbasa G, Moskal P, et al. Fixation beats: a novel marker for reaching the left bundle branch area during deep septal lead implantation. Heart Rhythm 2021;18(4):562–9.

33. Wang S, Wu S, Xu L, et al. Feasibility and efficacy of His bundle pacing or left bundle pacing combined with atrioventricular node ablation in patients with persistent atrial fibrillation and implantable cardioverter-defibrillator therapy. J Am Heart Assoc 2019;8(24):e014253.

34. Vijayaraman PSS, Cano O, Sharma PS, et al. Left bundle branch pacing for cardiac resynchronization therapy: results from international LBBP collaborative study group. JACC Clin Electrophysiol 2021; 7(2):135–47.

35. Upadhyay GA, Cherian T, Shatz DY, et al. Intracardiac delineation of septal conduction in left bundle-branch block patterns. Circulation 2019; 139(16):1876–88.

36. Ponnusamy SS, Pugazhendhi V. Axis deviation in non-ischemic cardiomyopathy with left bundle branch block: insights from left bundle branch pacing. J Cardiovasc Electrophysiol 2021. https://doi.org/10.1111/jce.15334.

37. Sharma PS, Naperkowski A, Bauch TD, et al. Permanent His bundle pacing for cardiac resynchronization therapy in patients with heart failure and right bundle branch block. Circ Arrhythm Electrophysiol 2018;11(9):e006613.

38. Vijayaraman PCO, Ponnusami SS, Molina-Lerma M, et al. Left bundle branch area pacing for cardiac resynchronization therapy in right bundle branch block: results from international LBBAP collaborative study group. Heart Rhythm 2021 (in press).

39. Cleland JG, Abraham WT, Linde C, et al. An individual patient meta-analysis of five randomized trials assessing the effects of cardiac resynchronization therapy on morbidity and mortality in patients with symptomatic heart failure. Eur Heart J 2013;34(46):3547–56.

40. Vijayaraman P, Herweg B, Ellenbogen KA, et al. His-optimized cardiac resynchronization therapy to maximize electrical resynchronization: a feasibility study. Circ Arrhythm Electrophysiol 2019;12(2):e006934.

41. Jastrzębski M, Moskal P, Huybrechts W, et al. Left bundle branch-optimized cardiac resynchronization therapy (LOT-CRT): results from an international

42. Rademakers LM, van Hunnik A, Kuiper M, et al. A possible role for pacing the left ventricular septum in cardiac resynchronization therapy. JACC Clin Electrophysiol 2016;2(4):413–22.

43. Keene D, Arnold AD, Jastrzębski M, et al. His bundle pacing, learning curve, procedure characteristics, safety, and feasibility: insights from a large international observational study. J Cardiovasc Electrophysiol 2019;30(10):1984–93.

44. Huang W, Chen X, Su L, et al. A beginner's guide to permanent left bundle branch pacing. Heart Rhythm 2019;16(12):1791–6.

45. Huang W, Wu S, Vijayaraman P, et al. Cardiac resynchronization therapy in patients with nonischemic cardiomyopathy using left bundle branch pacing. JACC Clin Electrophysiol 2020;6(7):849–58.

46. Wu S, Su L, Vijayaraman P, et al. Left bundle branch pacing for cardiac resynchronization therapy: nonrandomized on treatment comparison with His bundle pacing and biventricular pacing. Can J Cardiol 2021;37(2):319–28.

47. Orlov MV, Koulouridis I, Monin AJ, et al. Direct visualization of the His bundle pacing lead placement by 3-dimensional electroanatomic mapping: technique, anatomy, and practical considerations. Circ Arrhythm Electrophysiol 2019;12(2):e006801.

48. Vijayaraman P, Subzposh FA, Naperkowski A. Extraction of the permanent His bundle pacing lead: safety outcomes and feasibility of reimplantation. Heart Rhythm 2019;16(8):1196–203.

49. Vinther M, Risum N, Svendsen JH, et al. A randomized trial of His pacing versus biventricular pacing in symptomatic HF patients with left bundle branch block (His-Alternative). JACC Clin Electrophysiol 2021;7(11):1422–32.

50. Strauss DG, Selvester RH, Wagner GS. Defining left bundle branch block in the era of cardiac resynchronization therapy. Am J Cardiol 2011;107(6):927–34.

51. Yancy CW, Jessup M, Bozkurt B, et al. 2013 ACCF/AHA guideline for the management of heart failure: a report of the American College of Cardiology Foundation/American Heart Association Task Force on Practice Guidelines. J Am Coll Cardiol 2013; 62(16):e147–239.

52. Zweerink A, Zubarev S, Bakelants E, et al. His-optimized cardiac resynchronization therapy with ventricular fusion pacing for electrical resynchronization in heart failure. JACC Clin Electrophysiol 2021;7(7):881–92.

53. Deshmukh A, Sattur S, Bechtol T, et al. Sequential His bundle and left ventricular pacing for cardiac resynchronization. J Cardiovasc Electrophysiol 2020; 31(9):2448–54.

LBBAP collaborative study group. Heart Rhythm 2022;19(1):13–21.

His-Optimized and Left Bundle Branch-Optimized Cardiac Resynchronization Therapy: In Control of Fusion Pacing

Alwin Zweerink, MD, PhD[a,b], Haran Burri, MD[a,*]

KEYWORDS

- Cardiac resynchronization therapy (CRT) • Biventricular pacing (BiV) • His bundle pacing (HBP)
- His-optimized CRT (HOT-CRT)
- Left bundle branch optimized cardiac resynchronization therapy (LOT-CRT)
- Electrocardiographic imaging (ECGI) • Ventricular activation times

KEY POINTS

- Fusion pacing exploits intrinsic atrioventricular (AV) conduction to optimize cardiac resynchronization therapy (CRT), but requires automatic algorithms to provide continuous adaptation of the AV intervals, and is not applicable in case of AV block.
- His-optimized cardiac resynchronization therapy (HOT-CRT) and left-bundle branch optimized cardiac resynchronization therapy (LOT-CRT) provide constant timing between His-Purkinje activation (with partial correction or uncorrected bundle branch block (BBB)) and left ventricular or biventricular pacing (or right ventricular (RV) pacing in the setting of right bundle branch block (RBBB)), and are also applicable in case of AV block.
- HOT-CRT and LOT-CRT provide greater electrical resynchronization than biventricular pacing, but comparative studies with clinical outcomes are not as yet available.
- These emerging strategies deserve further study.

INTRODUCTION

Traditional cardiac resynchronization therapy (CRT) with biventricular pacing (BiV) results in the fusion of 2 non-physiological wavefronts, leaving a substantial degree of residual dyssynchrony.[1,2] Consequently, benefit from CRT is confined to patients with a wide QRS complex, whereas BiV in patients with a narrow QRS results in electrical desynchronization and increased risk of adverse events.[3] At present, merely two-third of patients implanted with CRT respond favorably to the therapy, whereas others are deemed nonresponders.[4] Fusion pacing is a potential strategy to improve electrical resynchronization and benefit from CRT by combining ventricular pacing (BiV, left ventricular [LV] or right ventricular [RV] -only) with intrinsic His-Purkinje activation. Intrinsic conduction and BiV pacing results in triple wavefront fusion creating a more homogenously activation pattern, whereas intrinsic conduction and LV-only pacing exploits spontaneous activation over the right bundle and avoids right ventricular (RV) pacing-induced dyssynchrony (**Fig. 1**). Of note, intrinsic conduction can also be fused with RV-only pacing, which offers a resynchronization strategy in patients with right bundle branch block (RBBB).

[a] Department of Cardiology, University Hospital of Geneva, Geneva, Switzerland; [b] Department of Cardiology and Amsterdam Cardiovascular Sciences (ACS), Amsterdam University Medical Centers (AUMC), Location VU Medical Center, Amsterdam, The Netherlands
* Corresponding author.
E-mail address: haran.burri@hcuge.ch

Card Electrophysiol Clin 14 (2022) 311–321
https://doi.org/10.1016/j.ccep.2021.12.006

Biventricular Pacing

HOT/LOT-CRT with BiV

HOT/LOT-CRT with LV

HOT/LOT-CRT with RV
(in setting of RBBB)

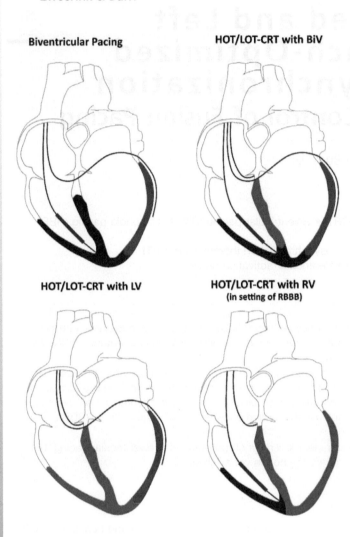

Fig. 1. Activation patterns with fusion pacing versus traditional CRT. Schematic representation of a patient in atrial fibrillation (no atrial lead) and complete atrioventricular block (no fusion with intrinsic conduction). *Top left panel:* BiV results in the fusion of two non-physiological wavefronts, leaving a substantial degree of residual dyssynchrony. *Top right panel:* HBPor LBBP without complete correction of left bundle branch activation. Triple wavefront fusion pacing with HOT/LOT-CRT homogenizes LV activation by combining His-Purkinje activation with BiV pacing. *Bottom left panel:* HOT-CRT with fusion between HBP and activation over the right bundle branch and LV pacing. With LBBP in LOT-CRT, RV activation occurs via transseptal myocardial propagation.[39] *Bottom right:* In the setting of right bundle branch block, LV activation occurs via conduction tissue, whereas correction of RV activation occurs by synchronized RV pacing (bifocal RV activation in the setting of LOT-CRT). BiV, biventricular; HOT-CRT, His-optimized cardiac resynchronization therapy; LOT-CRT, left bundle branch optimized resynchronization therapy; LV, left ventricle. RV, right ventricle.

FUSION-OPTIMIZED INTERVALS WITH STANDARD CARDIAC RESYNCHRONIZATION THERAPY

Synchronization of intrinsic His-Purkinje conduction with ventricular stimulation is key to optimize fusion pacing. Arbelo and colleagues[5] described a method of QRS-based CRT optimization of the atrioventricular (AV) and interventricular (VV) delays called fusion-optimized intervals (FOI). The first step with FOI is to find the longest AV interval with some ventricular capture. Subsequently, the AV interval is shortened by 20 ms decrements until there is full ventricular capture. Within this range, the interval with the narrowest QRS is chosen and subsequently, the VV offset is optimized (−30 ms; 0 ms; 30 ms). FOI resulted in improved acute hemodynamic performance. Subsequently, a randomized clinical trial by Trucco and colleagues[6] showed that device optimization based on FOI achieved greater LV remodeling compared with nominal settings. Lastly, Tamborero and

colleagues[7] showed in their study that ECG-based FOI was superior to echocardiographic optimization for achieving LV functional recovery. However, FOI at a given time point may not be sufficient to maintain constant fusion, as settings need to be constantly adjusted to accommodate for acute changes in AV conduction depending on the patient's activity, and with more gradual changes due to medication and evolution of native conduction properties. To overcome this problem, automatic device-based algorithms have been developed.

DYNAMIC FUSION ALGORITHMS FOR STANDARD CARDIAC RESYNCHRONIZATION THERAPY

Automatic device-based algorithms adjust the AV delay according to the intrinsic AV conduction times to obtain fusion pacing. Several manufactures have incorporated such algorithms in their devices, including Medtronic (AdaptivCRT);

Abbott (SyncAV/SyncAV plus); Boston Scientific (SmartDelay); and Biotronik (Autoadapt). As a general principle, the device regularly measures the intrinsic AV interval (from the right atrial [RA] to the RV lead) or P-wave duration (based on the unipolar atrial signal) and interventricular timing (RV to LV lead delay or far-field QRS width) and provides LV-only or BiV stimulation with an AV delay that is expected to result in fusion (usually around −50 ms or 70% of the intrinsic AV interval).[8,9] Some algorithms (AdaptivCRT, SyncAV/SyncAV plus and Autoadapt) repeatedly adjust the AV delay to pursue constant fusion pacing.

The Adaptive-CRT trial randomized 522 patients in a 2:1 ratio to CRT optimization with the AdaptivCRT algorithm versus echocardiography.[10] The algorithm provides optimized LV-only pacing in case of normal AV conduction, or BiV pacing otherwise, and resulted in a 44% absolute reduction in the percentage of RV pacing. The study met all their primary noninferiority endpoints with respect to clinical, structural, and functional parameters after 6 months. Moreover, a follow-up study of the Adaptive-CRT trial demonstrated better clinical outcomes with the algorithm compared with BiV pacing optimized by echocardiography in patients with normal AV conduction.[11]

The SyncAV algorithm also improves electrical synchrony (ie, QRS duration) beyond conventional CRT.[12,13]

Although results with automatic fusion algorithms are generally encouraging, several shortcomings have to be considered. First of all, these algorithms cannot be used in patients with complete AV block, atrial fibrillation, or may be limited by very prolonged AV intervals (AdaptivCRT). Moreover, abrupt changes in AV conduction may not be corrected in time as the algorithms' response has some delay which may result in temporary loss of capture (during accelerated AV conduction) or loss of fusion (slowing of AV conduction). Vacarescu and colleagues[14] prospectively included 55 patients with CRT who received LV-only fusion pacing and underwent exercise testing. They demonstrated that 20 (36%) patients had inadequate pacing or loss of LV capture during exercise testing. These drawbacks underline the need for an alternative that can cope with physiologic changes in AV conduction to provide constant fusion therapy.

CONSTANT FUSION WITH HIS-OPTIMIZED CARDIAC RESYNCHRONIZATION

His Bundle Pacing (HBP) has the potential to overcome bundle branch block (BBB) when the conduction disorder is located proximally within the bundle of His.[15] However, HBP may not, or only partially, normalize conduction abnormalities in case of distal BBB, or coexistence of intraventricular conduction delay (IVCD). Overall, approximately 25% of patients lack QRS narrowing with HBP.[15–17] Also, BBB correction may require a pacing output that is too high for clinical use. In these cases, HBP can be combined with stimulation from an additional ventricular lead (LV, RV, or both) to deliver His-optimized CRT (HOT-CRT). HOT-CRT allows for constant fusion between His-Purkinje and ventricular activation, and provides a new treatment option in patients with atrial fibrillation and patients with AV block.

Padeletti and colleagues[18] were the first to combine His pacing with LV pacing and performed pressure-volume loops in 11 patients with HF and LBBB, comparing HBP + LV pacing with BiV over a wide range of AV-intervals. Strictly speaking, this was not HOT-CRT, as HBP and LV pacing were simultaneous, without an optimization protocol. Nevertheless, combined pacing improved stroke work regardless of the AV delay, whereas BiV required an optimal timing of the AV delay to allow intrinsic conduction for fusion pacing. An advantage of HOT-CRT is that AV synchrony (ie, ventricular filling) can to a certain extent be optimized independently from the HBP-VP interval (while maintaining constant fusion). Although the study by Padeletti and colleagues[18] lacks clinical follow-up, acute changes in stroke work may translate into long-term benefit.[19] Boczar and colleagues[20] described a cohort of 12 out of 14 patients with HF with permanent AF who lacked BBB correction with HBP and received additional pacing from the LV lead or BiV pacing. Although this strategy was found feasible and resulted in significant narrowing of QRS width and improvement in echocardiographic LV function, no comparison was made with BiV pacing. Three other small-scale studies investigated electrical resynchronization with HOT-CRT and compared results with BiV pacing using standard 12-lead ECG recordings (**Table 1**). Vijayaraman and colleagues[21] retrospectively included 25 patients with HF and partial or uncorrected LBBB/IVCD or RVP and compared ECG parameters between HOT-CRT (HBP + LV) and BiV. The HBP-VP pacing interval was programmed equally to the HV or stimulus to ventricular interval (without any further optimization protocol). In this study, HOT-CRT resulted in a 26% shorter QRSd compared to BiV pacing. At follow-up, HOT-CRT resulted in high clinical (84%) and echocardiographic (92%) response rates, but these were not compared with BiV pacing. Coluccia and colleagues[22] performed an acute intrapatient comparison between

Table 1
Studies comparing His-optimized CRT (HOT-CRT) with biventricular pacing

Author	Sample Size	Selection Criteria	Study Design	Endpoints	Result HOT-CRT vs BiV
Padeletti [18]	n = 11	CRT indication and: • LBBB (all)	Prospective study with temporary HBP + LV vs BiV	Stroke Work derived from pressure-volume loops	HOT-CRT improved Stroke Work regardless of AV delay whereas BiV depends on optimal AV timing
Vijayaraman et al, [21] 2019	n = 25	CRT indication and: • LBBB (16) • IVCD (5) • RVP (4)	Retrospective study with permanent HBP + LV vs BiV	QRSd on 12-lead ECG	120 ± 16 ms (HOT-CRT) vs 162 ± 17 ms (BiV) (P < .05)
Coluccia et al, [22] 2020	n = 20	CRT indication and: • LBBB (9) • IVCD (3) • RVP (4) • Narrow QRS (3)	Prospective study with permanent HBP + LV/RV vs BiV	QRSd on 12-lead ECG	128 ± 14 ms (HOT-CRT) vs 153 ± 18 ms (BiV) (P < .01)
Deshmukh et al, [23] 2022	n = 21	CRT indication and: • LBBB (12) • IVCD (9)	Retrospective study with permanent HBP + LV vs BiV	QRSd on 12-lead ECG	110 ± 14 ms (HOT-CRT) vs 141 ± 15 ms. (BiV) (P < .0005)
				QRS area on vectorcardiography	39 ± 23 μVs (HOT-CRT) vs 68 ± 24 μVs (BiV) (P < .0005)
Zweerink et al, [27] 2021	n = 19	CRT indication and: • LBBB (8) • IVCD (2) • RBBB (6) • incomplete BBB (3)	Prospective study with permanent HBP + LV/RV vs BiV (including MPP)	QRSd on 12-lead ECG	126 ± 23 ms (HOT-CRT) 154 ± 18 ms (BiV) (P < .05)
				LVAT on ECGi	66 ± 17 ms (HOT-CRT) 90 ± 20 ms (BiV) (<0.01)
				RVAT on ECGi	68 ± 23 ms (HOT-CRT) 89 ± 18 ms (BiV) (<0.001)

Abbreviations: BBB, bundle branch block; BiV, biventricular pacing; CRT, cardiac resynchronization therapy; ECGi, ECG imaging; HBP, his bundle pacing; HOT-CRT, His-optimized CRT; IVCD, intraventricular conduction delay; LBBB, left bundle branch block; LV, left ventricular pacing; LVAT, left ventricular activation time; LV/RV left/right ventricular pacing; MPP, multi-point pacing; QRSd, QRS duration; RBBB, right bundle branch block; RVAT, right ventricular activation time; RVP, right ventricular pacing.

HOT-CRT (HBP + LV and HBP + BiV) and BiV pacing in 20 patients with various types of conduction disease. The HBP-VP interval was programmed to the interval between HBP stimulus and QRS onset (without further optimization). This study showed an 18% reduction in QRSd with HOT-CRT compared to BiV pacing, along with an improvement in echocardiographic dyssynchrony measurements. The optimal HOT-CRT configuration was HBP + LV in two-third of cases (HBP + BiV did not provide any additional benefit in most cases). Lastly, Deshmukh and colleagues[23] evaluated QRS reduction by HOT-CRT (HBP + LV) and BiV pacing among 21 patients with underlying BBB (LBBB or IVCD) which was incompletely corrected by HBP. In this study, both the interventricular (VV) interval with BiV pacing as well as the HBP-VP pacing interval with

HOT-CRT were optimized in order to minimize QRS duration. The narrowest paced QRS with sequential His bundle and LV pacing occurred at an HBP-VP offset of 42 ± 27 ms and reduced QRS duration to a greater extent than with BiV pacing by 22%. Moreover, additional vectorcardiography (VCG) analysis was performed (using digital 12-lead ECGs) in a subset of seventeen patients showing improved QRS area with HOT-CRT. Similar to the studies by Boczar[20] and Vijayaraman,[21] a majority of patients demonstrated improvement in echocardiographic and clinical parameters at follow-up (but was not compared to BiV). Very recently, Senes and colleagues[24] published results from a propensity-matched study, where 27 patients with HF and a CRT indication were implanted with HBP (n = 15) or HBP + LV (n = 12) and were compared with a historical cohort of 27 patients who had received traditional BiV pacing. Although QRS duration was reduced to a greater extend (14% shorter) with HBP/HOT-CRT, this did not result in improved echocardiographic or clinical outcomes compared to BiV pacing. However, this study suffers from major limitations. Most importantly, the study was underpowered to exclude any potential benefit from HBP or HOT-CRT. Moreover, attempted HBP resulted in para-Hisian capture in 10 (37%) patients, limiting true intrinsic His-Purkinje activation to only 16 patients.

Although the aforementioned studies indicate a positive effect of HOT-CRT on electrical resynchronization, QRSd measures total ventricular activation time and do not separately evaluate left ventricular electrical synchrony, which may be the predominant factor impacting pump function. This is suggested by data by Arnold and colleagues,[1] who compared HBP (with BBB correction) versus BiV pacing in 17 patients with HF and LBBB using ECG imaging (ECGI), and evaluated hemodynamic response by invasive and noninvasive blood pressure measurements. Reduction in LV activation time (LVAT) was correlated with an acute increase in blood pressure, whereas reduction in QRSd was not. Another study by Gage and colleagues[25] showed that the standard deviation of activation times measured with ECGi predicted CRT response better than QRS duration. ECGi allows for a detailed evaluation of left and RV activation times by combining electrical information from unipolar body surface mapping electrodes with anatomic information from the heart and torso using computed tomography. Recently, we performed a mechanistic proof-of-principle study to examine the acute effects of HOT-CRT compared to different BiV pacing modes (including multipoint pacing [MPP]) on ventricular activation using a novel ECGI system that measures epi- and endocardial activation (and includes the interventricular septum).[26] Nineteen patients with a standard CRT indication, implanted with HBP without the correction of BBB (eight LBBB; two IVCD; six RBBB; three incomplete BBB), combined with either BiV pacing, or RV pacing in the setting of RBBB, were prospectively enrolled. We optimized settings with ECGI to obtain minimum values of LVAT with each pacing configuration (BiV; MPP; HOT-CRT). The main finding of this study was that HOT-CRT outperforms BiV pacing (including MPP) for improving left ventricular synchrony in terms of LVAT, **Fig. 2**.[27] A typical example of ventricular activation with HOT-CRT is illustrated in **Fig. 3**. In the subgroup of patients with LBBB or IVCD, the optimal HOT-CRT setting for reducing LVAT was HBP + LV pacing in 9 out of 10 patients compared to HBP + BiV in only one patient (in line with results by Coluccia and colleagues[22]). Moreover, HBP + LV avoids RV desynchronization observed with BiV pacing and reduces battery drain. The median optimal HBP-VP pacing interval in the LBBB/IVCD subgroup was 40 ms (similar to the 42 ms found by Desmukh and colleagues[23]), which corresponded to 60% of the HBP to RV sensing (RVS) interval.

FUSION PACING WITH LEFT BUNDLE BRANCH-OPTIMIZED CRT (LOT-CRT)

Left bundle branch pacing (LBBP) is rapidly gaining interest as it has more favorable electrical parameters than HBP,[28,29] allows the recruitment of conduction tissue activation in more distal conduction disease, and may be easier to perform. Recently, LBBP has been combined with left ventricular or biventricular pacing to provide LOT-CRT, which results in significantly narrower QRS complexes compared to biventricular or LBBP (by 26 ms and 18 ms on average, respectively), with an improvement of left ventricular ejection fraction and functional class at follow-up.[30] The effect on LOT-CRT on RV synchrony has not been defined (whereas it has been shown that this parameter is preserved with HOT-CRT).[27] An example of a patient with LOT-CRT is shown in **Fig. 4**.

PATIENTS WITH RIGHT BUNDLE BRANCH BLOCK

Patients with RBBB have been shown to derive little clinical benefit from BiV pacing.[31,32] However, these patients may benefit from RV-only pacing to correct any right-sided conduction delay.

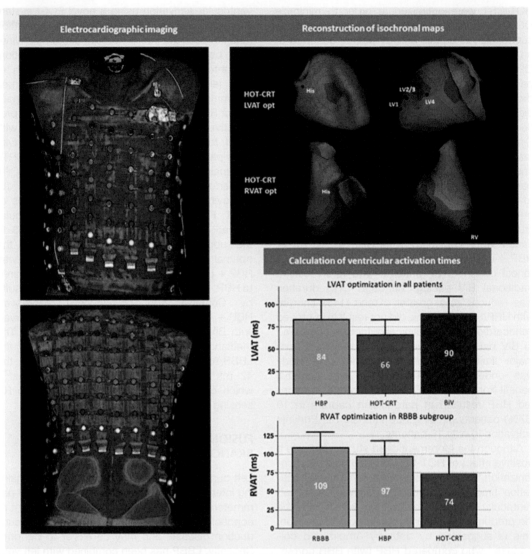

Fig. 2. Electrocardiographic imaging results with HOT-CRT. Patients implanted with HBP for a CRT indication underwent ECG imaging (ECGi) to calculate ventricular activation times. HBP with ventricular fusion pacing (ie, HOT-CRT) improved left ventricular activation times beyond BiV pacing in the total group.[27] Moreover, RVAT optimization with HOT-CRT improved right ventricular synchrony in a subselection of patients with RBBB. BiV, biventricular pacing; HBP, His bundle pacing; HOT-CRT, His-optimized cardiac resynchronization therapy; LVAT, left ventricular activation time; ms, milliseconds; RBBB, right bundle branch block; RVAT, right ventricular activation time. (*Adapted from* Zweerink A, Zubarev S, Bakelants E, et al. His-optimized cardiac resynchronization therapy with ventricular fusion pacing for electrical resynchronization in heart failure. JACC Clin Electrophysiol. 2021;7(7):881–92. https://doi.org/10.1016/j.jacep.2020.11.029; with permission.)

Giudici and colleagues[33] aimed to combine intrinsic conduction with RV pacing in 78 consecutive patients with RBBB who underwent pacemaker or ICD implantation. After implantation, patients underwent an AV-optimization protocol to maximize QRS narrowing which reduced the mean QRS width by 23% (baseline 147 ms). In a similar study, BiV fusion pacing using the SyncAV algorithm (allowing for triple wavefront activation)

improved electrical synchrony and LV ejection fraction in patients with RBBB.[34] Sharma and colleagues[35] reported that patients with RBBB respond favorably in terms of clinical and echographic response to HBP, either with the correction of BBB (n = 29) or with fusion pacing in patients with HBP and uncorrected RBB (n = 8) combining selective HBP with RV pacing (ie, HOT-CRT), or with nonselective His capture. Our

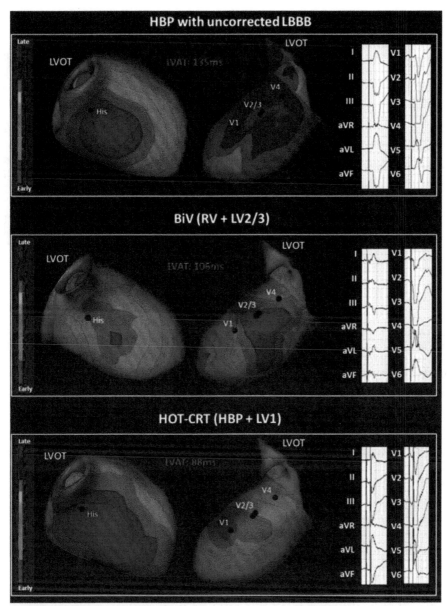

Fig. 3. ECGi left ventricular activation maps in a patient with His bundle pacing and uncorrected left bundle branch block (LBBB). Fusion of proximal His-Purkinje/right bundle branch activation with septal breakthrough and left ventricular activation during HOT-CRT reduced LVAT to a greater extent than BiV pacing. LVOT, left ventricular outflow tract. Other abbreviations same as in **Fig. 2.**

study[27] indicated that RV synchrony is actually worsened by BiV pacing, which is in agreement with a report by Varma and colleagues[36] which used ECGI. On the other hand, RV synchrony improved with HOT-CRT in patients with native RBBB, as illustrated in **Figs. 2** and **5**.

LOT-CRT has been performed in 11 patients with RBBB, but the outcome of this subgroup compared to patients with other types of conduction delay was not reported.[30]

PRACTICAL CONSIDERATIONS

Different configurations for connecting leads to the generator are shown in **Fig. 6**. In patients who are in chronic atrial fibrillation and are candidates for CRT, the atrial port (which is usually plugged) can simply be used to connect the HBP lead in combination with the LV and RV leads. This, however, requires specific programming considerations (eg, inactivation of ventricular safety

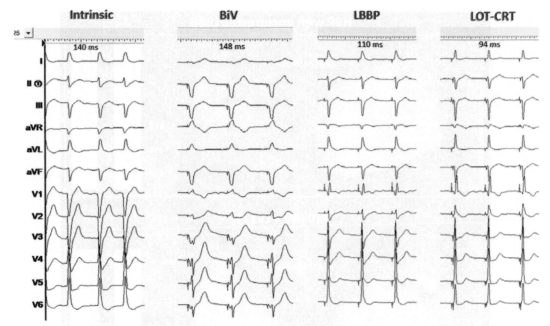

Fig. 4. Patient in atrial fibrillation with a biventricular defibrillator implanted with an additional LBBP lead (connected to the atrial port). LOT-CRT (combining LBBP + LV pacing with a delay of 30 ms) resulted in the shortest QRS duration. BiV, biventricular pacing; LBBP, left bundle branch pacing; LOT-CRT, left bundle branch optimized cardiac resynchronization therapy.

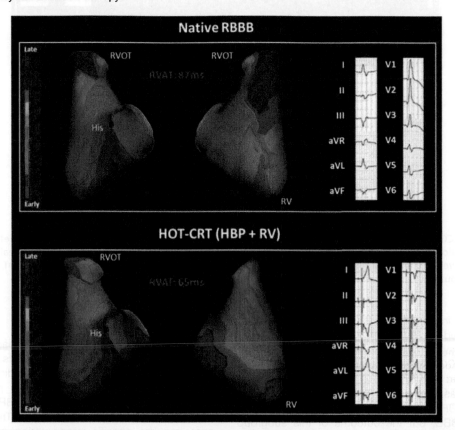

Fig. 5. ECGi right ventricular activation maps in a patient with right bundle branch block (RBBB). Regional activation at the His lead (ie, nonselective capture) combined with RV pacing reduced RVAT by 25% in this patient. RVOT, right ventricular outflow tract. Other abbreviations same as in **Fig. 2**.

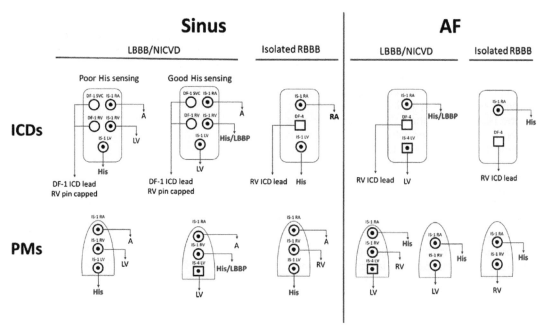

Fig. 6. Lead configurations for HOT-CRT and LOT-CRT. Configurations depend upon the presence of an atrial lead (patients in sinus rhythm), QRS morphology (requirement for RV and/or LV pacing), and whether the device is an ICD or PM. A DF-1 lead may be used in lieu of a DF-4 lead if preferred (not shown). In case of poor His sensing (high atrial or His potential amplitude/low ventricular amplitude), the LV lead can be connected to the RV port for sensing (with a risk of issues in case of LV lead dislodgment). In case of uncorrected RBBB with selective His capture (or high capture threshold for nonselective capture), fusion RV pacing may be delivered. A, atrial; AF, atrial fibrillation; HOT-CRT, His optimized cardiac resynchronization therapy; ICD, implantable cardioverter defibrillator; LBBB, left bundle branch block; LBBP, left bundle branch pacing; LOT-CRT, left bundle branch pacing optimized cardiac resynchronization therapy. LV, left ventricular; NIVCD, nonspecific intraventricular conduction delay; RBBB, right bundle branch block; RA, right atrium; RV, right ventricular.

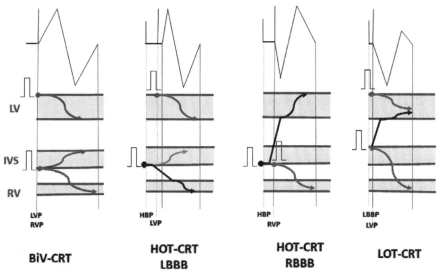

Fig. 7. Schematic representations of timing intervals with biventricular cardiac resynchronization therapy (BiV-CRT) without any fusion pacing, HOT-CRT in patients without the correction of bundle branch block with His bundle pacing (HBP), and LOT-CRT. With BiV-CRT, ventricular activation results entirely from ventricular capture. With HOT-CRT, ventricular activation results from a fusion of wavefronts via the His-Purkinje system and from ventricular pacing. In left bundle branch block (LBBB), HBP is delivered before left ventricular pacing (LVP), whereas in right bundle branch block (RBBB), HBP is delivered before right ventricular pacing (RVP). With LOT-CRT, LBBP is delivered slightly before LVP. Black arrows represent rapid activation via the intact His-Purkinje system. Green arrows represent activation via myocardial capture. Straight segments represent rapid conduction via the His-Purkinje system, whereas curved segments/arrows represent slower conduction via intramyocardial activation.

pacing) which are covered elsewhere.[37] The HBP/LBBP to RV/LV/BiV interval is limited by the minimum programmable AV delay (25–30 ms), which is nevertheless short enough. In patients with sinus rhythm (requiring an atrial lead), HOT-CRT can be delivered by connecting the LV lead to the RV port, and the HBP lead to the LV port (as ventricular sensing is usually better with the coronary sinus lead than the His lead). With LOT-CRT, as sensing is usually excellent, the LBBP lead can be connected to the RV port (without the need for an RV lead in pacemaker patients, as the RV is captured with LBBP). In patients with a CRT-D, a DF-1 ICD lead should be used, with the capping of the pace-sense pin (only the high voltage component of the lead is used).[38] Additional configurations using Y-adapters may also be used.[22]

It should be borne in mind that the factors impacting optimization and timing of activation wavefronts fusion are 1) delay of conduction via the His-Purkinje system 2) latency with ventricular pacing (ie, delay between pacing and QRS onset, usually greater with LV than with RV pacing) and 3) intramyocardial conduction (which is affected by factors such as fibrosis). This is illustrated in **Fig. 7.**

HOT-CRT can be empirically programmed with an HBP-ventricular pace interval corresponding to 60% of the HBP-RVS interval (with LV pacing in case of LBBB and RV pacing in case or RBBB). Alternatively, a 40 ms delay may be programmed in patients with LBBB and 60 ms in case of RBBB, but the effect on QRS narrowing should always be confirmed using a 12-lead ECG.

SUMMARY

HOT-CRT and LOT-CRT offer additional treatment options compared to BiV pacing alone and can be relatively simply implemented at the expense of implanting an extra lead. Whether HOT-CRT and LOT-CRT yield comparable results remains to be proven, as does their clinical benefit, which should be properly evaluated by prospective studies.

CLINICS CARE POINTS

- HOT CRT and LOT CRT combine conduction system pacing with appropriately timed left, right or biventricular pacing, with a synergistic effect.
- This strategy allows to provide constant fusion between activation wavefronts, and reduces ventricular activation times compared to biventricular pacing.

- HOT CRT can be empirically programmed with an interval from His pacing to LV pacing of 40 ms in patients with LBBB, and 60 ms to RV pacing in patients with RBBB, but should ideally be optimized individually for yielding the narrowest QRS.

REFERENCES

1. Arnold AD, Shun-Shin MJ, Keene D, et al. His resynchronization versus biventricular pacing in patients with heart failure and left bundle branch block. J Am Coll Cardiol 2018;72(24):3112–22.
2. Rickard J, Popovic Z, Verhaert D, et al. The QRS narrowing index predicts reverse left ventricular remodeling following cardiac resynchronization therapy. Pacing Clin Electrophysiol 2011;34(5):604–11.
3. Ruschitzka F, Abraham WT, Singh JP, et al. Cardiac-resynchronization therapy in heart failure with a narrow QRS complex. N Engl J Med 2013;369(15):1395–405.
4. Daubert C, Behar N, Martins RP, et al. Avoiding non-responders to cardiac resynchronization therapy: a practical guide. Eur Heart J 2017;38(19):1463–72.
5. Arbelo E, Tolosana JM, Trucco E, et al. Fusion-optimized intervals (FOI): a new method to achieve the narrowest QRS for optimization of the AV and VV intervals in patients undergoing cardiac resynchronization therapy. J Cardiovasc Electrophysiol 2014;25(3):283–92.
6. Trucco E, Tolosana JM, Arbelo E, et al. Improvement of reverse remodeling using electrocardiogram fusion-optimized intervals in cardiac resynchronization therapy: a randomized study. JACC Clin Electrophysiol 2018;4(2):181–9.
7. Tamborero D, Vidal B, Tolosana JM, et al. Electrocardiographic versus echocardiographic optimization of the interventricular pacing delay in patients undergoing cardiac resynchronization therapy. J Cardiovasc Electrophysiol 2011;22(10):1129–34.
8. Burri H, Prinzen FW, Gasparini M, et al. Left univentricular pacing for cardiac resynchronization therapy. Europace 2017;19(6):912–9.
9. Pujol-Lopez M, San Antonio R, Mont L, et al. Electrocardiographic optimization techniques in resynchronization therapy. Europace 2019;21(9):1286–96.
10. Martin DO, Lemke B, Birnie D, et al. Investigation of a novel algorithm for synchronized left-ventricular pacing and ambulatory optimization of cardiac resynchronization therapy: results of the adaptive CRT trial. Heart Rhythm 2012;9(11):1807–14.
11. Birnie D, Lemke B, Aonuma K, et al. Clinical outcomes with synchronized left ventricular pacing: analysis of the adaptive CRT trial. Heart Rhythm 2013;10(9):1368–74.

12. Thibault B, Ritter P, Bode K, et al. Dynamic programming of atrioventricular delay improves electrical synchrony in a multicenter cardiac resynchronization therapy study. Heart Rhythm 2019;16(7):1047–56.

13. Varma N, O'Donnell D, Bassiouny M, et al. Programming cardiac resynchronization therapy for electrical synchrony: reaching beyond left bundle branch block and left ventricular activation delay. J Am Heart Assoc 2018;7(3):e007489.

14. Vacarescu C, Cozma D, Petrescu L, et al. Exercise test is essential in LV-only fusion CRT pacing without right ventricle lead. Clin Interv Aging 2019;14:969–75.

15. Upadhyay GA, Cherian T, Shatz DY, et al. Intracardiac delineation of septal conduction in left bundle-branch block patterns. Circulation 2019;139(16):1876–88.

16. Lustgarten DL, Crespo EM, Arkhipova-Jenkins I, et al. His-bundle pacing versus biventricular pacing in cardiac resynchronization therapy patients: a crossover design comparison. Heart Rhythm 2015;12(7):1548–57.

17. Zweerink A, Bakelants E, Stettler C, et al. His bundle pacing to avoid electrical dyssynchrony with traditional right ventricular pacing: importance of heart size. Int J Cardiol 2020;311:54–7.

18. Padeletti L, Pieragnoli P, Ricciardi G, et al. Simultaneous his bundle and left ventricular pacing for optimal cardiac resynchronization therapy delivery: acute hemodynamic assessment by pressure-volume loops. Circ Arrhythm Electrophysiol 2016;9(5):e003793.

19. Zweerink A, Salden OAE, van Everdingen WM, et al. Hemodynamic optimization in cardiac resynchronization therapy: should we aim for dP/dtmax or stroke work? JACC Clin Electrophysiol 2019;5(9):1013–25.

20. Boczar K, Slawuta A, Zabek A, et al. Cardiac resynchronization therapy with his bundle pacing. Pacing Clin Electrophysiol 2019;42(3):374–80.

21. Vijayaraman P, Herweg B, Ellenbogen KA, et al. His-optimized cardiac resynchronization therapy to maximize electrical resynchronization: a feasibility study. Circ Arrhythm Electrophysiol 2019;12(2):e006934.

22. Coluccia G, Vitale E, Corallo S, et al. Additional benefits of nonconventional modalities of cardiac resynchronization therapy using His bundle pacing. J Cardiovasc Electrophysiol 2020;31(3):647–57.

23. Deshmukh A, Sattur S, Bechtol T, et al. Sequential His bundle and left ventricular pacing for cardiac resynchronization. J Cardiovasc Electrophysiol 2020; 31(9):2448–54.

24. Senes J, Mascia G, Bottoni N, et al. Is His-optimized superior to conventional cardiac resynchronization therapy in improving heart failure? Results from a propensity-matched study. Pacing Clin Electrophysiol 2021;44(9):1532–9.

25. Gage RM, Curtin AE, Burns KV, et al. Changes in electrical dyssynchrony by body surface mapping predict left ventricular remodeling in patients with cardiac resynchronization therapy. Heart Rhythm 2017;14(3):392–9.

26. Revishvili AS, Wissner E, Lebedev DS, et al. Validation of the mapping accuracy of a novel non-invasive epicardial and endocardial electrophysiology system. Europace 2015;17(8):1282–8.

27. Zweerink A, Zubarev S, Bakelants E, et al. His-optimized cardiac resynchronization therapy with ventricular fusion pacing for electrical resynchronization in heart failure. JACC Clin Electrophysiol 2021 Jul;7(7): 881–92.

28. Qian Z, Qiu Y, Wang Y, et al. Lead performance and clinical outcomes of patients with permanent His-Purkinje system pacing: a single-centre experience. Europace 2020;22(Suppl_2):ii45–53.

29. Hua W, Fan X, Li X, et al. Comparison of left bundle branch and his bundle pacing in bradycardia patients. JACC Clin Electrophysiol 2020;6(10):1291–9.

30. Jastrzebski M, Moskal P, Huybrechts W, et al. Left bundle branch-optimized cardiac resynchronization therapy (LOT-CRT): results from an international LBBAP collaborative study group. Heart Rhythm 2022 Jan;19(1):13–21.

31. Birnie DH, Ha A, Higginson L, et al. Impact of QRS morphology and duration on outcomes after cardiac resynchronization therapy: results from the Resynchronization-Defibrillation for Ambulatory Heart Failure Trial (RAFT). Circ Heart Fail 2013;6(6):1190–8.

32. Zareba W, Klein H, Cygankiewicz I, et al. Effectiveness of cardiac resynchronization therapy by QRS morphology in the multicenter automatic defibrillation implantation trial-cardiac resynchronization therapy (MADIT-CRT). Circulation 2011;123(10):1061–72.

33. Giudici MC, Abu-El-Haija B, Schrumpf PE, et al. Right ventricular septal pacing in patients with right bundle branch block. J Electrocardiol 2015;48(4):626–9.

34. AlTurki A, Lima PY, Vidal A, et al. Fusion pacing in patients with right bundle branch block who undergo cardiac resynchronization therapy. J Electrocardiol 2021;64:66–71.

35. Sharma PS, Naperkowski A, Bauch TD, et al. Permanent his bundle pacing for cardiac resynchronization therapy in patients with heart failure and right bundle branch block. Circ Arrhythm Electrophysiol 2018; 11(9):e006613.

36. Varma N, Jia P, Ramanathan C, et al. RV electrical activation in heart failure during right, left, and biventricular pacing. JACC Cardiovasc Imaging 2010; 3(6):567–75.

37. Burri H, Keene D, Whinnett Z, et al. Device programming for his bundle pacing. Circ Arrhythm Electrophysiol 2019;12(2):e006816.

38. Zweerink A, Bakelants E, Stettler C, et al. Cryoablation vs. radiofrequency ablation of the atrioventricular node in patients with His-bundle pacing. Europace 2021;23(3):421–30.

39. Jastrzębski M, Burri H, Kiełbasa G, et al. The V6-V1 interpeak interval: a novel criterion for the diagnosis of left bundle branch capture. Europace 2021.

Status and Update on Cardiac Resynchronization Therapy Trials

Angelo Auricchio, MD, PhD*, Tardu Özkartal, MD

KEYWORDS

- Cardiac resynchronization therapy • Implantable cardioverter-defibrillator • Pacemaker
- Implantation • Cardiac imaging • Clinical studies

KEY POINTS

- Since the early 1990s, a large number of prospective controlled trials showed remarkably consistent positive benefit in cardiac resynchronization therapy (CRT)-treated patients.
- These studies demonstrate that CRT, by restoring systolic synchronicity and enhancing both atrial and ventricular function, improves clinical symptoms in most patients (often dramatically), reverses left ventricular remodeling, and reduces the frequency of hospitalization as well as the number of deaths.
- Many registries and large observational cohort studies have helped in quantifying the clinical benefit and prolongation of survival in different classes of patients with chronic heart failure (HF), thus identifying patients who benefit most from CRT.
- In the most recent years, advancements in diagnostic capability to select patients with HF who may derive a significant benefit by CRT, and technological improvements in CRT delivery, device and lead optimization, and programming occurred.
- We present studies completed since the publication of the most recent EHRA/ESC clinical practice guidelines or ongoing studies in different areas of CRT research, which include patient selection by novel diagnostic tools, studies investigating extension of clinical criteria for CRT, left ventricular lead positioning and pacing site selection, optimization of CRT delivery and programming, and selection of device type.

INTRODUCTION

Since the early 1990s, a large number of prospective controlled trials showed remarkably consistent positive benefit in cardiac resynchronization therapy (CRT)-treated patients. Together, these studies demonstrate that CRT, by restoring systolic synchronicity and enhancing both atrial and ventricular function, improves clinical symptoms in most patients (often dramatically), reverses left ventricular (LV) remodeling, and reduces the frequency of hospitalization as well as the number of deaths. Many registries and large observational cohort studies have helped in quantifying the clinical benefit and prolongation of survival in different classes of patients with chronic heart failure (HF), thus identifying patients who benefit most from CRT.[1–9]

According to most recent clinical practice guidelines issued by international scientific societies,[10,11] CRT is recommended—in addition to guideline-directed medical therapy—in only defined subsets of the HF patient population, the majority being patients with symptomatic HF in sinus rhythm with reduced left ventricular ejection fraction (LVEF) and a QRS duration greater than or equal to 130 milliseconds. Other HF patient groups that may be considered for CRT include

Cardiocentro Ticino Institute, Ente Ospedaliero Cantonale, Via Tesserete 48, 6900 Lugano, Switzerland
* Corresponding author. Cardiocentro Ticino Institute, Ente Ospedaliero Cantonale, Via Tesserete 48, 6900 Lugano, Switzerland.
E-mail address: angelo.auricchio@eoc.ch

Card Electrophysiol Clin 14 (2022) 323–343
https://doi.org/10.1016/j.ccep.2021.12.007
1877-9182/22/© 2021 Elsevier Inc. All rights reserved.

very symptomatic patients with atrial fibrillation (AF), reduced LVEF, and a QRS duration of 130 milliseconds or more. Finally, patients who develop worsening of HF due to high rate of right ventricular (RV) pacing represent another group that may benefit from CRT.

Although CRT is considered an established nonpharmacologic treatment of HF, clinical research efforts continue with the goal to further improve CRT clinical efficacy. A first key attempt in this direction is to change the definition of CRT clinical efficacy.[12] Over the years, the response to CRT has been arbitrarily defined using a binary approach—response/nonresponse. Using this binary approach, disease nonprogression would fall into the category of nonresponse. However, from clinical standpoint, the definition is misleading. Indeed, in analogy to the efficacy of oncology therapy, where the important concept of disease "remission" and "nonprogression" is commonly accepted, the slowing of HF progression shall be considered an equally positive outcome in a CRT-treated patient. A recent joint position statement from the Heart Failure Association, European Heart Rhythm Association (EHRA), and European Association of Cardiovascular Imaging of the European Society of Cardiology (ESC) calls to stop the current binary approach of CRT response, but rather it suggests that CRT should be classified as a treatment for "disease modification."[13]

More recently, advancements in diagnostic capability to select patients with HF who may derive a significant benefit by CRT and technological improvements in CRT delivery, device and lead optimization, and programming occurred. This article presents studies completed since the publication of the most recent EHRA/ESC clinical practice guidelines or ongoing studies in different areas of CRT research, which include patient selection by (1) novel diagnostic tools, (2) extension of clinical criteria, (3) LV lead positioning and pacing site selection, (4) optimization of CRT delivery and programming, and (5) selection of device type. We do not consider studies already included in recent clinical practice guidelines for cardiac pacing and CRT by the ESC.[10] Studies comparing conventional CRT with alternative pacing sites, such as His bundle or left bundle branch pacing are covered elsewhere in this issue.

Novel Diagnostic Tools for Cardiac Resynchronization Therapy Patient Selection

QRS duration and left bundle branch block (LBBB) morphology are currently considered the most reliable biomarkers for selecting CRT candidates.

However, electrocardiography (ECG) criteria to classify LBBB significantly differ among scientific organizations, investigators, trials, and guidelines,[14] which may pose uncertainty in meta-analytical investigations and comparison of outcomes. Notably, ECG definitions for LBBB have never been designed to predict response to CRT. Owing to a large number of potential limitations of surface ECG in precisely defining bundle branch block and reliable prediction of CRT clinical efficacy,[12] other approaches may be worth considering. The MARC-2 (Markers and Response to CRT in Non-LBBB) is a multicenter, exploratory, prospective, interventional postmarket release, nonrandomized trial and evaluates the relation of QRS area, determined by vectorcardiography, and response to CRT in patients with wide QRS complex without typical LBBB on a hierarchical clinical composite end point (death, HF hospitalizations, HF complaints, and cardiac function). The study will enroll 800 patients with symptomatic HF (New York Heart Association [NYHA] functional class I to IV) with a reduced LVEF and a prolonged QRS duration greater than or equal to 130 milliseconds as measured before implantation of a CRT device (Table 1). All patients will be followed for 1 year after implant. Each patient will visit the clinical site at baseline and at 6-month and 12 month follow-ups. The total study duration will be 3 years.

Other studies included in Table 1 are dealing with different cardiac imaging modalities or with novel diagnostic tools, such as CardioInsight to better define patients who may benefit from CRT or improve patient's outcome.

Extension of Clinical Criteria

There is robust evidence that patients in sinus rhythm, reduced LVEF, QRS duration greater than or equal to 150 ms, and LBBB benefit most from CRT. In contrast, clinical practice guidelines have a lower level of evidence for patients with non-LBBB morphology or patients in AF. Indeed, evidence for these patient groups is mostly given by posthoc analysis of large randomized trials or large observational clinical registries in the absence of prospectively designed clinical trials in these patients. Non-LBBB is, however, a very heterogeneous patient cohort including patients with right bundle branch block or diffuse ventricular conduction disturbance (IVCD) with a QRS duration greater than 120 milliseconds. Studies listed in Table 2 cover several areas in which evidence is modest. Worth mentioning is the NICD-CRT trial (Assessment of Cardiac Resynchronization Therapy in Patients with Wide QRS and Non-specific Intraventricular Conduction Delay: a Randomized Trial).

Table 1
Novel diagnostic tools for cardiac resynchronization therapy patient selection

Study Name or Acronym	NCT #	Status	Type of Study	No. Patient	Tested Hypothesis	Outcome Measurements							
						NYHA Class	QoL	Rev Rem	HFH	CV Death	Mort.	CCRS	Other Outcomes
MARC-2: Markers And Response to CRT in Non-LBBB	04120909	OG	M, P, O	800	Assessing role of QRS area, as well as other electrocardiographic, echocardiographic, and blood and clinical markers in predicting CRT response	Y	-	Y	Y*	-	Y*	Y*	-
ANIMATION: Cardiac Non Invasive Mapping in Resynchronization	04347109	OG	P, O	50	Noninvasive mapping with the Cardio Insight system in patients with heart failure requiring CRT to optimize therapy, and to understand mechanisms underlying pacing-induced cardiomyopathy and ventricular arrhythmias	-	Y*	Y*	Y*	-	Y*	-	-
CRID-CRT: Contractile Reserve in Dyssynchrony: A Novel Principle to Identify Candidates for Cardiac Resynchronization Therapy	02525185	N.A.	P, O	200	Assessing if myocardial work, measured by echocardiography in combination with viability assessment by LGE-CMR can predict CRT response	Y	Y*	Y	Y	-	Y	-	-
WORK-CRT: Myocardial Work and Metabolism in CRT	02537782	N.A.	M, P, O	200	Evaluation of regional myocardial workload and metabolism via apical rocking and other noninvasive measures of LV mechanical dyssynchrony to determine their predictive value in CRT response	Y	Y*	Y	Y	-	Y	-	-

(continued on next page)

Table 1
(continued)

Study Name or Acronym	NCT #	Status	Type of Study	No. Patient	Tested Hypothesis	Outcome Measurements								
						NYHA Class	QoL	Rev Rem	HFH	CV Death	Death	Mort.	CCRS	Other Outcomes
MIBGinCRT: SPECT-based Prediction and Evaluation of CRT Efficacy in CHF	03667989	C	P, O	60	Assessing the state of the cardiac sympathetic activity and severity of ventricular dyssynchrony in patients with chronic heart failure via SPECT and its capabilities in predicting prognosis	-	-	Y*	-	-	-	-	-	-
BIO-2-HEART - Identification of Biomarkers in T2DM and Heart Failure	03323216	OG	P, O	200	Aiming to identify biomarkers, determined prior to CRT implantation, to differentiate between responders and non-responders and to better understand the role of type 2 diabetes mellitus in heart failure	-	-	-	-	-	-	-	-	biomarkers[a]
BIOCRT: Biomarkers to Predict CRT Response in Patients With HF	01949246	N.A.	P, O	496	Assessing role of biomarkers for prediction of response to CRT and their effect on left ventricular remodelling	-	-	-	Y*	-	Y*	Y	-	-

Abbreviations: C, completed; CCRS, composite clinical response score; CMR, cardiac magnetic resonance; CV death, number of cardiovascular death; HFH, frequency of heart failure hospitalization; HFrEF, heart failure with reduced ejection fraction; LGE, late gadolinium enhancement; LV, left ventricle or ventricular; LVESV, left ventricular end-systolic volume; M, multicenter; Mort., all-cause mortality; MSP, multisite pacing; N.A., not available; NCT, National Clinical Trial number; NYHA, change in New York Heart Association class; O, observational trial; OG, ongoing; P, prospective; QoL, quality-of-life; R, randomized; Rev Rem, echocardiographic assessment of reverse remodeling; RV, right ventricle or ventricular; SPECT, single-photon emission computed tomography; Y, yes.
* Primary outcome.

Table 2
Extension of clinical criteria for cardiac resynchronization therapy

Study Name or Acronym	NCT #	Status	Type of Study	No. Patient	Tested Hypothesis	Outcome Measurements								
						NYHA Class	QoL	Rev Rem	HFH	CV Death	Death	Mort.	CCRS	Other Outcome
NICD-CRT: Assessment of Cardiac Resynchronization Therapy in Patients With Wide QRS and Non-specific Intraventricular Conduction Delay: a Randomized Trial	02454439	OG	M, P, 1:1	200	Assessing whether patients implanted with CRT who have an intrinsic QRS > 130 ms and NICD benefit from CRT	Y	Y	Y	Y*	Y	Y*	Y*	Y	-
Narrow QRS HF Patients Assessed by ECG Belt	03367104	C	P, O	10	Aiming to quantitate electrical dyssynchrony in patients with HF with QRS complexes ≤ 130 ms using the ECG belt to provide data that can be used in designing and implementing prospective CRT studies in patients with narrow QRS selected and optimized with the ECG belt	-	-	-	-	-	-	-	-	Quantification of electrical dyssynchrony*
PREFECTUS - Cardiac Resynchronisation Therapy vs Rate-responsive Pacing in Heart Failure With Preserved Ejection Fraction	03338374	OG	P, O	10	Assessing the incremental benefit of CRT over and above rate response pacing in patients with preserved left ventricular ejection fraction and chronotropic insufficiency	Y	-	-	-	-	-	-	-	Diastolic and systolic reserve index*

(continued on next page)

Table 2
(continued)

Study Name or Acronym	NCT #	Status	Type of Study	No. Patient	Tested Hypothesis	Outcome Measurements							
						NYHA Class	QoL	Rev Rem	HFH	CV Death	Mort.	CCRS	Other Outcome
REAL-CRT - A randomized controlled trial of cardiac resynchronization therapy in patients with prolonged atrioventricular interval	02150538	N.A.	P, 1:1	82	Investigate whether CRT is superior to right ventricular pacing in patients with left ventricular ejection fraction > 35% and PR interval ≥ 220 ms	Y	Y	Y*	-	-	-	-	
Metabolic Mapping and Cardiac Resynchronization	03420833	OG	P, 1:1	100	Assessing safety and effectiveness of CRT in patients with mild heart failure (left ventricular ejection fraction 36%–50%) and left bundle branch block (QRS ≥ 130 ms)	-	-	Y*	Y	-	Y	-	
RAFT-PermAF: Resynchronization/Defibrillation for Ambulatory Heart Failure Trial in Patients With Permanent Atrial Fibrillation	01994252	OG	M, P, 1:1	200	Determine whether CRT will reduce LVESV in patients with HF with permanent atrial fibrillation, mild to moderate heart failure, left ventricular ejection fraction ≤ 35%, and prolonged QRS duration, when compared with implantable cardioverter-defibrillator	-	Y	Y*	Y	Y	Y	-	

(continued on next page)

Table 2
(continued)

Study Name or Acronym	NCT #	Status	Type of Study	No. Patient	Tested Hypothesis	NYHA Class	QoL	Rev Rem	HFH	CV Death	Mort.	CCRS	Other Outcome
CAAN-AF: Cardiac Resynchronisation Therapy and AV Nodal Ablation Trial in Atrial Fibrillation Patients	01522898	C	M, P, 1:1	145	Assessing benefit of atrioventricular junction ablation when compared with medical rate control in patients with persistent or permanent atrial fibrillation and CRT	-	Y	Y	Y*	Y	Y*	-	
Budapest Upgrade CRT Study: Effect of Biventricular Upgrade on Left Ventricular Reverse Remodeling and Clinical Outcomes in Patient With Left Ventricular Dysfunction and Intermittent or Permanent Apical/Septal Right Ventricular Pacing	02270840, N.A.		M, P, 3:2	360	Aiming to compare the efficacy and safety of CRT upgrade from conventional pacemaker or implantable cardioverter-defibrillator therapy in patients with intermittent or permanent right ventricular septal/apical pacing, reduced left ventricular ejection fraction, and symptomatic heart failure	Y*	-	Y*	Y*	Y*	Y*	-	

Abbreviation: NICD, nonspecific intraventricular conduction delay. n:n, randomized trial with mode of randomization.
* primary outcome.

This is a multicenter, prospective, double-blind, randomized, study comparing effects of CRT in patients with IVCD as recorded on 12-lead ECG. IVCD is defined as a QRS duration greater than 130 ms without criteria for LBBB or the presence of right bundle branch block according to the AHA/ACCF/HRS recommendations.[15] The patients are randomized to either CRT on or CRT off. Primary end point is a composite of all-cause mortality and percentage of HF hospitalizations at 12 months. The investigators plan to enroll 200 patients, and study completion is expected to be July 2023.

AF is one of the most common comorbidities in patients receiving CRT. The vast majority of CRT studies including patients with history of paroxysmal or persistent AF have shown a similar outcome of these patients with those in sinus rhythm. Accordingly, clinical practice guidelines do not give specific recommendations for patients with history of AF. In contrast, strong evidence of clinical benefit in patients with permanent AF is still missing. Shortly after the publication of the ESC 2021 guidelines for pacing and CRT,[10] Brignole and colleagues[16] published the results of atrioventricular (AV) junction (AVJ) ablation and cardiac resynchronization for patients with permanent AF and narrow QRS: the APAF-CRT mortality trial. APAF-CRT mortality trial prospectively tested the effects of AVJ ablation with CRT implantation in patients with symptomatic AF when compared with pharmacologic rate control alone.[16] The trial was stopped prematurely after a median follow-up of 29 months because of a significant reduction in all-cause mortality for patients randomized to AVJ ablation and CRT implantation (hazard ratio 0.29; 95% confidence interval [CI] 0.10–0.65; $P = .004$) compared with patients assigned to pharmacologic therapy. Interestingly, the reduction in mortality and HF hospitalization with the ablation and CRT strategy was achieved irrespective of patient's baseline EF. The CAAN-AF trial (Cardiac Resynchronisation Therapy and AV Nodal Ablation Trial in Atrial Fibrillation Patients) recently completed recruitment (August 2020), and its results should be published soon. It is the first multicenter, prospective, randomized, controlled trial comparing AVJ ablation versus medical ventricular rate control with a target heart rate less than 90 bpm in 145 patients with already implanted CRT and persistent (≥ 1 month) or permanent AF. The primary outcome is a composite of all-cause mortality and nonfatal HF events.

Several studies have demonstrated the deleterious effect of chronic RV pacing with respect to increased risk of worsening of HF symptoms and HF hospitalizations, which may be reduced by the use of CRT device. The benefit of CRT upgrade has been investigated only in observational small studies. Importantly, patients referred for a CRT upgrade differ from patients referred for de novo CRT implantation: they are older, mainly male patients, and have more comorbidities. The BUDAPEST-CRT Upgrade study (Effect of Biventricular Upgrade on Left Ventricular Reverse Remodeling and Clinical Outcomes in Patient with Left Ventricular Dysfunction and Intermittent or Permanent Apical/Septal Right Ventricular Pacing) is the first prospective, randomized, multicenter trial, and its rationale and design were published in 2017 in Europace.[17] The study is enrolling patients with heart failure with reduced ejection fraction less than or equal to 35%, paced QRS greater than or equal to 150 ms, and RV pacing greater than or equal to 20%. Patients are randomized to CRT-D versus ICD. The primary end point consists of a composite of all-cause mortality, first HF event, or less than 15% reduction in LV end-systolic volume at 12 months. The results of this study might alter the indication for CRT upgrade. The study was supposed to be completed by the end of 2018.

Left Ventricular Lead Positioning, and Possible Pacing Configurations

An area of intense research has always been the investigation of the most optimal LV lead positioning and whether a mechanical or electrical target shall be aimed. Several studies have shown that pacing the LV in a region of late activation results in larger LV reverse remodeling, better quality of life, and improved survival of patients on CRT. In clinical practice, electrophysiologists either target a preprocedurally and noninvasively determined area with late peak shortening, or the location at the LV wall with the longest electrical delay when compared with the RV lead (RV-LV interval) or the Q wave on surface electrocardiogram (ECG; QLV interval), both of which are determined invasively and during the implant procedure. Clearly, determination of the best LV pacing location before the implant procedure in a noninvasive manner is to be preferred, but this can only be achieved if late mechanical activation also coincides with late electrical activation. Few studies that have until now investigated the agreement between the area of late electrical and late mechanical activation reported conflicting results. A recent study by Maffessanti and colleagues[18] indicated that the relation between electrical and mechanical activation is variable and particularly weak in hearts with scar. Importantly, the effects of scar seemed independent of the distance between scar and latest activated region, implying that scar also affects the electromechanical coupling remote from the scar.

Limited data exist on CRT effectiveness in patients with non-LBBB. Clinicians generally deliver CRT through an anatomic implantation approach; however, targeting the QLV may serve as an individualized implantation strategy in patients with non-LBBB. The ENHANCE CRT study enrolled 248 subjects at 29 US centers. Subjects were randomized in a 2:1 ratio between a QLV-based implantation approach and anatomic implantation approach. The primary end point was the clinical composite score after 12 months of follow-up. The study analyzed 191 available subjects at 12 months of follow-up. The responder rate at 12 months measured by the clinical composite score was 67.2% in the QLV arm and 73.0% in the control arm ($P = .506$). The study's conclusion was that although patient-tailored LV lead placement guided by QLV is promising, no difference in outcome between the QLV-based implantation approach and the conventional anatomically guided implantation approach was observed in patients with non-LBBB. More recently, Borgquist and colleagues[19,20] published the results of the CRT Clinic (Combining Myocardial Strain and Cardiac CT to Optimize Left Ventricular Lead Placement in CRT Treatment), which tested the hypothesis that, by combining cardiac imaging using radial strain echocardiography, cardiac computed tomography, and cardiac magnetic resonance imaging with gadolinium contrast, the responder rates should increase. Patients were randomized to either optimal LV lead location (defined as the latest mechanically activated available segment, free of transmural scar), determined by radial strain echocardiography, or conventional approach. The study originally planned to recruit 144 patients but was terminated early after an interim analysis indicated that the main result was neutral between the 2 groups.[19]

Table 3 summarizes the hypothesis tested in each of the ongoing studies, the number of patients that each study will enroll, and the expected outcome measurements. Most of these studies use a multimodality imaging approach for scar evaluation and venous anatomy assessment. The blinded, multicenter, randomized controlled ADVISE trial (Image Supported Lead Placement in CRT), for instance, is assessing the efficacy of real-time guidance by means of cardiac magnetic resonance and fluoroscopy-fusion imaging. The participating centers are currently recruiting and plan to enroll 130 patients until 2023. Other studies are investigating the still open question whether LV lead positioning guided either by electrical delay

(the latest electrical activation recorded) or by mechanical dyssynchrony is as effective as anatomic LV lead position, that is, guided by anatomic vein availability. The DANISH-CRT study (Does Electric Targeted LV Lead Positioning Improve Outcome in Patients with Heart Failure and Prolonged QRS) randomizes patients with CRT indication to receive either standard LV lead placement or placement at the latest electrical activation recorded by electrical mapping of the coronary sinus during the implantation. Primary outcome is death or first unplanned HF hospitalization. The study plans to recruit 1000 patients and is supposed to be completed in November 2023.

During the last decade, improved physiologic knowledge and significant technological advancement have resulted in LV placement guided by multimodality imaging, more appropriate selection of LV epicardial pacing sites via the coronary sinus, possible multiple site pacing, and multipoint LV pacing. According to common terminology, multisite pacing is obtained by using 2 leads in 2 different coronary veins or 2 separate RV sites, whereas multipoint pacing is delivered using multiple electrodes on a single LV lead. The concept of multisite-multipoint pacing is based on the hypothesis that pacing at multiple locations within the ventricles electrically engages a larger ventricular mass and will therefore improve cardiac resynchronization.[21–24] Although a recent meta-analysis[25] including 7 studies with a total of 1390 patients and a follow-up of greater than 6 months showed that in nonrandomized trials multisite pacing was associated with a greater probability of echocardiographic improvement when compared with standard CRT (odds ratio 5.33, 95% CI 3.05–9.33; $P < .01$); the benefit could not be confirmed in randomized trials.[21,23,26–28] There was no difference in terms of NYHA class improvement or left ventricular end-systolic volume reduction. At present, there are a large number of ongoing clinical trials, which are summarized in **Table 4**. The outcome of these studies will help in shedding further light onto the still open issue of multisite pacing. The recently completed SMART-MSP (presented at APHRS 2021) was designed to examine the safety and effectiveness of patients who are nonresponsive to conventional CRT. The trial is a prospective, observational study that enrolled 584 CRT recipients at 52 sites in the United States. CRT recipients were assessed at 6-month follow-up using the clinical composite score. Nonresponders had the LV multisite pacing feature turned on and were followed until 12 months. In a typical modern CRT population, 75% of patients were considered responders to CRT; the remaining 137 patients were classified

Table 3
Imaging or electric guidance of left ventricular lead positioning and pacing site selection

Study Name or Acronym	NCT #	Status	Type of Study	No. Patient	Tested Hypothesis/Results	Outcome Measurements							
						NYHA Class	QoL	Rev Rem	HFH	CV Death	Mort.	CCRS	Other Outcome
ADVISE: Image supported lead placement in CRT	05053568	OG	M, P, O	130	Efficacy of real-time guidance of left ventricular lead placement by cardiac resonance imaging and fluoroscopy-fusion imaging	Y	Y	Y	-	Y	Y	Y	% of successful LV lead implantation*
GUIDE-CRT: Image fusion of SPECT MPI and fluoroscopy venography to guide LV lead placement for improved CRT response	03125720	OG	M, P, 1:1	300	Guiding LV lead placement by fusion single-photon emission computed tomography-myocardial perfusion imaging and fluoroscopy venogram	Y	Y*	Y	-	Y	Y	-	-
ECHO-CRT: Prediction of Response to Cardiac Resynchronization Therapy by New Echocardiographic Methods	02986633	OG	P, O	1000	Identifying echocardiographic parameters, including speckle tracking strain, to predict CRT response and better outcome	-	Y*	-	-	Y	-	-	-
DANISH-CRT: Does Electric Targeted LV Lead Positioning Improve Outcome in Patients With Heart Failure and Prolonged QRS	03280862	OG	M, P, 1:1	1000	Testing whether targeting left ventricular lead positioning toward latest electrically activated segment improves outcome when compared with standard left ventricular lead implant	Y	Y	Y*	Y	Y*	-	-	-

(continued on next page)

Table 3
(continued)

Study Name or Acronym	NCT #	Status	Type of Study	No. Patient Results	Tested Hypothesis/ Results			Outcome Measurements						
						NYHA Class	QoL	Rev Rem	HFH	CV Death	Mort.	CCRS	Other Outcome	
ECG Belt for CRT Response	03504020	OG	M, P, 1:1	498	The ECG belt will be used at implant and follow-up to help choose a suitable left ventricular pacing site and optimize pacing vector/ timing parameters	-	-	Y*	-	-	-	-	-	
Optimization of CRT Using an ECG Vest	02699944	C	P, O	56	Assessing the potential benefit of the ECG vest as part of CRT optimization strategy	-	-	Y*	-	-	-	-	-	

* primary outcome.

Table 4
Multisite pacing

Study Name or Acronym	NCT #	Status	Type of Study	No. Patient	Tested Hypothesis	Outcome Measurements							
						NYHA Class	QoL	Rev Rem	CV HFH	Death	Mort.	CCRS	Other Outcome
MORE-CRT MPP - More Response on Cardiac Resynchronization Therapy With MultiPoint Pacing	02006069	N.A.	M, P, 1:1	6898	Assessing impact of multipoint pacing at 12 months in CRT nonresponders	Y	Y	Y*	-	-	-	Y	-
MPP-VARR: The Effect of MultiPoint pacing on reverse remodeling and the incidence of ventricular arrhythmias	-	N.A.	M, P, 1:1	282	Assessing benefit of CRT with multipoint pacing in terms of LV remodeling and reduction of ventricular arrhythmias	-	-	Y*	-	-	-	-	-
MPP-PMS - MultiPoint Pacing Post Market Study	02832622	C	M, P, O	2169	Postmarket study to characterize the real-world use of multipoint pacing in CRT patients	Y	Y	Y	Y	-	Y	Y*	-
SCOPE-CRT - Simultaneous or Sequential Multipoint Pacing	03301363	OG	P, O	50	Assessing if sequential multipoint is superior to simultaneous LV MSP in reducing QRS duration and acute hemodynamic changes	-	-	-	-	-	-	-	QRS duration changes*
COMPACT-MPP - Comparison of Multi-point Pacing and Conventional CRT Through Non-invasive Hemodynamics Measurement and Global Longitudinal Strain Assessment	04299360	C	M, P, O	52	Comparing multipoint pacing with conventional CRT through noninvasive hemodynamics measurement and global longitudinal strain assessment	Y	-	-	-	-	-	-	dP/dT and global strain improvement*

(continued on next page)

Table 4
(continued)

Study Name or Acronym	NCT #	Status	Type of Study	No. Patient	Tested Hypothesis	NYHA Class	QoL	Rev Rem	HFH	CV Death	Mort.	CCRS	Other Outcome
						____ Outcome Measurements ____							
IMAGE-CRT: Impact of MultiPoint Pacing Technology in CRT Patients With Reduced RV-to-LV Delay	02713308	OG	P, O	248	Assessing CRT responder rate in patients with multipoint pacing in presence of RV-to-LV delay < 80 ms	-	-	Y*	-	-	-	-	-
TRIPLEAD: Prospective Randomized Trial Comparing TRIPLE Site Ventricular Stimulation vs Conventional Pacing in CRT Candidates	02962791	N.A.	P, 1:1	166	Comparing triple-site pacing (2 pacing sites in the RV + LV pacing) with standard CRT	-	-	Y*	-	-	Y	-	-
IRON-MPP: Italian Registry On Multipoint Left Ventricular Pacing	02606071	N.A.	M, P, O	436	Registry designed to collect clinical and device data from a large cohort of CRT-D patients implanted with a device capable of delivering multipoint pacing	-	-	Y*	Y	-	-	-	-

* primary outcome.

Table 5
Optimization of cardiac resynchronization therapy response

Study Name or Acronym	NCT #	Status	Type of Study	No. Patient	Tested Hypothesis	Outcome Measurements								
						NYHA Class	QoL	Rev Rem	HFH	CV Death	Death	Mort.	CCRS	Other outcome
METEOR-CRT: Multi-lead ECG to Effectively Optimize Resynchronization Devices: New CRT Recipients	04083690	OG	M, P, 1:1	120	Comparison of standard CRT programming with simultaneous biventricular pacing and fixed AV delay vs ECG-guided programming optimization	-	-	Y*	-	-	-	-	-	-
BIO|Adapt: Evaluation of the BIOTRONIK AutoAdapt Algorithm for Continuous Automatic Adaptive Cardiac Resynchronization	04774523	OG	P, O	350	Assessment of BIOTRONIK's AutoAdapt feature that optimizes atrioventricular delay and sets pacing configuration to biventricular or left ventricular only, based on intracardiac conduction times	Y*	-	Y	Y*	-	-	Y*	Y*	-
Tailoring Pacemaker Output to Physiology in Chronic Heart Failure	03781427	OG	P, 1:1	70	Assessing benefit of high pacing output programming when compared with standard programming	-	Y	Y	-	-	-	Y	-	-
Effects of CRT Optimization as Assessed by Cardiac MR	04763460	OG	M, P, 1:1	40	Assessing whether CRT optimization guided by ECG parameters is superior to standard programming, assessed by cardiac	-	Y	Y*	-	-	-	-	-	-

(continued on next page)

Table 5 (*continued*)

Study Name or Acronym	NCT #	Status	Type of Study	No. Patient	Tested Hypothesis	NYHA Class	QoL	Rev Rem	HFH	CV Death	Death	Mort.	CCRS	Other outcome
					magnetic resonance imaging									
AdaptResponse Clinical Trial	02205359	N.A.	M, P, 1:1	3700	Assessing long-term benefit of AdaptivCRT algorithm, which provides RV synchronized LV pacing or biventricular pacing with adjustment of atrioventricular and ventriculo-ventricular intervals in CRT patients	Y	Y	-	Y*	-	Y*	Y	-	-
SyncAV Post-Market Trial	04100148	OG	M, P, 1:1	1400	Assessing long-term benefit of SyncAV algorithm that automatically adapts AV interval to maximize biventricular pacing in CRT	-	-	Y*	-	-	-	-	-	-
Crusty Plus	-	OG	M, P, 1:1	722	Assessing whether CRT using automatic continuous AV delay optimization via Abbott's SyncAV Plus algorithm is superior to CRT with conventional biventricular pacing	Y	Y	Y*	Y	Y	Y	Y	-	-
Electrical Activation Mapping Guided Tailor Made Approach for Cardiac Resynchronization Therapy	03356652	OG	P, O	93	Assessing benefit of patient-tailored CRT delivery through noninvasive electrical mapping system	Y	Y	Y*	-	-	-	-	-	-

(continued on next page)

Table 5
(continued)

Study Name or Acronym	NCT #	Status	Type of Study	No. Patient	Tested Hypothesis	Outcome Measurements							
						NYHA Class	QoL	Rev Rem	HFH	CV Death	Mort.	CCRS	Other outcome
SMART CRT: Strategic Management to Optimize Response To Cardiac Resynchronization Therapy	03089281	C	M, P, 1:1	699	Assessing benefit of SmartDelay algorithm in patients with a prolonged RV-LV interval when compared with fixed atrioventricular delay programming	-	-	Y*	-	-	-	-	-
BIO|MASTER.Edora Family Study	03091322	C	M, P, O	120	Evaluating AV Opt and LV VectorOpt features in Biotronik Edora devices	-	-	-	-	-	-	-	usability of the algorithms*
Mid-Q Response Study	04180696	OG	M, P, 1:1	232	Assessing whether AdaptivCRT algorithm is superior to standard CRT therapy in CRT patients with moderate QRS duration (120–149 ms)	Y	Y	Y	Y	Y	Y	Y*	-

* primary outcome.

Table 6
Choice of device

Study Name or Acronym	NCT #	Status	Type of Study	No. Patient	Tested Hypothesis	NYHA Class	QoL	Rev Rem	HFH	CV Death	Mort.	CCRS	Other Outcome
RESET-CRT - Re-evaluation of Optimal Re-synchronization Therapy in Patients With Chronic Heart Failure	03494933	OG	M, P, 1:1	1356	Head-to-head comparison of CRT-P vs CRT-D in patients with primary CRT indication	-	Y	-	Y	Y	Y*	-	-
CRT-REALITY: CRT-P or CRT-D in Dilated Cardiomyopathy	04139460	OG	M, P, 1:1	924	Head-to-head comparison of CRT-P vs CRT-D in patients with primary CRT indication, nonischemic cardiomyopathy, and absence of LV midwall fibrosis on LGE-CMR	-	Y	-	Y*	Y*	-	-	-
Cardiac Resynchronization in the Elderly	03031847	C	M, P, 1:1	103	Head-to-head comparison of CRT-P vs CRT-D in elderly patients > 75 years with primary CRT indication	-	Y	-	-	-	-	-	cost of care
BioCONTINUE: Assessment of Ventricular Arrhythmia Risk After CRT-D Replacement for Patients With Primary Prevention Indication	02323503	C	M, P, O	289	Aiming to determine the relevance of defibrillator backup after generator replacement of the first CRT-D in a primary prevention population	-	-	-	-	-	-	-	Rate of patients with at least one sustained VT after replacement*

* primary outcome.

Table 7
Miscellaneous

Study Name or Acronym	NCT #	Status	Type of Study	No. Patient	Tested Hypothesis/Results	NYHA Class	QoL	Rev Rem	HFH	CV Death	Mort.	CCRS	Other Outcome
RECOVER - Reduction of Extension of Conduction Time With Ventricular Electromechanical Remodeling	04397224	OG	M, P, O	100	Aiming to detect serial changes in ventriculo-ventricular conduction times according to cardiac resynchronization therapy response	-	-	-	-	-	-	-	Change in ventriculo-ventricular conduction times*
Sleep Apnea and CRT Upgrading	01970423	C	P, 1:1	56	Aiming to test whether CRT does improve sleep apnea and if preexisting sleep apnea predicts CRT response in patients with conventional RV pacing undergoing CRT upgrade	-	Y	-	-	-	-	-	Improvement of sleep apnea*
BIO|STREAM HF: Observation of Clinical Routine Care for Heart Failure Patients Implanted With BIOTRONIK CRT Devices	03366545	OG	M, P, O	3000	Assessing outcome, efficacy, and residual safety aspects of CRT based on long-term data from an unselected, real-world population	Y*	-	Y*	Y*	Y*	Y*	-	-
COGNI-CRT: How is Cognitive Function Affected by Cardiac Resynchronisation Therapy?	03755570	OG	P, O	198	Assessing the effect of CRT on cognitive function in heart failure patients with an LVEF ≤ 35%	Y	-	Y	-	-	-	-	Change in cognitive battery test*

* primary outcome.

as nonresponders and LV multisite pacing was enabled in 102 subjects. At 12 month follow-up, the conversion rate from nonresponder to responder was 50%; these patients had a significantly lower risk of HF decompensation at the subsequent 6-month follow-up. The SMART-CRT results provided several important messages, including considering turning on LV multisite pacing in case of CRT nonresponse and when possible to incorporate the most proximal LV electrode for pacing. By doing so, multisite pacing can convert a significant proportion of CRT nonresponders into responders with a minimal impact on battery longevity.

Optimization of Cardiac Resynchronization Delivery and Programming

Failing hearts depend more on properly timed atrial contraction than normal hearts. This property clarifies why optimal timing of atrial and ventricular stimulation is of special interest in patients with HF. Well established is the concept that pacemakers can actually improve the coupling between atria and ventricles over that without pacing. This issue applies to patients with excessively long PQ times where the hemodynamic benefit was achieved with AV sequential pacing at a physiologic interval. These beneficial effects are striking, because these studies were performed before the era of resynchronization therapy and the RV apex was used as ventricular pacing site. Although the role of the atrial contraction in patients with dilated ventricles and low ejection fraction varies among individuals, the importance of appropriate AV timing in improving cardiac output in patients receiving CRT is undoubted. Therefore, all device manufacturers have developed and implemented algorithms to automatically manage AV coupling. Some of these algorithms are currently tested in prospective multicenter studies, as shown in **Table 5**.

Device Selection

The mortality benefit of CRT-D over CRT-P is still unclear, mostly because no head-to-head comparison study has been conducted to compare the two treatment modalities. COMPANION is the only prospective clinical trial to randomize patients to CRT-D and CRT-P. CRT-P was associated with a marginally nonsignificant reduction in the risk of all-cause mortality, whereas CRT-D was associated with a significant, 36% risk reduction.[8] A large multicenter registry including more than 50,000 patients indicated that CRT-D was associated with a significantly lower

mortality. This finding is consistent with a propensity-matched cohort study,[29] as well as with the CeRtiTuDe cohort study.[30] Notably, some recent large observational studies and the DANISH study highlighted the importance of cause of HF in the assessment of potential benefits of CRT-D over CRT-P. Notably, most of the trials and registries have been conducted before sacubitril-valsartan or sodium glucose transport protein 2 (SGLT 2) inhibitors were available or not yet considered standard of care.[31] It is possible that improved HF therapy might improve LV remodeling and hence reduce the risk of malignant arrhythmias and sudden cardiac death. Important novel information on the issue of CRT-D versus CRT-P in patients with HF treated with modern medical therapy is expected to come from an ongoing trial, Re-evaluation of Optimal Re-synchronization Therapy in Patients with Heart Failure (RESET-CRT). RESET-CRT is a prospective, multicenter study currently randomizing patients with symptomatic HF with reduced LVEF less than or equal to 35%, who are on optimal medical treatment and have a CRT primary prevention indication, to receive either CRT-P or CRT-D. Aim of the study is to demonstrate noninferiority of CRT-P over CRT-D. No distinction is made regarding ischemic or nonischemic cause of HF for inclusion to the study. The researchers plan to include more than 1300 patients with an estimated median follow-up period of 29 to 40 months. The primary end point is time to all-cause death, and the study is estimated to be complete by August 2024. Other important studies in better defining patients who may benefit most from CRT-D are listed in **Table 6**.

Finally, there are several ongoing studies investigating special situations around CRT investigating the changes in electromechanical remodeling after CRT or the role of sleep apnea in patients with CRT and vice versa (**Table 7**).

SUMMARY

After decades of clinical use, CRT can be considered an established therapy. Despite that, there are still multiple open questions to be addressed that shall further improve the proportion of patients who respond to CRT. Progress in better understanding the profound relationship between electrical and mechanical disorder in patients with HF with ventricular conduction abnormalities is of paramount importance. Similarly of great clinical importance is the understanding of choice of the most appropriate device and of optimal programming and pacing site.

CLINICS CARE POINTS

- QRS duration and LBBB morphology are currently considered the most reliable biomarkers for selecting CRT candidates. However, ECG criteria to classify LBBB significantly differ among scientific organizations, investigators, trials, and guidelines, which may pose uncertainty in meta-analytical investigations and comparison of outcomes. Novel biomarkers are therefore investigated.

- There is robust evidence that patients in sinus rhythm, reduced LVEF, QRS duration greater than 150 ms, and LBBB benefit most from CRT. In contrast, clinical practice guidelines have a lower level of evidence for patients with non-LBBB morphology or patients in AF. Several ongoing trials are now focused to evaluate novel approaches to improve outcome of patients with non-LBBB QRS morphology.

- An area of intense research has always been the investigation of the most optimal LV lead positioning and whether a mechanical or electrical target shall be aimed. Several studies have shown that pacing the LV in a region of late activation results in larger LV reverse remodeling, better quality of life, and improved survival of patients on CRT. Multimodality cardiac imaging approaches to select target area for lead placement are currently tested in several prospective controlled trials.

- The mortality benefit of CRT-D over CRT-P is still unclear, mostly because no head-to-head comparison study has been conducted to compare the two treatment modalities. Important novel information on the issue of CRT-D versus CRT-P in patients with HF treated with modern medical therapy is expected to come from an ongoing trial.

DISCLOSURE

A. Auricchio: consultant to Boston Scientific, Backbeat, Biosense Webster, Cairdac, Corvia, Microport CRM, EPD-Philips, Radcliffe Publisher. He received speaker fees from Abbott, Boston Scientific, Medtronic, and Microport. He participates in clinical trials sponsored by Boston Scientific, Medtronic, EPD-Philips. He has intellectual properties with Boston Scientific, Biosense Webster, and Microport CRM. T. Özkartal: nothing to disclose.

REFERENCES

1. Cazeau S, Leclercq C, Lavergne T, et al. Multisite Stimulation in Cardiomyopathies (MUSTIC) Study Investigators. Effects of multisite biventricular pacing in patients with heart failure and intraventricular conduction delay. N Engl J Med 2001;344(12):873–80.

2. Tang AS, Wells GA, Talajic M, et al. Resynchronization-defibrillation for ambulatory heart failure trial investigators. Cardiac-resynchronization therapy for mild-to-moderate heart failure. N Engl J Med 2010; 363(25):2385–95.

3. Linde C, Leclercq C, Rex S, et al. Long-term benefits of biventricular pacing in congestive heart failure: results from the MUltisite STimulation in cardiomyopathy (MUSTIC) study. J Am Coll Cardiol 2002;40(1): 111–8.

4. Auricchio A, Stellbrink C, Sack S, et al. Pacing Therapies in Congestive Heart Failure (PATH-CHF) Study Group. Long-term clinical effect of hemodynamically optimized cardiac resynchronization therapy in patients with heart failure and ventricular conduction delay. J Am Coll Cardiol 2002;39(12):2026–33.

5. Young JB, Abraham WT, Smith AL, et al. Multicenter InSync ICD randomized clinical evaluation (MIRACLE ICD) trial investigators. Combined cardiac resynchronization and implantable cardioversion defibrillation in advanced chronic heart failure: the MIRACLE ICD Trial. JAMA 2003;289(20):2685–94.

6. Moss AJ, Hall WJ, Cannom DS, et al. MADIT-CRT Trial Investigators. Cardiac-resynchronization therapy for the prevention of heart-failure events. N Engl J Med 2009;361(14):1329–38.

7. Abraham WT, Young JB, León AR, et al. Multicenter InSync ICD II Study Group. Effects of cardiac resynchronization on disease progression in patients with left ventricular systolic dysfunction, an indication for an implantable cardioverter-defibrillator, and mildly symptomatic chronic heart failure. Circulation 2004;110(18):2864–8.

8. Bristow MR, Saxon LA, Boehmer J, et al. Comparison of medical therapy, pacing, and defibrillation in heart failure (COMPANION) Investigators. Cardiac-resynchronization therapy with or without an implantable defibrillator in advanced chronic heart failure. N Engl J Med 2004;350(21):2140–50.

9. Cleland JG, Daubert JC, Erdmann E, et al. Cardiac Resynchronization-Heart Failure (CARE-HF) Study Investigators. The effect of cardiac resynchronization on morbidity and mortality in heart failure. N Engl J Med 2005;352(15):1539–49.

10. Glikson M, Nielsen JC, Kronborg MB, et al, ESC Scientific Document Group. 2021 ESC Guidelines on cardiac pacing and cardiac resynchronization therapy. Eur Heart J 2021;42(35):3427–520.

11. Kusumoto FM, Schoenfeld MH, Barrett C, et al. 2018 ACC/AHA/HRS guideline on the evaluation and

management of patients with bradycardia and cardiac conduction delay: a report of the American College of Cardiology/American Heart Association Task Force on Clinical Practice Guidelines and the Heart Rhythm Society. Circulation 2019;140(8):e382–482 [Erratum appears in Circulation 2019;140(8):e506-e508].

12. Auricchio A, Prinzen FW. Enhancing response in the cardiac resynchronization therapy patient: the 3B perspective-bench, bits, and bedside. JACC Clin Electrophysiol 2017;3(11):1203–19.

13. Mullens W, Auricchio A, Martens P, et al. Optimized implementation of cardiac resynchronization therapy: a call for action for referral and optimization of care: a joint position statement from the Heart Failure Association (HFA), European Heart Rhythm Association (EHRA), and European Association of Cardiovascular Imaging (EACVI) of the European Society of Cardiology. Eur J Heart Fail 2020;22(12):2349–69.

14. Caputo ML, van Stipdonk A, Illner A, et al. The definition of left bundle branch block influences the response to cardiac resynchronization therapy. Int J Cardiol 2018;269:165–9.

15. Surawicz B, Childers R, Deal BJ, et al. American Heart Association Electrocardiography and Arrhythmias Committee, Council on Clinical Cardiology; American College of Cardiology Foundation; Heart Rhythm Society. AHA/ACCF/HRS recommendations for the standardization and interpretation of the electrocardiogram: part III: intraventricular conduction disturbances: a scientific statement from the American Heart Association Electrocardiography and Arrhythmias Committee, Council on Clinical Cardiology; the American College of Cardiology Foundation; and the Heart Rhythm Society. Endorsed by the International Society for Computerized Electrocardiology. J Am Coll Cardiol 2009; 53(11):976–81.

16. Brignole M, Pentimalli F, Palmisano P, et al. AV junction ablation and cardiac resynchronization for patients with permanent atrial fibrillation and narrow QRS: the APAF-CRT mortality trial. Eur Heart J 2021; ehab569. https://doi.org/10.1093/eurheartj/ehab569.

17. Merkely B, Kosztin A, Roka A, et al. Rationale and design of the BUDAPEST-CRT Upgrade Study: a prospective, randomized, multicentre clinical trial. Europace 2017;19(9):1549–55.

18. Maffessanti F, Jadczyk T, Kurzelowski R, et al. The influence of scar on the spatio-temporal relationship between electrical and mechanical activation in heart failure patients. Europace. 2020 May 1;22(5):777-786. [Erratum in:Europace 2020;22(5):786].

19. Borgquist R, Carlsson M, Markstad H, et al. Cardiac resynchronization therapy guided by echocardiography, MRI, and CT Imaging: a Randomized Controlled Study. JACC Clin Electrophysiol 2020; 6(10):1300–9.

20. Singh JP, Berger RD, Doshi RN, et al, ENHANCE CRT Study Group. Targeted left ventricular lead implantation strategy for non-left bundle branch block patients: the ENHANCE CRT Study. JACC Clin Electrophysiol 2020;6(9):1171–81.

21. Niazi I, Baker J 2nd, Corbisiero R, et al. MPP investigators. safety and efficacy of multipoint pacing in cardiac resynchronization therapy: the MultiPoint Pacing Trial. JACC Clin Electrophysiol 2017;3(13):1510–8.

22. Leclercq C, Gadler F, Kranig W, et al. TRIP-HF (triple resynchronization in paced heart failure patients) Study Group. A randomized comparison of triple-site versus dual-site ventricular stimulation in patients with congestive heart failure. J Am Coll Cardiol 2008;51(15):1455–62.

23. Pappone C, Ćalović Ž, Vicedomini G, et al. Improving cardiac resynchronization therapy response with multipoint left ventricular pacing: twelve-month follow-up study. Heart Rhythm 2015;12(6):1250–8.

24. Osca J, Alonso P, Cano O, et al. The use of multisite left ventricular pacing via quadripolar lead improves acute haemodynamics and mechanical dyssynchrony assessed by radial strain speckle tracking: initial results. Europace 2016;18(4):560–7.

25. Mehta VS, Elliott MK, Sidhu BS, et al. Multipoint pacing for cardiac resynchronisation therapy in patients with heart failure: a systematic review and meta-analysis. J Cardiovasc Electrophysiol 2021;32(9):2577–89.

26. Leclercq C, Burri H, Curnis A, et al. Cardiac resynchronization therapy non-responder to responder conversion rate in the more response to cardiac resynchronization therapy with MultiPoint Pacing (MORE-CRT MPP) study: results from Phase I. Eur Heart J 2019;40(35):2979–87.

27. Almusaad A, Sweidan R, Alanazi H, et al. Long-term reverse remodeling and clinical improvement by MultiPoint Pacing in a randomized, international, middle Eastern heart failure study. J Interv Card Electrophysiol 2021. https://doi.org/10.1007/s10840-020-00928-2. Epub ahead of print.

28. Nunes Ferreira A, Antonio PS, Aguiar-Ricardo I, et al. P578Multipoint pacing in cardiac resynchronization therapy - how to improve remodeling criteria and its impact in quality of life. EP Europace 2020;22(Suppl_1). https://doi.org/10.1093/europace/euaa162.085.

29. Leyva F, Zegard A, Okafor O, et al. Survival after cardiac resynchronization therapy: results from 50 084 implantations. Europace 2019;21(5):754–62.

30. Marijon E, Leclercq C, Narayanan K, et al. CeRtiTuDe Investigators. Causes-of-death analysis of patients with cardiac resynchronization therapy: an analysis of the CeRtiTuDe cohort study. Eur Heart J 2015;36(41):2767–76.

31. McDonagh TA, Metra M, Adamo M, et al, ESC Scientific Document Group. 2021 ESC Guidelines for the diagnosis and treatment of acute and chronic heart failure. Eur Heart J 2021;42(36):3599–726.

Generating Evidence to Support the Physiologic Promise of Conduction System Pacing

Status and Update on Conduction System Pacing Trials

Nandita Kaza, MBChB, Daniel Keene, PhD*, Zachary I. Whinnett, PhD

KEYWORDS

- His bundle pacing • Left bundle branch area pacing • Physiologic pacing
- Randomized controlled trials

KEY POINTS

- Conduction system pacing (CSP) approaches using His bundle or left bundle branch area pacing have been demonstrated to be technically feasible with a favorable safety profile.
- Modestly sized clinical trials have explored the physiologic benefits offered by conduction system pacing across using key imaging and hemodynamic parameters.
- Future trials focusing on clinical end points will further establish the role of CSP as an alternative to RV pacing for bradycardia and biventricular CRT for patients with heart failure, and for those with AF following AV node ablation.
- A large body of observational data supports the use of CSP for patients with bradycardia, suggesting its role in avoiding the potentially deleterious effects of right ventricular (RV) pacing.
- Randomized evidence is needed to establish CSP approaches as the standard of care in eligible patients with bradycardia indications.

INTRODUCTION

Conduction system pacing (CSP) includes pacing at either the His bundle or left bundle locations, which is termed left bundle pacing or left bundle area pacing (LBAP). The technique of His bundle pacing (HBP) has developed over the past 20 years, whereas left bundle pacing was first reported less than 5 years ago. Both approaches target locations within the heart's intrinsic conduction system to deliver rapid ventricular activation. The aim of CSP is to avoid the potential deleterious effects associated with nonphysiologic electrical activation from right ventricular (RV) pacing, or to provide cardiac resynchronization to patients with heart failure.

Increasing numbers of cardiologists around the world have taken up CSP, producing observational data demonstrating safety and feasibility, as well as the suggestion of improved clinical outcomes.[1–4] There is much less data available from randomized controlled trials (RCTs).[5–8] These RCTs have focused on physiologic (imaging or hemodynamic) end points. There are several ongoing and planned trials that are designed to assess the effect of CSP when used for various clinical

N. Kaza and D. Keene are joint first authors.

National Heart and Lung Institute, Imperial College London, Hammersmith Hospital, London W12 0HS, UK

* Corresponding author.

E-mail address: d.keene@imperial.ac.uk

Card Electrophysiol Clin 14 (2022) 345–355
https://doi.org/10.1016/j.ccep.2022.01.002
1877-9182/22/© 2022 Elsevier Inc. All rights reserved.

indications; these include the treatment of brady-cardia andheart failure (as an alternative to biventricular pacing) as well as a method for delivering ventricular pacing following atrioventricular node ablation.

In this review we outline the main findings from observational studies and the available prospective data and provide an overview of the current ongoing trials. We have also set out areas where we believe further RCTs are required.

Evidence of Safety and Feasibility: A mandatory requirement for large-scale clinical trials.

Observational datasets have provided evidence that both HBP and LBAP can be safely delivered with relatively high implant success rates using currently available tools. These studies report HBP implantation success rates of ~86% (range 59%–100%).[1–4,8–13] There is evidence of a learning curve, with an increase in implant success rates with greater operator experience in HBP.[14] Another factor that seems to influence implant success rate is the pacing indication, with infra-Hisian block and left bundle branch block being more challenging than other indications.[14] Lead reintervention rates are similar to those seen with coronary sinus pacing leads (~7%), but higher than those observed with conventional RV pacing (~3%).[15,16] The main reported reason for reintervention is increase in capture thresholds, rather than macrodisplacement of the lead. The observation of late threshold increases during HBP, using currently available leads and implantation tools, provided the stimulus to target more distal sites within the conduction system.

LBAP using a transseptal approach has been shown to be feasible, with high implant success rates (81%–94%) and low complication rates reported in several observational studies.[17–25] LBAP has also been found to have a learning curve (~50 cases).[26] Given its relative novelty, no prolonged follow-up data are available. However, the data from the ~1200 cases published are encouraging: stable capture thresholds and low rates of lead dislodgement (1%); but septal perforation (2%) has been reported.[27]

Therefore there is a growing body of evidence from observational studies which suggests that CSP is technically feasible in many patients using existing tools. On the basis of these observational data and the potential physiologic advantages, a growing number of implanters worldwide have taken up CSP in recent years. However, CSP still constitutes only a small proportion of the pacemakers implanted worldwide every year.

One of the barriers to greater uptake is the need for data from prospective studies and RCTs. Observational data are susceptible to the potential

for reporting bias. Many operators are therefore waiting for randomized evidence demonstrating improved outcomes with CSP compared with conventional pacing approaches, before they change practice.

Conduction System Pacing: A Suitable Treatment for Bradycardia?

RV pacing produces nonphysiologic ventricular activation, which is believed to be the mechanism for pacing-induced cardiomyopathy, which occurs in approximately 25% (12%–37%) of patients, as judged by clinical event rates in RCTs.[2,16,28] The observation that the incidence of heart failure increases, as RV pacing percentage increases, supports the concept that dyssynchronous ventricular activation is the trigger for pacing-induced cardiomyopathy in susceptible individuals.[28] In some patients, a deterioration in cardiac function or symptoms is noted within weeks to months; however, for many patients, these deleterious effects may take years to manifest.[29]

The desire to avoid the harmful effects of nonphysiologic ventricular activation has been one of the main drivers in the development of CSP. Data from randomized CSP studies with physiologic end points support the concept that preserving normal physiologic activation produces positive effects on ventricular function.[30–32] In a randomized hemodynamic study, Kronborg and colleagues[30] observed improved mean left ventricular (LV) ejection fraction (LVEF) (55% ± 10% vs 50% ± 11%) and reduced LVESV (42 ± 21 mL vs 49 ± 26 mL) after 12 months of HBP compared with those randomized to RVP. LBAP has been shown to offer similar mechanical synchrony to that achieved with both HBP (assessed through myocardial perfusion imaging) and native conduction.[33–35]

Randomized Controlled Clinical Outcome Trials

No randomized controlled clinical outcome trial of CSP in this population currently exists. There are currently 8 registered RCTs (**Table 1**), aiming to address this gap in evidence for CSP. Many of the trials listed on clinicaltrials.gov focus on LBAP (only 2 for HBP) and rely on imaging end points or upgrade to biventricular pacing as trial end points. The aim of using these end points is to minimize the duration of follow-up and patient numbers required in these studies. Although these studies will be of immense value to the field, we believe that wholly clinical end point RCTs will be required to stimulate a global change in practice away from RV pacing as the default pacing method for patients with a bradycardia indication.

For a CSP trial to show definitive reductions in mortality and heart failure events, we anticipate that a future study would need a median follow-up of 4 years and in excess of 2000 patients.

Abbreviations: AV, atrioventricular; AVB, HFH, LVESI; NYHA, New York Heart Association; PI, principal investigator; PICM.

Thus far, results from randomized hemodynamic studies are consistent with finding from observational studies. Favorable effects have been observed with CSP; a meta-analysis of 1438 patients from observational studies found that patients who began with normal LV function had preservation of LV function and those who began with reduced LV function actually had an increase of ~11 percentage points with HBP ($P < .001$).[3] This observation is in contrast to known deleterious effects of RVP on LV function.[6] Meta-analyses have also documented significant improvements in New York Heart Association (NYHA) class, paced QRS duration, measures of ventricular dyssynchrony, and 6-minute walk test duration with CSP over RVP.[4,10] Whether these multiple favorable mechanistic indicators translate into reduced mortality and morbidity now needs to be tested in adequately powered RCTs.

Observational studies with clinical end points have reported lower morbidity and mortality with CSP compared with RVP. The largest report shows a hazard ratio of 0.65 (25.3% vs 35.6%, $P = .02$) for mortality and heart failure hospitalization.[36]

However, only an RCT can test whether this is a genuine mechanistic causation or merely a reflection of undocumented differences between patient groups or operators.

Improving the Ablate-and-Pace Treatment Approach?

Deshmukh and colleagues[37] first described the effects of HBP in patients with heart failure and atrial fibrillation undergoing AVN ablation. Observations included improved LVEF, LV dimensions, and exercise capacity. A randomized crossover trial conducted by Occhetta and colleagues[38] demonstrated significant improvement in NYHA class and exercise tolerance with HBP pacing compared with RVP. Similar positive outcomes in LVEF and NYHA class have since been reported in observational studies with no signal of significant harm, although it is noted that ablation sites close to the HBP lead tip can lead to increased capture threshold.[39–43]

The recent APAF-CRT trial showed a 74% relative risk reduction in mortality with biventricular pacing and AVN ablation compared with rate control strategies alone[44,45]; this was in patients with narrow QRS duration at recruitment, in whom the paced QRS duration was subsequently prolonged with biventricular pacing. The mechanism of benefit is likely due to ventricular rate regularization and control, but BVP is known to produce ventricular electrical dyssynchrony compared with normal intrinsic ventricular activation, which has the potential to offset some of the beneficial effects.

The recent ALTERNATIVE trial randomized patients with persistent AF, LV impairment, and narrow QRS duration to either LBAP or BVP pacing. Symptomatic improvement was observed with both pacing approaches, but LBAP delivered additional improvements in left ventricular ejection fraction.[46]

The His-PAAF study (NCT04512586) is currently recruiting patients with AF and heart failure (LVEF<35%) across 4 centers in Sweden. The study aims to randomize 90 patients to either pulmonary vein isolation or AVN ablation combined with HBP, evaluating quality of life as the primary outcome.

Patient-reported outcomes are becoming increasingly important in trial design and are important end points to consider particularly when comparing CSP with biventricular pacing where differences in clinical end points are likely to be smaller than those observed when comparing CSP with RV pacing. An additional advantage of CSP compared with BVP is that it can be delivered with a single lead.

Conduction System Pacing for Heart Failure

His bundle pacing for cardiac resynchronization therapy

Biventricular pacing is a very well-established treatment of patients with heart failure and evidence of electrical ventricular dyssynchrony (particularly left bundle branch block [LBBB]). Multiple large, randomized studies have demonstrated improvements in cardiac function and importantly, reductions in morbidity and mortality.[47,48]

Despite its established role in delivering cardiac resynchronization therapy (CRT), biventricular pacing has potential limitations. First, it is not always possible to successfully implant an LV lead; second, it may deliver incomplete ventricular resynchronization and as a result may not be delivering the maximum potential improvements in cardiac function; and finally, it may not be best suited

Table 1
Summary of registered trials investigating conduction system pacing for bradycardia consistency between observational and randomized controlled trial data

Trial Name, Status, & PI	Inclusion	Intervention & Comparator	Design	Recruitment Target (n)	Primary Outcome(s)	Follow-up Duration (months)
His-PACE NCT04672408 Not yet recruiting Single center, Haran Burri (PI)	Bradycardia indication with expected rate of ventricular pacing >20, LVEF >40%	His bundle pacing and RV pacing	Randomized, crossover, double blind	50	LVEF	6 mo
HIS-PrEF NCT04529577 Recruiting 3 centers, Rasmus Borgquist (PI)	Second- or third-degree AV block with high expected rate of ventricular pacing, LVEF 40%–55%	His bundle pacing and RV pacing	Randomized, crossover, double blind	40	LVEF	12 mo
LEAP Trial -NL Netherlands Trial Registry 9672 Recruiting Justin Luermans (PI)	Bradycardia indication including second- or third-degree AVB or atrial arrhythmia with slow ventricular conduction and expected ventricular pacing percentage >20%, LVEF >35%	LV septal pacing vs RV pacing	Randomized, double blind,	470	Composite of all-cause mortality, HFH, and 10% decrease in LVEF leading to LVEF <50% at follow-up	12 mo
OptimPacing NCT04624763 Not yet recruiting 11 centers, Jiangang Zou (PI)	Bradycardia indication (second- or third-degree AV block or AF with mean ventricular rate <50 bpm and associated symptoms), NYHA class I–III, LVEF >35%	Left bundle branch pacing vs RV pacing	Randomized, double blind	683	Composite of all-cause mortality, HFH, and PICM at 6, 12, 24, and 36 mo	36 mo

LEFT-HF NCT 05015660 Not yet recruitingSingle centre, Jacqueline Joza (PI)	Bradycardia indication where expected ventricular pacing rate is >90%, LVEF >50%	Left bundle pacing vs RV pacing	Randomized, single blind	100	LVESI, successful implant and feasibility of recruitment	24 mo
ChiCTR200003433 5 Recruiting	AV block	Left bundle branch area pacing vs RV apical pacing	Randomized, single blind	210	LVEF	Unknown

to delivering treatment to patients with alternative, non-LBBB electrical treatment targets. These reasons have prompted the evaluation of alternative methods for delivering cardiac resynchronization. CSP already shows considerable promise as an alternative to BVP in patients with LBBB, as well as a potential method for expanding indications for pacing therapy for heart failure beyond LBBB to alternative electrical conduction abnormalities.

Three RCTs have been published; one has been completed and is awaiting publication and one is in the planning/recruiting stages according to clinicaltrials.gov (a further trial is registered in the Chinese Online Registry of Clinical Trials) (Table 2).

The first trial comparing HBP with biventricular pacing was published in 2015.[5] This trial was conducted while HBP experience and tools were limited. In this small feasibility trial, 29 patients (median age 71 years, 34% female, mean ejection fraction [EF] 26.5%) were recruited to undergo implantation of devices capable of providing both biventricular pacing and HBP. Patients experienced 6-month periods in each pacing mode in a crossover fashion with only 12 patients completing the trial. Patients predominantly exited the trial due to inability to deploy a His lead or lack of QRS narrowing with HBP. Of patients completing the trial protocol, clinical response was similar to BiV pacing: QoL, left ventricular EF, NYHA class, and 6-minute walk test showed similar improvements with no significant difference observed between the two.

More recently, the His-Sync RCT compared HBP with biventricular pacing for patients with typical CRT heart failure indications.[6] This small trial randomized 41 patients (age 64 ± 13 years, 38% female, EF = 28%) to conventional BiV-CRT or HBP-CRT. Intention-to-treat analysis did not reveal significant differences (for QRS shortening, LVEF improvement, or cardiovascular morbidity).

Interpretation of His-Sync requires consideration of the mandated crossover rules and crossover rates to better appreciate the potential patient benefits when HBP is successfully delivered. Of the 21 patients randomized to His-CRT, only 11 received successful HBP implantation, (obligated to achieve QRS narrowing by >20% or QRS width of ≤130 ms). Those who did not fulfill these criteria or those who demonstrated high correction thresholds (>5 V at 1 ms) were mandated to crossover to BiV-CRT. It is worth noting that approximately half of the patients who crossed from HBP to biventricular had non-LBBB at baseline. Of note in parallel, unfavorable coronary sinus anatomy meant that 26% of patients intended for biventricular pacing crossed over to receive HBP.

In the per-protocol analysis, which provides insight for the potential benefit that could be expected when HBP is successfully delivered, QRS narrowing was greater (124 ± 19 ms vs 162 ± 24 ms; P < .001) and there was a trend toward higher rate of echocardiographic response (91% vs 54%, P = .078).

Once HBP was delivered, it was safe and reliable with no lead displacements during the follow-up period. These findings suggest that as a minimum HBP is an acceptable bailout for failed left ventricular lead implantation if it can be delivered with shortening of the QRS duration. Based on per-protocol analysis, the findings are hypothesis generating that its effect could be superior.[7]

The most recent trial assessing CSP for delivering CRT included 50 patients (age 65.7 years, 18% female, EF 30%) with typical LBBB pattern and LVEF less than 35% and randomized patients to either BiV CRT or His-CRT.[8]

When compared with the His-Sync study, the His-Alternative trial included a more select population of CRT-eligible patients, that is, only those with typical LBBB. The primary outcome was successful His lead implantation, capture of the left bundle, and maintenance of this for 6 months; this was achieved in 72% of those assigned to His-CRT. Seven patients crossed over from the His-CRT group to BiV-CRT and one patient crossed over from BiV-CRT to His-CRT. After 6 month no significant difference in LVEF was seen between the groups following intention-to-treat analysis. Per-protocol analysis, however, revealed a significantly higher LVEF (48% vs 42%, P < .05) in the His-CRT group as well as a lower LVESV (65 mL vs 83 mL, P < .05), although at the expense of higher pacing thresholds (2.2 ± 1.2 V vs 1.1 ± 0.7 V; P < .001). Although a single-center study limited by a small sample size, this trial found electrocardiographic and echocardiographic improvements conferred by successful HBP for CRT, which provides further support for future trials to evaluate clinical outcomes to secure its role as a guideline-indicated alternative to BiV-CRT.

These prospective studies of HBP in CRT-eligible patients (as opposed to those with bradycardia indications) report 52% to 72% implant success rates.[5–8] Lead complication rates were low in these studies with only 1 lead-related complication reported in the His-Alternative study (with 1 lead-related complication noted with BiV pacing as well) and no lead complications in the His- Sync study, although follow-up duration was short (6 months).[5–8]

Table 2

Summary of published and registered trials investigating conduction system pacing for heart failure published randomized controlled trials

Trial Name, Status & Principal Investigator	Year	Intervention and Comparator	Design	Sample Size Recruitment Target (n)	Follow-up (months)
Daniel Lustgarten Published	2015	His bundle pacing and biventricular pacing (CRT indications)	Randomized crossover, patient blinded	29 (12 completing crossover analysis)	12
His-Sync Guarav Upadhyay Published	2019	His bundle pacing and biventricular pacing (CRT indications)	Randomized, double blind	41	6
His-Alternative Michael Vinther Published	2021	His bundle pacing and biventricular pacing (LBBB indications)	Randomized, double blind	50	6
Hope-HF Zachary Whinnett Completed awaiting publication	2021	AV-optimized His pacing or backup pacing only (prolonged PR indication)	Randomized crossover, double blind	167	12
LBBP-RESYNC (NCT04110431) Jiangang Zou Recruiting	2021 (expected completion)	Left bundle pacing and biventricular pacing	Randomized, double blind	40	6
ChiCTR2000028726 Yongqang Wu Recruiting	2022 (Expected completion)	Left bundle area pacing and biventricular pacing	Randomized	180	18

Based on the findings of currently available data, His-CRT has now been included in international guidelines (ESC and AHA), in case of failure to implant an LV lead.[49,50]

Left Bundle Area Pacing for Cardiac Resynchronization Therapy

Observational studies have reported impressive reductions in QRS duration and improved mechanical synchrony when LBAP is delivered to patients with heart failure and LBBB.[34–36]

Data from 4 observational studies (n = 100) suggest that ventricular resynchronization delivered with LBAP translates into improvements in cardiac function.[17–20] In a meta-analysis of these observational studies, combined with 2 single-arm studies of LBAP for CRT (LBAP n = 174), average baseline LVEF increased from 30.2% ± 1.7% to 48.8% ± 4.8% at follow-up (P < .0001).[21] This meta-analysis also reported improvements in BNP, NYHA class. Since the publication of this meta-analysis, 3 further observational studies have been published exploring the role of LBAP for heart failure.[22–24] These studies report similar findings, with greater improvements in QRS duration brought about by LBAP; however, there was no significant difference in echocardiographic response compared with BiV pacing.

Therefore observational data suggest that LBAP-CRT is an effective treatment of patients with LBBB and heart failure, which supports further investigation in randomized controlled studies to assess the efficacy of LBAP compared with BiV pacing for CRT. The following 2 clinical trials in progress are seeking to answer this question.

LBBP-RESYNC (NCT04110431) has randomized 40 patients with LVEF less than 35% and typical LBBB to either left bundle or BiV pacing; the primary outcome is change in LVEF, LVESV, and LVEDV compared with baseline after 6 months follow-up. Cheng and colleagues[51] are performing a randomized single-center noninferiority trial, again focusing on LVEF as their primary outcome.

The His-Alt investigators are currently recruiting to a further trial (His-Alt_2, NCT 04409119), randomizing 80 patients to His/LBAP and 45 patients to BiV pacing. His-Alt_2 aims to evaluate noninferiority for His or LBAP for the primary binary end point of a change in LVESV, defined as a decrease of greater than 15% from baseline.

Although these studies are recruiting small numbers of patients and focusing on surrogate (echo) end points, these studies will be pivotal in further demonstrating the feasibility of LBAP-CRT

in prospective studies. If the findings are positive then they will provide the justification for further larger studies assessing clinical end points, which we believe are required in order for CSP to be recommended as a first-line treatment of CRT in international guidelines.

Expanding Heart Failure Cardiac Resynchronization Therapy Indications

BiV pacing seems to be most beneficial in patients with heart failure and LBBB.[52] However, many patients with heart failure do not have LBBB, and there is therefore interest in determining whether pacing therapy for heart failure can deliver improvements in patients who have alternative electrical treatment targets. CSP may be a more suitable method, than BVP, for treating these potential alternative treatment targets.

Right Bundle Branch Block

Patients with right bundle branch block (RBBB) are a group of patients who have been shown to have limited benefit from biventricular pacing.[53] BVP may prolong left ventricular activation relative to intrinsic conduction in patients with RBBB, whereas HBP can preserve normal physiologic left ventricular activation and correct RBBB and as a result has the potential to deliver more effective ventricular resynchronization. An observational study of HBP has shown benefit in this group when compared with baseline.[12] HBP corrected RBBB in 78% of patients and improved NYHA class and LVEF from 31% ± 10% to 39 ± 13% (P = .004).[23] No RCT to date has focused on this group of patients.

Prolonged PR

A prolonged PR interval has been shown to be an adverse prognostic marker in heart failure.[54] The multicenter double-blind HOPE-HF trial, randomized 167 patients with LV impairment, narrow QRS, or RBBB with a prolonged PR interval (>200 ms) to AV-optimized His pacing or backup pacing only.[55] This trial is the largest multicenter CSP randomized trial that has been conducted to date. Results presented at AHA 2021 report that HBP maintained ventricular synchrony (in contrast to other forms of pacing, which prolong ventricular activation relative to intrinsic conduction), and although no significant improvement in MVO2 was observed (primary outcome), there was a significant improvement in blinded QOL measured using the Minnesota Living With Heart Failure Questionnaire and most participants preferred the His pacing period.[56]

SUMMARY

CSP is becoming an increasingly popular form of pacing, with increasing numbers of implanters worldwide. CSP has been included in international guidelines, based on the evidence of safety and feasibility obtained from observational studies and small randomized studies. There is, however, still a need for large-scale randomized trials, focusing on clinical end points, to better define the role of CSP. Positive trials will trigger a step change in implant behavior, whereas negative trials are likely to temper the enthusiasm brought about by the physiologic promise of these approaches.

CLINICS CARE POINTS

- International guidelines for cardiac pacing now include recommendations on the use of CSP, providing a basis for cardiologists to incorporate the technique into their clinical practice where appropriate.

- Acquiring skills for delivering CSP can provide a pacing approach that delivers a solution for several indications across the spectrum of patients presenting with bradycardia and/or heart failure.

- CSP provides an option for delivering CRT to patients in whom biventricular pacing has not been successful (within the same patient visit).

- Clinicians adopting CSP into their practice for the first time should be aware there is a well-documented learning curve (30–50 cases) across CSP approaches.

DISCLOSURE

D. Keene and Z.I. Whinnett receive honorarium from Medtronic for teaching.

REFERENCES

1. Barakat AF, Inashvili A, Alkukhun L, et al. Use trends and adverse reports of selectsecure 3830 lead implantations in the United States: implications for his bundle pacing. Circ Arrhythm Electrophysiol 2020; 13(7):e008577.

2. Abdelrahman M, Subzposh FA, Beer D, et al. Clinical outcomes of his bundle pacing compared to right ventricular pacing. J Am Coll Cardiol 2018; 71(20):2319–30.

3. Zanon F, Ellenbogen KA, Dandamudi G, et al. Permanent His-bundle pacing: a systematic literature review and meta-analysis. Europace 2018;20(11): 1819–26.

4. Yu Z, Chen R, Su Y, et al. Integrative and quantitive evaluation of the efficacy of his bundle related pacing in comparison with conventional right ventricular pacing: a meta-analysis. BMC Cardiovasc Disord 2017;17(1):221.

5. Lustgarten D, Crespo E, Arkhipova-Jenkins I. His bundle pacing versus biventricular pacing in cardiac resynchronisation therapy patients: a crossover design comparison. Heart Rhythm 2015;12:7.

6. Upadhyay GA, Vijayraman P, Nayak HM. His corrective pacing or biventricular pacing for conduction system pacing in heart failure. J Am Coll Cardiol 2019;74(1):157–66.

7. Upadhyay GA, Vijayaraman P, Nayak HM, et al. On-treatment comparison between corrective His bundle pacing and biventricular pacing for cardiacresynchronization: a secondary analysis of His-SYNC. Heart Rhythm 2019;16(12):1797–807.

8. Vinther M Risum N, Hastrup J. A randomized trial of his pacing versus biventricular pacing in symptomatic HF patients with left bundle branch block (His-ALT). J Am Coll Cardiol.2021;7(11):1422–1432.

9. Vijayaraman P, Naperkowski A, Subzposh FA, et al. Permanent His-bundle pacing: Long-term lead performance and clinical outcomes. Heart Rhythm 2018;15(5):696–702.

10. Slotwiner DJ, Raitt MH, Del-Carpio Munoz F, et al. Impact of physiologic pacing versus right ventricular pacing among patients with left ventricular ejection fraction greater than 35%: a systematic review for the 2018 ACC/AHA/HRS guideline on the evaluation and management of patients with bradycardia and cardiac conduction delay: a report of the american college of cardiology/american heart association task force on clinical practice guidelines and the heart rhythm society. J Am Coll Cardiol 2019;74(7): 988–1008.

11. Fernandes GC, Knijnik L, Lopez J, et al. Network meta-analysis of His bundle, biventricular, or right ventricular pacing as a primary strategy for advanced atrioventricular conduction disease with normal or mildly reduced ejection fraction. J Cardiovasc Electrophysiol 2020;31(6):1482–92.

12. Sharma P, Naperkowski A, Bauch T, et al. Permanent his bundle pacing for cardiac resynchronisation therapy in patients with heart failure and right bundle branch block. Circ Arrhythm Electrophysiol 2018;11: e006613.

13. Lewis AJ, Foley P, Whinnet ZI. His bundle pacing: a New strategy for physiological ventricular activation 2019;8(6):e010972.

14. Keene D, Arnold AD, Jastrzębski M, et al. His bundle pacing, learning curve, procedure

characteristics, safety, and feasibility: insights from a large international observational study. J Cardiovasc Electrophysiol 2019;30(10):1984–93.

15. Gamble J, Herring N, Ginks M, et al. Procedural success of left ventricular lead placement for cardiac resynchronisation therapy: a meta-analysis. JACC Clin EP 2016;2(1):69–77.

16. Curtis AB, Worley SJ, Adamson PB, et al. Biventricular pacing for atrioventricular block and systolic dysfunction. N Engl J Med 2013;368(17):1585–93.

17. Guo J, Li L, Xiao G, et al. Remarkable response to cardiac resynchronisation therapy via left bundle branch pacing in patients with true left bundle branch block. Clin Cardiol 2020;43:1460–8.

18. Huang W, Wu S, Vijayaraman P, et al. Cardiac resynchronsiation therapy in patients with nonischaemic cardiomyopathy using left bundle branch pacing. JACC Clin Electrophysiol 2020;6:849–58.

19. Li X, Qiu C, Xie R, et al. Left bundle branch area pacing delivery of cardiac resynchronisation therapy and comparison with biventricular pacing. ESC Heart Fail 2020;7:1711–22.

20. Wang Y, Gu K, Qian Z, et al. The efficacy of left bundle branch area pacing compared with biventricular pacing in patients with heart failure: a matched case-control study. J Cardiovasc Electrophysiol 2020;31:2068–77.

21. Zhong C, Xu W, Shi Shunyi, et al. Left bundle branch pacing for cardiac resynchronisation therapy: a systematic literature review and meta-analysis. PACE 2021;44:497–505.

22. Liu W, Hu C, Wang Y, et al. Mechanical synchrony and myocardial Work in heart failure patients with left bundle branch area pacing and comparison with biventricular pacing. Front Cardiovasc Med 2021;8:727611.

23. Zu L, Zhang J, Wang L. Cardiac resynchronisation therapy performed by LBBAP-CRT in patients with cardic insufficiency and left bundle branch block. Ann Noninvasive Electrocardiol 2021;00:e12898.

24. Vijayraman P, Ponnusamy S, Cano O. Left bundle branch pacing for cardiac resynchronisation therapy: results from the international LBBAP Collaborative study group. JACC Clin Electrophysiol 2021; 7(2):135–47.

25. Padala SK, Master VM, Terricabras M, et al. Initial experience, safety, and feasibility of left bundle branch area pacing: a multicenter prospective study. JACC Clin Electrophysiol 2020;6(14):1773–82.

26. Wang Z, Zhu H, Li X, et al. Comparison of procedure and Fluoroscopy time between left bundle branch area pacing and right ventricular pacing for bradycardia: the learning curve for the novel pacing strategy. Front Cardiovasc Med 2021;8:695531.

27. Padala S, Ellenbogen K. Left bundle branch pacing is the best approach to physiological pacing. Heart Rhythm Soc 2020;1(1):59–67.

28. Kiehl EL, Makki T, Kumar R, et al. Incidence and predictors of right ventricular pacing-induced cardiomyopathy in patients with complete atrioventricular block and preserved left ventricular systolic function. Heart Rhythm 2016;13(12):2272–8.

29. Merchant FM, Hoskins MH, Musat DL, et al. Incidence and time Course for developing heart failure with high-Burden right ventricular pacing. Circ Cardiovasc Qual Outcomes 2017;10(6):e003564.

30. Kronborg MB, Mortensen PT, Poulsen SH, et al. His or para-His pacing preserves left ventricular function in atrioventricular block: a double-blind, randomized, crossover study. Europace 2014;16(8): 1189–96.

31. Occhetta E, Bortnik M, Magnani A, et al. Prevention of ventricular desynchronization by permanent para-Hisian pacing after atrioventricular node ablation in chronic atrial fibrillation: a crossover, blinded, randomized study versus apical right ventricular pacing. J Am Coll Cardiol 2006;47(10):1938–45.

32. Wang J, Liang Y, Wang W, et al. Left bundle branch area pacing is superior to right ventricular septum pacing concerning depolarization-repolarization reserve. J Cardiovasc Electrophysiol 2020;31(1): 313–22.

33. Hou X, Qian Z, Wang Y, et al. Feasibility and cardiac synchrony of permanent left bundle branch pacing through the interventricular septum. Europace 2019;21:1694–702.

34. Cai B, Huang X, Li L, et al. Evaluation of cardiac synchrony in left bundle branch pacing: insights from echocardiographic research. J Cardiovasc Electrophysiol 2020;31:560–9.

35. Huang W, Su L, Wu S, et al. A novel pacing strategy with low and stable output: pacing the left bundle branch immediately beyond the conduction block. Can J Cardiol 2017;33:1736.e1-3.

36. Zanon F, Abdelrahman M, Marcantoni L, et al. Long term performance and safety of His bundle pacing: a multicenter experience. J Cardiovasc Electrophysiol 2019;30(9):1594–601.

37. Deshmukh P, Casavat DA, Romanyshyn M, et al. Permanent, direct His bundle pacing: a novel approach to cardiac pacing in patients with normal His-Purkinje activation. Circulation 2000;101: 869–77.

38. Occhetta E, Bortnik M, Mangani A, et al. Prevention of ventricular dyssynchronisation by permanent para-Hisian pacing after atrioventricular node ablation in chronic atrial fibrillation: a crossover, blinded randomized study versus apical right ventricular pacing. J Am Coll Cardiol 2006;47:1938–45.

39. Vijayaraman P, Subzposh FA, Naperkowski. Atrioventricular node ablation and His bundle pacing. Europace 2017;19:10–6.

40. Huang W, Su L, Wu S, et al. Benefits of permanent His bundle pacing combined with atrioventricular

node ablation in atrial fibrillation patients with heart failure with both preserved and reduced left ventricular ejection fraction. J Am Heart Assoc 2017;6: e005309.

41. Deshmukh P, Romanyshyn M. Direct his bundle pacing: present and future. Pacing Clin Electrophysiol 2014;27:862–70.

42. Žižek D, Antolič B, Mežnar AZ, et al. Biventricular versus His bundle pacing after atrioventricular node ablation in heart failure patients with narrow QRS. Acta Cardiol 2021;2:1–9.

43. Su L, Cai M, Wu S, et al. Long-term performance and risk factors analysis after permanent His-bundle pacing and atrioventricular node ablation in patients with atrial fibrillation and heart failure. Europace 2020. 22ii19–ii26.

44. Brignole M, Pokushalov E, Pentimalli F, et al. A randomized controlled trial of atrioventricular junction ablation and cardiac resynchronization therapy in patients with permanent atrial fibrillation and narrow QRS. Eur Heart J 2018;39(45):3999–4008.

45. Brignole M, Pentimalli F, Palmisano P, et al. AV junction ablation and cardiac resynchronization for patients with permanent atrial fibrillation and narrow QRS: the APAF-CRT mortality trial. European Heart Journal 2021;42(46):4731–9.

46. Huang W, Su L, Wang S, et al. Comparison of his bundle pacing and Bi-ventricular pacing in heart failure patients with atrial fibrillation who need atrial-ventricular node ablation: the ALTERNATIVE study. Circulation 2021;144:A13774.

47. Sohaib S, Chen Z, Whinnett ZI, et al. Meta-analysis of symptomatic response attributable to the pacing component of cardiac resynchronization therapy. Eur J Heart Fail 2013;15:1419–28.

48. Cleland JG, Abraham WT, Linde C, et al. An individual patient meta-analysis of five randomized trials assessing the effects of cardiac resynchronization therapy on morbidity and mortality in patients with symptomatic heart failure. Eur Heart J 2013;34: 3547–56.

49. Vijayraman P, Dandamudi G, Zanon F, et al. Permanent his bundle pacing: recommendations from a multicenter his bundle pacing Collaborative Working group for standardization of definitions, implant measurements, and follow-up. Heart Rhythm 2018; 15:460–8.

50. Glikson M, Nielsen JC, Jroborg MB, et al. 2021 ESC Guidelines on cardiac pacing and cardiac resynchronization therapy: developed by the Task Force on cardiac pacing and cardiac resynchronization therapy of the European Society of Cardiology (ESC) with the special contribution of the European Heart Rhythm Association (EHRA). Eur Heart J 2021. https://doi.org/10.1093/eurheartj/ehab364. ehab364.

51. Chen L, Zhang J, Wang Z, et al. Efficacy and safety of left bundle branch pacing versus biventricular pacing in heart failure patients with left bundle branch block: study protocol for a randomized controlled trial. BMJ Open 2020;10:e036972.

52. Moss AJ, Jackson W, Cannon D. Cardiac resynchronisation therapy for the prevention of heart failure events. N Engl J Med 2009;361:1329–38.

53. Sipahi I, Chou J, Hyden M. Effect of QRS morphology on clinical event reduction with cardiac resynchronisation therapy: meta-analysis of randomized controlled trials. Am Heart J 2012;163(2):260–7.

54. Nikolaidou T, Pellicori P, Zhang J, et al. Prevalence, predictors, and prognostic implications of PR interval prolongation in patients with heart failure. Clin Res Cardiol 2018;107(2):108–19.

55. Keene D, Arnold A, Shun-Shin M. Rationale and design of the randomized multicentre his optimised pacing evaluated for heart failure. ESC Heart Fail 2018;5(5):965–76.

56. Whinnett Z, Shun-Shin MJ, Tanner M et al. His-optimised pacing in patients with a Long PR interval, narrow QRS and heart failure: results of the Hope-HF clinical trial. Presented at the American Heart Association Scientific Sessions 2021.